Psychopharmacology
An Introduction to Experimental and Clinical Principles

Spectrum Monographs in Modern Neurobiology

PSYCHOPHARMACOLOGY
An Introduction to Experimental and Clinical Principles
Luigi Valzelli

NEUROCHEMISTRY OF CEREBRAL ELECTROSHOCK
Walter B. Essman

**CURRENT BIOCHEMICAL APPROACHES
TO LEARNING AND MEMORY**
Edited by Walter B. Essman and Shinshu Nakajima

Psychopharmacology
An Introduction to Experimental and Clinical Principles

By Luigi Valzelli,
Chief, Neuropsychopharmacology
Mario Negri Institute for Pharmacological Research
Milan, Italy

Edited by Walter B. Essman
Queens College of the City University of New York

SPECTRUM PUBLICATIONS, INC.
Flushing, New York

DISTRIBUTED BY THE HALSTED PRESS DIVISION OF

JOHN WILEY & SONS
New York   Toronto   London   Sydney

Spectrum Publications, Inc.
75-31 192 Street, Flushing, New York 11366

Distributed solely by Halsted Press Division, John Wiley & Sons, Inc., New York.

ISBN 0-470-89783X

Library of Congress Catalog Card Number: 73-3848

Printed in the United States of America

PREFACE

As with other branches of the medical sciences, psychopharmacology becomes a concrete entity only if and when the many sources and roots, which converge into it, are recognized, analyzed, and inserted into a harmonically tuned picture. In other words, psychopharmacology is not intended to be a single and privileged appendage of either pharmacology, biochemistry, neuroanatomy, psychology or psychiatry, but it can take up its full sense only when such different specialities are integrated with each other in completing the psychopharmacological knowlege.

Such a standpoint represents the basic ground upon which this book has been developed, with the aim of giving a sequence of information that, proceeding along the course of a common thread, may allow the reader an overview of the entire field. This formulation may, perhaps, represent a certain advantage point in the face of other excellent and more specialized and extended textbooks on psychopharmacology. The present book is of relevance to those who are not especially acquainted with the manifold aspects of this fascinating area. It becomes obvious that a compensatory feature to such a scheme must be present: this is represented by a list of references wide enough to accommodate the possibility of deepening single, specialized interests in the several areas treated.

I do not know to what extent I succeeded in accomplishing all the tasks which this book implies. But, I know how much indebted I am to Professor Walter B. Essman, who greatly contributed to this work with his extremely helpful and enthusiastic participation and with his deep knowlege of the field.

Likewise, it is my pleasure to take this occasion to express my gratitude to my secretary, Miss Loredana Morgese, for her precious collaboration, as well as to warmly thank Miss Vanna Pistotti, Librarian of the Mario Negri Institute, for her well qualified help.

As a last, but not least, point, my acknowledgments to SPECTRUM PUBLICATIONS, INC., and to its staff for their accuracy and solicitude in printing the text.

Luigi Valzelli

Milan, Italy
November 27, 1972

CONTENTS

ix   CONTENTS

x CONTENTS

INTRODUCTION

Psychopharmocology, although one of the newest branches of the pharmacological sciences, may, in a less pragmatic sense, be concurrently considered as one of the most ancient and almost instinctive efforts by man to search for a new dimension of the human mind. In this regard, primitive man was certainly extraordinarily skillful in deriving a virtually inexhaustible supply of psychoactive substances from natural sources so that, throughout several centuries, drug use became an important aspect of magical rituals and religious ceremonies.

Moreover, in a more or less directed way, man has searched for means to better understand and to potentiate his own mental abilties, with the intentions of becoming fully self-mastering and to prevail over his own environment and contemporaries.

BERGER (1966), who is responsible for the development of meprobamate, one of the most important psychoactive drugs, recently said that "since time immemorial man has been interested in means that would enable him to control the mind of others"; many have and still believe that this task may be accomplished by employing suitable drugs.

The emphases upon the application of the psychopharmaca for the social, intellectual, and perceptual improvement of man should not necessarily be viewed as a position that occupies only historical significance for pre-20th century science. Even in this century, and quite recently, psychotechnology, of which psychopharmacology occupies a prominent position, has been invoked as a means of coping with social and political problems. In his presidential address to the American Psychological Association, KENNETH B. CLARK has said:

> The work on the effects of direct stimulation of certain areas of the brain; the role of specific areas of the midbrain in controlling certain affects; the effects of certain drugs on exciting, tranquilizing, or depressing the emotional and motivational levels of the individual; and the effects of externally induced behavioral changes on internal biochemistry of the organism suggest that we might be on the threshold of that type of scientific biochemical intervention which could stabilize and make dominant the moral and ethical propensities of man and

1

subordinate, if not eliminate, his negative and primitive behavioral tendencies (CLARK, 1971).

In a classical work of the 16th century, "Historia general de làs cosas de Nueva España" by the Franciscan Friar Bernardino de Sahagun, and in another collection of papers by Toribio of Benavente, mention is made of numerous drugs which were employed in magical and religious ceremonies to achieve "divine ecstasy". Prominent among these were peyotl, theonanacatl, and ololiuqui which are now again being given considerable scientific attention. Moreover, Francisco Hernandez, a Spanish physician appointed by Philip the 2nd to study Mexican flora and fauna, described the hallucinatory syndromes observed in Indian priests when they drank the "sacred potions" in order to communicate with the deities.

The term "psychopharmakon" itself is not as recent as one may believe. In fact, in 1548 a book was published in Germany by Reinhardus Lorichius, dedicated to the Count Ludwig von Stolberg, Lord of Epstein, the title of which was, "Psychopharmakon: hoc est medicina animae, non aegrotis solum aut cum morte conflictantibus, sed etiam iis qui prospera valetudine praediti sunt, admodum utilis ac necessaria". This detailed treatise, more or less intentionally by the author, was surprisingly concerned with psychopharmacology of the present era. As a matter of fact, today psychopharmacology concerns the study of those drugs which act upon higher functions of the central nervous system, both in normal and under altered conditions.

However, as far as its present status and controlled therapeutic uses are concerned, modern psychopharmacology can probably be considered no more than twenty years old; its "official" birth is usually taken to be coincident with the introduction, for therapeutic use, of chlorpromazine and reserpine in the early 1950's.

The rapid evolution of psychopharmacology is a corollary of both of its intrinsic functions—the chemotherapy of behavior disorders, as well as, the study of brain functions utilizing biochemical and behavioral methodologies. This concept appears to be more readily apparent when one considers that only an extension of our knowledge concerning brain structures and their functions can permit a better understanding of the causes of behavioral alterations, which can lead, in turn, to the study of psychotropic drug derivatives. To accomplish this, psychoactive drugs are frequently employed more actively and selectively in laboratory animals, as a means of inducing behavioral modifications, the possible biochemical correlates of such modifications as well as the specialized brain functions involved therein are thereby studied. As a consequence, psychopharmacology brings together the interests of chemist, biochemist, pharmacologist, physiologist, and clinician; even mathematicians and physicists, have proposed models for brain functions based upon electronic analogies, circuit theory, or computer systems, such as to allow possible mathematical extrapolations of the basic schemes of cerebral activity.

As a final point, it seems to be useful to emphasize that although our present knowledge in this discipline is incomparably more advanced than, for instance, that of twenty years ago, the complexity of some of the issues, data, and mechanisms illustrates how extensive the exploratory requirements of this field are.

REFERENCES

Berger, F. M., (1966) Amer. J. Pharm. **138**, 51.
Clark, K. B., (1971) Amer. Psychol. **26**, 1047.

Chapter I

THE BRAIN

The brain is certainly the most complex organ of the animal structure, not only from anatomical and physiological standpoints, but also from a functional one, as may be verified by the extremely wide range of activities which are under its control. It is not within the scope of this book to review the evolutionary stages of the central nervous system, beginning with the simplest organism to the more complex ones including higher mammals and man, although relevant and important data could emerge from such an examination. In this context however, a sentence from CUSHING (1932) would be highly appropriate, he said, speaking about the hypothalamus, that in the medial and older regions of this small brain area lies the fulcrum of the instinctual, vegetative, and affective expressions of life which man strives to cover under a cortex of inhibitions.

The earliest descriptions of the nuclei and of brain structures, can be found in the work, "De humanis corporis Fabrica" by VESALIO, published in 1543. The validity of these descriptions has evolved significantly into contemporary neuromorphology with a series of major contributions, the most important of which are represented by the work of COSTANZO VAROLIO (1573), THOMAS WILLIS (1664), VIEUSSENS (1685), SPALTEHOLTZ (1895), and of several others. It seems, however, important to note the discrepancy between the accuracy of empirical data and the sparsity of information about the functions and the activities to which different brain structures are relegated. The entire cerebral organization is therefore an extremely complex one and the earliest concept of "functional centers" was gradually transformed into the present conception of "functional circuits", which takes into account the integrated aspects of the brain. In accord with this last point, different brain regions are thought to actively and functionally cooperate; it is certainly easier to assign the participation of such brain regions to one or another activity rather than to single out and specify a graded functional sequence. From an extremely simplified point of view, four main functional circuits may be outlined: the motor inputs, activation of which leads to a motor response mediated through the pyramidal and extrapyramidal pathways; the sensory inputs,

5

which receive the afferents from the inner and outside environment; the emotional inputs, which elaborate behavioral responses, coloring them with affective nuances; and the associative or secondary projection inputs, whose integrated functions are to a great extent, not yet well understood.

These general systems are summarized in a very diagrammatic way in Figure 1.

Past consideration of the neocortex, for example, has assigned that brain area as generally serving the intellective functions such as intelligence, memory, decisional, and discriminative abilities; but, it has become obvious that all of these cerebral processes are much more dependent upon a series of integrated functions than on a strictly delimited cerebral zone or area. Hence, as far as psychopharmacology is concerned, it seems too simple to ascribe the activity of a specific psychoactive drug to, for example, its effect upon a specialized cerebral nucleus without taking into account all of the numerous modifications which take place at the level of the integrated circuits and functions to which such a hypothetical nucleus pertains. Moreover, consideration should also be given to the position that all brain functions are in turn dependent upon modifications of nerve impulses and their propagation from one neuron to another. In this respect one may deal further with the subject at a more complex level, several aspects of which are still a matter of extensive investigation.

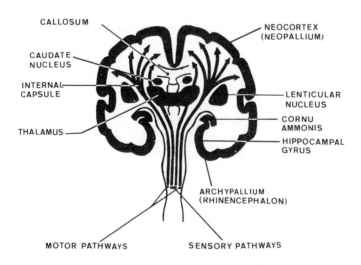

Fig. 1. Schema of general brain organization.

A) BRAIN COMPLEXITY

An absolute touchstone which provides an exact measure of brain complexity and activity does not exist; such a gauge perhaps depends upon several aspects of brain function which still remain obscure. An approximate and general picture, however, may be developed from the simple enumeration of some data, in part empirical and in part the result of computer performances, the circuits of which suggest a number of cerebral analogies.

The brain contains about thirty million neurons (HART et al., 1970), these represent its working units. The neurons are interconnected in multiple ways, so that the possible operational stages, which are dependent upon these neuronal interconnections can reach numbers as large as $1.5 \times 10^{3,000,000,000}$ (BLINKOV and GLEZER, 1968). Reaction times dependent upon the transmission of nerve impulse are in the millisecond range with amplitude excursions of between three and ten volts, and the entire system operates with a potency of about 100 watts; frequencies vary from 0.5 to 4 cycles per second for the δ rhythm (corresponding to the sleep phase), from 14 to 18 cycles per second for the β rhythm (characteristic of intense cerebral arousal). However, brain frequencies can reach much more elevated levels (GOZZANO, 1935) and even activity of 200 to 1400 cycles per second have been described (LION et al., 1950; TRABKA, 1962); the firing pattern of the nerve impulse in a simple neuron is about 1000 to 2000 cycles per second.

Considering that oxygen is one of the essential requirements for brain function, the brain burns it at a medium rate of 0.033 ml/g of tissue per minute (KETY, 1960). Taking a modern computer as an analogy, it would consume the power output of a generating station designed to serve a community of about 200,000 people, if it had to activate the same number of transistors similar to one of the brain cells. Insofar as the concept of memory is concerned, the capacity of the brain to retain information may be considered to constitute as much as 60,000 items, each about as complex as the basic multiplication tables, while a computer is able to store only 1000 such items. In terms of bits, or binary digits (where it is assumed that a bit corresponds to an elementary signal or information unit which leads only to a positive or negative outcome or response), a modern computer can take up no more than 3 million such bits while the human brain can store 10 million bits, 4 million of which are taken up visually, some hundred thousand through audition and olfaction and the rest through the cutaneous senses, mainly tactile. It is astonishing to realize that the brain acquires such bits at an average of one every twenty seconds. Nevertheless, the brain does not become saturated as one may suppose, possibly because of discrimination processes which abolish those environmental informational stimuli that are either not useful or may be irrelevant for that cerebral activity peculiar to a certain specific event; also possibly because the ribonucleic acid complex (RNA) of nerve cells, which may be directly involved, as has been hypothesized, in the memory storage mechanisms (DINGMAN and SPORN, 1961; HYDÉN and EGYHÁZI, 1964; UNGAR, 1968), is capable of incorporating more than 10 million units, so, every single neuron can be considered as an archive of enormous capacity. Moreover, the brain can be considered a sequential machine, when this term is applied to a syncronous system with a finite number of inputs, a finite number of internal operational states, and a finite number of outputs. In fact, the brain is constituted: (a) by a finite number of active elements (the neurons), which are at any moment in a finite number of stages of activity, where (b) the number of sensory inputs and signals, even though extremely wide, is finite and (c) the number of output channels is finite and only a finite number of different signals pass through them.

More specifically, the brain can be considered as a monosequential machine as it can interpret, from time to time, only a unique sequence of information units, working upon a unique sequence of elaboration and providing a unique sequence of responses, as the commonest computers do. By contrast, more recently developed computers, having two or more central ruling units operating simultaneously, can be considered as true multisequential machines, as they are able to elaborate two or more sequences of information at the same time using different sections of the apparatus, without any mutual interference (VACCA, 1965). Based upon these considerations, mathematical theories of the central nervous system have been developed such as that proposed by LANDAHL in 1962 and, subsequently new fields of study, such as biophysics, cybernetics, and bionics have evolved. Models of some single cerebral functions have been proposed for the response of the nervous system to sensory stimuli (ROSENBLITH, 1959), for the transmission of nerve impulses in the cerebral cortex (HENDRIX, 1965; CIHAK, 1965; PAVLIDIS, 1965), for schema within which the neuron is considered as an oscillator; models such as these have led to the further elaboration of elementary models of the entire brain (GALAMBOS, 1961; DEUTSCH, 1967).

The area of models for specific cerebral units or functions is still quite recent and rapidly evolving and it may certainly be considered as a promising probe for a better understanding of certain basic brain functions.

B) THE LIMBIC SYSTEM

The limbic system is a typical example of those functional circuits which have been previously mentioned. It brings together several nuclei, associative pathways and cerebral areas to form a specialized section of the components, modulating in the broadest way differing aspects of animal behavior. This system was therefore defined by FULTON (1951) as the neuroanatomical substrate of emotional expressions or, according to PAPEZ (1958), the coordinator of the sensory inputs with the visceral responses of the body.

The view that emotional processes are dependent upon a neuroanatomical substrate, was proposed by PAPEZ in 1937 in such a precise way that the sequence of different levels which participate in the constitution of the limbic system have also been referred to as the "Papez Circuit". The cortical areas of this system derive from the rhinencephalon or archipallium (see Fig. 1), which is also called the "Visceral Brain" (MacLEAN, 1949), and is associated with oral, visual, acoustic, olfactory, sexual, and visceral inputs. ANAND (1957) has said that what an individual feels depends upon the limbic system, while what he knows is a function of his neocortex.

The principal structures involved in the limbic system are schematically represented in Figure 2.

From a physiological as well as behavioral point of view, the major anatomical aspect of the limbic system is represented by the fact that it is phylogenetically a very old structure, its components, except for the hypothalamus, deriving from the embryonic olfactory areas of the brain (PAPEZ, 1958). The development and the organization of the limbic system is the same in all mammals (MacLEAN, 1958a), with only some minor differences in the extent of associated anatomical processes, according to the species considered (Fig. 3); this system can be considered a useful common

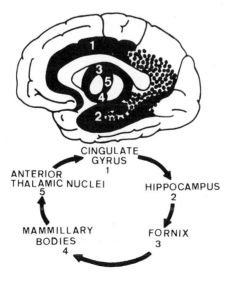

Fig. 2. Limbic system.

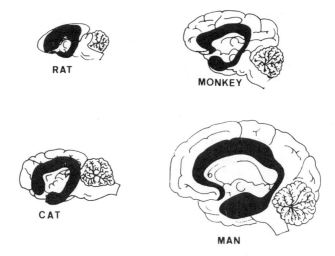

Fig. 3. The extent of limbic system in different animal species.

denominator, mainly of the emotional modulation of behavior and the basic drives which may be elaborated to motivational significance in the development of basic psychological processes, both in animal and man (ANAND, 1957).

A series of experimental investigations (MacLEAN, 1955) have led to specification of a number of specific activities attributable to different sections of the limbic system. For instance, the *fronto-temporal zone* governs the functions of the so-called oral coordination or, in other words, the behavioral aspects of attack, defense, fighting, nutrition and search for food, and it also influences the secretion of adrenocorticotropic hormone (ACTH) which follows a stressful situation (MacLEAN, 1955) in such a way to participate in the hormonal control of the body. The *parieto-occipital zone* regulates the secretion of sexual hormones as well as sexual activity, so that stimulation of this zone leads to the activation of sexual behavior. The *medial occipito-temporal zone,* which is mainly represented by hippocampus, seems to play a prominent role in affective experiences, primarily in connection with memory. Recently, the importance of hippocampus was underlined in the organization of orienting reactions (KARMOS et al., 1965). The *medial temporo-frontal zone* remains as the least well known, although it is recognized as playing an integrated and extremely important role with the previously cited zones (Fig. 4).

Different functions governed by the limbic system may converge to regulate two essential aspects of living organisms, those of *species preservation* and of *self-preservation*. In species preservation, interpreted in terms of

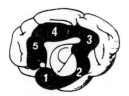 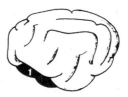

Fig. 4. Limbic system functions. (1) Fronto-temporal zone: attack, defense, nutrition. (2) Parieto-occipital zone: sexual activity. (3) Occipito-temporal zone: affective experiences, memory. (4) and (5) Temporal and frontal-medial zones; not well known: emotional behavior?

reproductive functions, the rhinencephalon and the olfactory routes play an important role in animals, but are also important in man. In fact, a diminution of olfactory perception can result in conflict behavior associated with sexual activity (ROSENBAUM, 1959) and, moreover, alterations of the sense of smell are known to be present, to some extent, in different psychopathological syndromes (DE MAIO, 1966). Some experimental data have indicated that some limbic structures such as the septal area, the hippocampus, the amygdala, and the cingulate gyrus, are involved in mimicking and expressive behavior and in the activation of internal feelings; both merge into the preliminaries of intercourse and into social behavior (MacLEAN, 1958a,b). Hypersexual activity (KLÜVER and BUCY, 1939), as well as sexual deviations (MacLEAN, 1958b; SCHREINER and KLING, 1953), has been observed as a consequence of lesions of these cerebral areas, both in animals and in man (ERICKSON, 1945).

As far as social behavior is concerned, ablation of the olfactory bulbs as well as the lesions of the olfactory boundaries or of the prepyriform cortex in laboratory rats can lead to the induction of an extremely intense and compulsive aggressive behavior (KARLI, 1960; VERGNES and KARLI 1963); these findings will be discussed in more detail later on.

The second important function in which the limbic structures participate, the *preservation of self,* derives from and is strictly linked to the first function so that aggression or flight behavior, the competition for social rank, reproduction and food, the effect of previous emotional experiences with frustrating or rewarding content, fear, and defense are all behavioral patterns that are dependent upon the limbic system (FULTON, 1951; HERRICK, 1948; MacLEAN, 1958a,b; MacLEAN and DELGADO, 1953).

In conclusion, we agree with COBB (1950), that the boundaries between the limbic system and the neocortex represent the ground upon which man rules out his intellectual activities, supporting in this way what FREUD

(1933) defined as biological psychiatry when he spoke of the psychological roots of biological processes.

Finally, it is also apparent that a wide number of emotional effects can influence the peripheral equilibrium of the body to the point of inducing not only momentary variations but also stable alterations leading to the induction of somatic changes such as peptic ulceration (SEND and ANAND, 1957), hypertensive illness, etc.

C) THE MEMORY CIRCUITS

As an initial task it might be appropriate to define the term "memory"; the meaning of this word is so diffuse, that when the term is applied to the ability to retain and retrieve specific information when necessary, all the anatomical functions of the nervous system may possibly also be included. As a consequence, the regulation of heart rate, blood pressure, respiration, and many other functions depends upon both central control and numerous responses regulating peripheral homostasis; these may be put into the category of an automatic memory, so that every single neuron as well as the whole brain can be considered as the residence of selective and specialized memories.

According to JARVIK (1964), memory can be defined as a process by means of which the effect of an experience persists and becomes operant on animal behavior during the following period of time. In this context, the process of memory can be divided into three essential steps, the first one represented by *registration* of the information and the others by its *storage* and *retrieval* whenever called upon (WOODWORTH, 1938; WOODWORTH and SCHLOSBERG, 1954).

During the past ten years, several experimental approaches have taken a number of biological, neurophysiological, psychological, semantic, and environmental factors into consideration which may in several respects modify memory processes, (HYDÉN and EGYHÁZI, 1962, 1964; JOHN 1965, 1967; ROZEBOOM, 1965; SCHMITT, 1965; ESSMAN, 1970, 1971). However, from an anatomical point of view a series of observations allows for specification of a sequence of brain structures, areas, and nuclei which are directly involved in memory mechanisms (OJEMANN, 1966) (Fig. 5).

In this context, the neocortex is functionally important for learning and memory processes involving visual, auditory, and tactile stimuli, for word meaning, and for mathematical figures and concepts (ADAMS et al., 1961), but these behaviors are integrated by subcortical structures which mainly lie within the limbic system. Consequently, such a situation implies that several

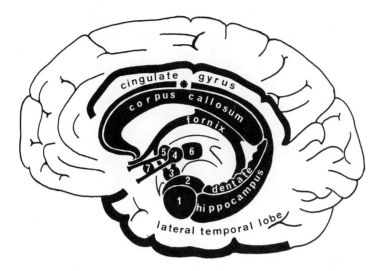

Fig. 5. Anatomical substrates of memory: (*) cingulum; (1) amygdala; (2) uncus; (3) mammillary bodies; (4) dorso-medial nucleus of the thalamus; (5) anterior nucleus of the thalamus; (6) pulvinar; (7) anterior commissure.

emotional components can positively or negatively affect memory processes and possibly explains how earlier frustrating or rewarding experiences may profoundly influence animal behavior.

On the basis of extensive observation, JAMES (1890) hypothesized the two types of memory which he defined as "primary" and "secondary", anticipating what has now been respectively labeled as recent, immediate or short-term memory (BROWN, 1964; CONRAD and HILLE, 1958; KEPPEL and UNDERWOOD, 1962; MELTON, 1963) and as old, distant, or long-term memory (KEPPEL and UNDERWOOD, 1962; MELTON, 1963; WEIS-KRANTZ et al., 1962). In this regard, there are many theories of memory and several pschoanalytic interpretation of related responses and functions; (NEIDERLAND, 1965; RAPAPORT and LEWY, 1944; SALZMAN, 1966) such theories are certainly important and interesting but do not pertain to the content of this book.

As far as neuroanatomy is concerned, data derived from clinical observations seems to indicate that the hippocampal area is principally involved in memory processes (DRACHMAN and ARBIT, 1966; PENFIELD and MIL-NER, 1958) and there are considerable data showing that the uncus, amygdala, and the anterior two thirds of the hippocampus are highly relevant to the mechanisms of recent or short-term memory (SCOVILLE, 1954; SCOVILLE and MILNER, 1957; MILNER, 1959). Another such area implicated in short-term memory is the cortex of the lateral temporal lobe

(ADAMS et al., 1961). The anatomical areas related to long-term memory seem, instead, to be located in the tip of the temporal lobe (TERZIAN and DALLE ORE, 1955) but they have still not been very well defined (OJE-MANN, 1966) and the problem perhaps requires redefinition in terms of functional interactions among different nuclei and associative pathways rather than relegation to a strictly specialized area.

Moreover at a molecular level, memory processes can be considered in terms of modification of macromolecular protein structure (KATZ and HALSTEAD, 1950), so that the theoretical emphasis obtains not only at this level but also relates directly to subcellular constituents. In a general sense, an external stimulus can be considered as an input capable of inducing an internal transition from one stage to another, with relatively small energy consumption; this stage variation must persist long enough to permit the imprinting and the storage of the input itself. The first step involved in the memory of an event seems therefore to be represented by a brief neuronal current change, as a response to the stimulus, which is followed by a long-lasting imprinting on subcellular levels (KATCHALSKY and OPLATKA, 1966a,b). In this case, some authors (ANKER, 1960; SMITH, 1962; SZILARD, 1964) have suggested that this process is linked to an enzymatic mechanism, while others have demonstrated a correlation between both the quantitative and structural aspects of ribonucleic acid (RNA) in the cell nucleus and the learning processes in several mammals (HYDÉN and EGYHÁZI, 1962). McCONNELL et al. (1959) as well as CORNING and JOHN (1961) were also able to demonstrate several potential relationships between RNA and the processes of learning, while the experiments of FLEXNER et al. (1962, 1963, 1965), AGRANOFF and KLINGER (1964), and DAVIS et al. (1965a,b) have emphasized the significance of protein synthesis for memory.

In conclusion, a great deal of experimental work suggests that memory fixation implies changes in the previous structure of macromolecular complexes or, in other words, is, by analogy, linked to a true engraving process of the information on biopolymers as a consequence of a variation in the steric structure of these macromolecules. From this point of view biopolymers behave like a magnetic tape endowed with hysteresis sufficient to permanently retain the engraving (ENDERBY, 1955; KATCHALSKY and OPLATKA, 1966a,b; MACOVSCHI, 1966).

D) SLEEP MECHANISMS

Sleep is one of the major functions of the central nervous system, however it is also one of the least well known. From a simple descriptive point of view, the sleep phenomenon can be defined as an expression of a transient, reversible, and rhythmic interruption of consciousness together with persistent activity, at a reduced level, of those servomechanisms which regulate vegetative activities. In this context, only the subconscious remains alert and active and, according to psychoanalytical interpretations, releases the valences which elaborate the mechanisms of dreaming.

Most of our knowledge regarding sleep is mainly descriptive so that, not so many years ago, COBB (1959) said that, though man spends about one third of his entire life in sleep, we know practically nothing about the processes which regulate fluctuations between waking and sleeping. The use of electroencephalographic methods, such as the studies of RHEIN-BERGER and JASPER (1937) and subsequently by the measurement of changes, reflecting the transitional phase between the waking and sleeping state (DEMENT, 1958), it was possible to demonstrate other differences corresponding to stages of sleep (SIMON and EMMONS, 1956) (Fig. 6).

There are several theories concerned with sleep but such theoretical emphasis perhaps explains why no one of these is sufficiently explanatory to deal with and interrelate all aspects of the phenomenon. For example, PAVLOV (1928) described sleep as dependent upon a spreading cortical inhibition, while KLEITMAN (1955) interpreted cortical inhibition as a result of a reduction of afferent impulses, mainly coming from the muscles, which reach the sensory areas; thus, sleep was viewed as a reflex originating from the body periphery. Other authors (HESS, 1929) have advanced the hypothesis that sleep is a consequence of activation of some centers of the central nervous system and this introduces the concept of structural loci involved in sleep mechanism.

MAUTHNER in 1890 and later VON ECONOMO in 1929 and 1930 discussed sleep in terms of cerebral localization, mainly suggesting the importance of the anterior hypothalamus; this position has been more recently confirmed by AKERT and HESS (1962). Other brain structures such as the medial thalamus (KRAYENBÜHL et al., 1964), and those of the limbic mesencephalic and pontine nuclei, were also recognized as playing a role in sleep behavior (CAMPBELL and BIGGART, 1939).

Although experimental evidence demonstrates that the functional integration of different neural circuits and the participation of various brain structures in sleep behavior can be neuroanatomically represented, the integrated functions by which sleep is regulated are still not completely understood.

The major anatomical structures and nuclei which participate in this circuit are the thalamic nuclei lateral to the massa intermedia (HESS, 1944), the intralaminar thalamic nuclei (JASPER, 1949; MORISON and DEMP-SEY, 1942), their associative pathways (POWELL and COWAN, 1956), the caudate nucleus (AKERT and ANDERSSON, 1951; BUCHWALD et al.,

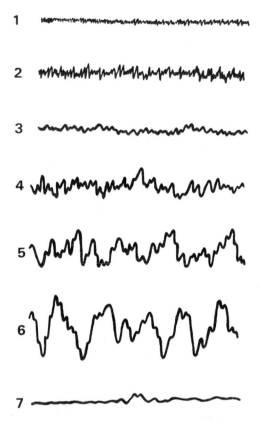

Fig. 6. Schema of the sleep electroencephalographic patterns: (1) alertness; (2) somnolence; (3) sleep (transitional phase); (4)
sleep (initial phase); (5) sleep (median
phase); (6) deep sleep; (7) paradoxical
sleep (REM phase).

1961), the preoptic area (HERNÁNDEZ-PEÓN and CHÁVEZ-IBARRA,
1963; STERMAN and CLEMENTE, 1962), the cortical and subcortical
zones of the limbic system (PARMEGGIANI, 1960), the region of the
nucleus of the tractus solitarius (BONVALLET and ALLEN, 1963), the
ascending reticular formation (MORUZZI, 1963), the frontal areas
(JOUVET, 1961), and the medial nuclei of the mesencephalic raphé
(JOUVET, 1968; KOSTOWSKI et al., 1968).

Although it is difficult to outline the sequence and the stages followed
by sleep in terms of neurophysiological representation and spread through

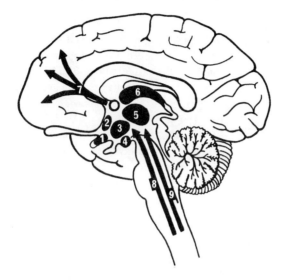

Fig. 7. Anatomical substrates of sleep: (1) supraoptical
        nuclei; (2) preoptical nuclei; (3) hypothalamus;
        (4) mammillary bodies; (5) thalamus; (6) caudate
        nucleus;(7) frontal projections;(8) mesencephalic
        raphe; (9) reticular system.

various areas of the brain, it now seems possible to trace a schema of the
anatomical structures involved in this process. It should be emphasized that
this has been intended as only a tentative schematic representation
(Fig. 7).

The integration of those anatomical circuits, which will be treated later
in more detail, has now been more recently hypothesized as a neurochemi-
cally dependent process, so that some more basic biological principles seem
to play an important role in the definition of sleep mechanisms. This
development is obviously related to what DUBOIS suggested in 1901
speaking of a "sleep hormone"; this at subsequent times, has been identified
as lactic acid, cholesterol, and other hypothetical substances such as so-
called hypnotoxin, leucomaines, etc.

The significance and functional utility of sleep has been emphasized in
experiments in man demonstrating that sleep is critically necessary for the
functional equilibrium of the brain rather than for other tissues in the rest
of the body (BEST and TAYLOR, 1955; KLEITMAN, 1954). The sleeping
process acts as a stabilizing mechanism which allows the recovery of central

nervous system activities; as a consequence, sleep disturbances can have a considerable importance on the general status of an individual as well as upon his psychological equilibrium, while in turn, many psychological disturbances can negatively reflect upon sleep (SULLIVAN et al., 1956).

The effects of forced and prolonged sleep deprivation are extremely dramatic, so that subsequent to the early work of PATRICK and GILBERT in this area (1896) many investigators emphasized the appearance of schizo-phrenic-like syndromes (TYLER, 1947) and of more generalized psychotic symptomatologies (BERGER and OSWALD, 1962; WEST et al., 1962). These aspects appear anatomically related to the structures shared with the limbic system which are thought to be involved with sleep mechanisms. In this regard, the emotional components and the dream phase of sleep are believed to be of great importance as a restorative effect on sleep.

In fact, the experimental deprivation of the sleep-dream phase, which is characterized by rapid eye movement (REM) results in a series of anxiety-associated symptoms, accompanied by signs of irritability and concentration difficulties; short-lasting periods of depersonalization, memory disturbances, and aggressive behavior have also been observed (SAMPSON, 1966; DEMENT, 1960; FISHER, 1965; SNYDER, 1963). Therefore, among the several brain activities related to sleep behavior the dream state appears to be a fundamental one; this observation provides a new source of interest in the dream theory which FREUD formulated in 1900.

REFERENCES

Adams, R. D., Collins, G. H., and Victor, M., (1961) in "Physiologie de l'Hippo-campe," Paris, C. N. R. S., p. 273.

Agranoff, B. W. and Klinger, P. D., (1964) Science 146, 952.

Akert, K. and Andersson, B., (1951) Acta Physiol. Scand. 22, 281.

Akert, K. and Hess, W. R., (1962) Schweiz. Med. Wschr. 92, 1524.

Anand, B. K., (1957) Indian J. Physiol. Pharmacol. 1, 149.

Anker, H. S., (1960) Nature 188, 938.

Berger, R. J. and Oswald, I., (1962) J. Ment. Sci. 108, 457.

Best, C. H. and Taylor, N. B., (1955) "The Physiological Basis of Medical Practice," 6th ed., Williams & Wilkins, Baltimore, p. 1966.

Blinkov, S. M. and Glezer, I. I., (1968) "The Human Brain in Figures and Tables," Basic Books Inc. Publ. and Plenum Press, New York.

Bonvallet, M. and Allen M. B., Jr., (1963) Electroenceph. Clin. Neurophysiol. 15, 969.

Brown, J., (1964) Brit. Med. Bull., 20, 8.

Buchwald, N. A., Wyers, E. J., Okuma, T., and Heuser G., (1961) Electroenceph. Clin. Neurophysiol. 13, 509.

Campbell, A. C. P. and Biggart, J. H., (1939) J. Pathol. Bacteriol. 48, 245.

Cihak, P., (1965) Acta Physiol. Acad. Sci. Hung. 26, 143.

Cobb, S., (1950) "Emotions and Clinical Medicine," Norton Publ., New York, p. 25.
Cobb, S., (1959) in "American Handbook of Psychiatry," vol. 2, Basic Books, New York, p. 1646.
Conrad, R. and Hille, B. A., (1958) Can. J. Psychol. 12, 1.
Corning, W. C. and John, E. R., (1961) Science 134, 1363.
Cushing, H. V., (1932) Surg. Gyn. Obstetr. 55, 1.
Davis, R. E. and Agranoff, B. W., (1965a) Fed. Proc. 24, 328.
Davis, R. E., Bright, P. J., and Agranoff, B. W., (1965b) J. Comp. Physiol. Psychol. 60, 162.
De Maio, D., (1966) "Le Allucinazioni Olfattive dei Malati Psichici," Quaderni di Acta Neurologica, Napoli, N. XXV.
Dement, W., (1958) Electroenceph. Clin. Neurophysiol. 10, 291.
Dement, W. C., (1960) Science 131, 1705.
Deutsch, S., (1967) "Models of the Nervous System," Wiley, New York.
Dingman, W. and Sporn, M. B., (1961) J. Psychiat. Res. 1, 1.
Drachman, D. A. and Arbit, J., (1966) Arch. Neurol. 15, 52.
Dubois, R., (1901) Compt. Rend. Soc. Biol. 53, 229.
Enderby, J. A., (1955) Trans. Faraday Soc. 51, 835.
Erickson, T. C., (1945) Arch. Neurol. Psychiat. 53, 226.
Essman, W. B., (1970) Trans. N. Y. Acad. Sci. 32, 948.
Essman, W. B., (1971) Int. J. Neuroscience 2, 199.
Fisher, C., (1965) J. Amer. Psychoanal. Assoc. 13, 197.
Flexner, J. B., Flexner, L. B., Stellar, E., De La Haba, G., and Roberts, R. B., (1962) J. Neurochem., 9, 595.
Flexner, J. B., Flexner, L. B., and Stellar, E., (1963) Science 141, 57.
Flexner, L. B., Flexner, J. B., and Stellar, E., (1965) Exper. Neurol. 13, 264.
Freud, S., (1900) "Traumdeutung," Deuticke, Lipzig, Wien.
Freud, S., (1933) in "New Introductory Lectures on Psychoanalysis," Norton Publ., New York, p. 132.
Fulton, J. F., (1951) in "Frontal Lobotomy and Affective Behavior a Neurophysiological Approach," Norton. Publ., New York, p. 32.
Galambos, R., (1961) in "Brain and Behavior," vol. 1, Brazier M. A. B., Ed., Amer. Inst. Biol. Sci., Washington D.C., p. 171.
Gozzano, M., (1935) Riv. Neurol. 8, 212.
Hart, E. M., Csermely, T. J., Beek, B., and Lindsay, (1970) J. Theoret. Biol. 26, 93.
Hendrix, C. E., (1965) Bull. Mathemat. Biophys. 27, 197.
Hernández-Peón, R. and Chávez-Ibarra, G., (1963) Electroenceph. Clin. Neurophysiol. (Suppl.) 24, 188.
Herrick, C. J., (1948) "The Brain of Tiger Salamander," Chicago Univ. Press, Chicago.
Hess, W. R., (1929) Amer. J. Physiol. 90, 386.
Hess, W. R., (1944) Helv. Physiol. Pharmacol. Acta 2, 305.
Hydén, H. and Egyházi, E., (1962) Proc. Nat. Acad. Sci. 48, 1366.
Hydén, H. and Egyházi, E., (1964) Proc. Nat. Acad. Sci. 52, 1030.
James, W., (1890) "The Principles of Psychology," Holt, New York.
Jarvik, M. E., (1964) in "Animal Behavior and Drug Action," Ciba Foundation Symp., Churchill, Ltd., London, p. 44.
Jasper, H. H., (1949) Electroenceph. Clin. Neurophysiol. 1, 405.
John, E. R., (1965) Perspect. Biol. Med. 9, 35.
John, E. R., (1967) "Mechanisms of Memory," Academic Press, New York.
Jouvet, M., (1961) in "The Nature of Sleep," Ciba Foundation Symp., Churchill Ltd., London, p. 188.

Jouvet, M., (1968) in "Advances in Pharmacology," Garattini, S. and Shore, P.A., Eds., Vol. 6B, Academic Press, New York, p. 265.

Karli, P., (1960) Compt. Rend. Soc. Biol. **154,** 1079.

Karmos, G., Grástyan, E., Losonczy, H., Vereczkey L., and Grósz, J., (1965) Acta Physiol. Acad. Sci. Hung. **26,** 131.

Katchalsky, A. and Oplatka, A., (1966a) Israel J. Med. Sci. **2,** 4.

Katchalsky, A. and Oplatka, A., (1966b) Neurosciences Res. Progr. Bull. (Suppl.) **4,** 71.

Katz. J. J. and Halstead, W. C., (1950) Comp. Psychol. Monogr. **20,** 1.

Keppel, G. and Underwood, B. J., (1962) J. Verb. Learn. Verb. Behav. **1,** 153.

Kety, S. S., (1960) in "Handbook of Physiology, Section 1: Neurophysiology," Vol. 3, American Physiological Society, Washington D.C., p. 1751.

Kleitman, N., (1954) in "The Cyclopedia of Medicine, Surgery, Specialities," Vol. 12, Davis Publ., Philadelphia, p. 733.

Kleitman, N., (1955) in "The Physiological Basis of Medical Practice" Best, C. and Taylor, N. B., Eds., Williams and Wilkins, Baltimore.

Klüver, H. and Bucy, P. C., (1939) A. M. A. Arch. Neurol. Psychiat. **42,** 979.

Kostowski, W., Giacalone, E., Garanttini, S., and Valzelli, L., (1968) Europ. J. Pharmacol. **4,** 371.

Krayenbühl, H., Akert, K., Hartmann, K., and Yasargil, M. G., (1964) Neurochirurgie **10,** 397.

Landahl, H. D., (1962) Ann. N. Y. Acad. Sci. **96,** 1056.

Lion, K. S., Winter, D. F., and Levin, E., (1950) Electroenceph. Clin. Neurophysiol. **2,** 205.

MacLean, P. D., (1949) Psychosom. Med. **11,** 338.

MacLean, P. D., (1955) Psychosom, Med. **17,** 355.

MacLean, P. D., (1958a) Amer. J. Med. **25,** 611.

MacLean, P. D., (1958b) J. Nerv. Ment. Dis. **127,** 1.

MacLean, P. D. and Delgado, J. M. R., (1953) Electroencephalogr. **5,** 91.

Macovschi, E., (1966) Rev. Roum. Biochim. **3,** 249.

Mauthner, L., (1890) Wiener Klin. Wschr. **3,** 445.

McConnell, J. V., Jacobson, A. L., and Kimble, D. P., (1959) J. Comp. Physiol. Psychol. **52,** 1.

Melton, A. W., (1963) J. Verb. Learn. Verb. Behav. **2,** 1.

Milner, B., (1959) N. L. M. Psychiat. Res. Rep. **11,** 43.

Morison, R. S. and Dempsey, E. W., (1942) Amer. J. Physiol. **135,** 281.

Moruzzi, G., (1963) Harvey Lect. **58,** 233.

Neiderland, W. G., (1965) J. Amer. Psychoanal. Assoc. **13,** 624.

Ojemann, R. G., (1966) Neurosciences Res. Progr. Bull. (Suppl.) **4,** 1.

Papez, J. W., (1937) A. M. A. Arch. Neurol. Psychiat. **38,** 725.

Papez, J. W., (1958) J. Nerv. Ment. Dis. **126,** 40.

Parmeggiani, P. L., (1960) Helv. Physiol. Pharmacol. Acta **18,** 523.

Patrick, G. T. W. and Gilbert, J. A., (1896) Psychol. Rev. **3,** 469.

Pavlidis, T., (1965) Bull. Mathemat. Biophys. **27,** 215.

Pavlov, I. P., (1928) in "Lectures on Conditioned Reflexes," International Publishers, New York, p. 305.

Penfield, W. I. and Milner, B., (1958) A. M. A. Arch. Neurol. Psychiat. **79,** 475.

Powell, T. P. S. and Cowan, W. M., (1956) Brain **79,** 364.

Rapaport, D. and Lewy, E., (1944) Psychoanal. Quart. **13,** 16.

Rheinberger, M. and Jasper, H. H., (1937) cited by Magoun, H. W. in "The Waking Brain," Thomas, Springfield, Ill. (1958) p. 64.

Rosenbaum, J. B., (1959) Amer. Psychoanal. Assoc. Meeting, New York, December 4-6.
Rosenblith, W. A., (1959) in "Biophysical Science: A Study Program," Oncley, J. L., Schmitt, F. O., Williams, R. C., Rosenberg, M. D., and Bolt, R. H., Eds., Wiley, New York, p. 532.
Rozeboom, W. W., (1965) Psychol. Rec. 15, 329.
Salzman, L., (1966) Brit. J. Med. Psychol. 39, 197.
Sampson, H., (1966) J. Nerv. Ment. Dis. 143, 305.
Schmitt, F. O., (1965) Science 149, 931.
Schreiner, L. and Kling, A., (1953) J. Neurophysiol. 16, 643.
Scoville, W. B., (1954) J. Neurosurg. 11, 64.
Scoville, W. B. and Milner, B., (1957) J. Neurol. Neurosurg. Psychiat. 20, 11.
Send, R. N. and Anand, B. K., (1957) Indian J. Med. Res. 45, 515.
Simon, C. W. and Emmons, W. H., (1956) Science 124, 1066.
Smith, C. E., (1962) Science 138, 889.
Snyder, F., (1963) Arch. Gen. Psychiat. 8, 381.
Spalteholtz, W. (1895) "Manuale Atlante di Anatomia Umana," Amsterdam.
Sterman, M. B. and Clemente, C. D., (1962) Exper. Neurol. 6, 103.
Sullivan, H. S. et al., (1956) "Clinical Studies in Psychiatry," Norton, New York.
Szilard, L., (1964) Proc. Nat. Acad. Sci. 51, 1092.
Terzian, H. and Dalle Ore, G., (1955) Neurology 5, 373.
Trabka, J., (1962) Electroenceph. Clin. Neurophysiol. 14, 453.
Tyler, D. B., (1947) Amer. J. Physiol. 150, 253.
Ungar, G., (1968) Perspect. Biol. Med. 11, 217.
Vacca, R., (1965) "Esempi di Avvenire," Rizzoli, Milano.
Varolio, C., (1573) "De Nervis Opticis," Padova.
Vergnes, M. and Karli, P., (1963) Compt. Rend. Soc. Biol. 157, 176.
Vesalio, A., (1543) "De humani Corporis Fabrica libri Septem," Oporinus, Basilea.
Vieussens, R., (1685) "Nervographia universalis: oc est, omnium corporis humani nervorum, simul et cerebri, medullaeque spinalis descriptio anatomica," Lugduni.
Von Economo, C., (1929) "Die Encephalitis lethargica, ihre Nachkrankheiten und ihre Behandlung," Urban and Schwarzenberg, Berlin und Wien, p. 251.
Von Economo, C., (1930) J. Nerv. Ment. Dis. 7, 249.
Weiskrantz, L., Mihailovic, L., and Gross, C. G., (1962) Brain 85, 487.
West, L. J., Janszen, H. H., Lester, B. K., and Cornelisson, F. S., Jr., (1962) Ann. N. Y. Acad. Sci. 96, 66.
Willis, T., (1664) "Cerebri anatome, cui accessit nervorum descriptio et usus," Flesher, London.
Woodworth, R. S., (1938) "Experimental Psychology," Holt, New York.
Woodworth, R. S. and Scholsberg, H., (1954) "Experimental Psychology," rev. ed., Holt, New York.

Chapter II

THE NEURON

Several functions of the brain depend almost totally upon the physiological integration of some of those various specialized cerebral circuits and specific nuclei already mentioned. Their activity is ultimately the result of the contribution of each single neuron representing an operative unit of the central nervous system.

The first anatomical description of nerve cells were made by DUTROCHET (1824) and EHRENBERG (1833), while PURKINJE (1838) and REMAK (1837) completed the first systematic studies of axons, dendrites, and their connections with the cell body for which DEITERS in 1865 provided a complete descriptive picture; this description separated the neuron, dividing it morphologically from earlier generic descriptions and bundles and nervous fibers as defined in 1718 by VAN LEEUWENHOEK. Through a series of subsequent steps, it was possible to describe the shape of the neuron, so that it still holds contemporary validity, even when analyzed by means of optical techniques incomparably more precise in their power of resolution as, for instance, with the electron microscope; this has enabled the visualization of select subcellular elements, not visible with more traditional microscopic methods.

The neuron is essentially constituted by a cell body which includes the nucleus, the nucleoli, and GOLGI reticular apparatus (1898), by a series of branchings, the dendrites, and by a main extension, the axon (Fig. 8).

The size of the neuron may vary considerably as a function of the cerebral area within which it is located; in this respect it is possible to consider neuronal surfaces ranging from 300 μ^2 to almost 4,000 μ^2. In a similar manner, the number of dendrites of each neuron can vary (from 18 to 83) as may their length, which can range from 1,000 μ to 5,000 μ (BLINKOV and GLEZER, 1968). However, a key-point of functional significance, is represented by the synapses or intraneuronal junctions (see Fig. 8) which represent the points of contact among neurons. The synapses regulate the functional activity of the neurons, allowing the conduction of the nerve impulse from one element to another.

The number of central synapses is quite extensive, with as many as

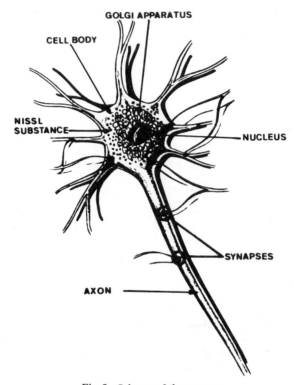

Fig. 8. Schema of the neuron.

almost ten thousand for each neuron; thus the overall potential for the shunting of nervous impulses can reach an extremely large number. According to the functional state of a specific cerebral region at a given moment, the synaptic network may allow for the possibility of an extremely rapid transmission of a signal to a receptor region or for the shifting of it through secondary "circuits"; in this way a true system of relays endowed with a differential and variable impedence is constituted. From both systematic and morphological viewpoints, it is possible to recognize axodentritic (DE ROBERTIS, 1959; GRAY, 1961; INOUYE et al., 1963; PATTERSON and FINEAN, 1961), as well as axosomatic (BODIAN, 1964; DE ROBERTIS, 1962; McMAHAN, 1964), dendrodendritic (VAN DER LOOS, 1964), and axoaxonic, synapses (BODIAN, 1962; GRAY, 1962; SZENTAGOTHAI, 1963). Central synapses are extremely complex and therefore make it difficult to make morphological generalizations, even though functionally different synapses have certain structural similarities.

A) THE SUBCELLULAR COMPONENTS

The fundamental components of the fine structure of the neuron have been described by PALAY and PALADE (1955) in their classical paper. Several subcellular elements, present in the neuron, assume not only morphological importance but may serve as substrates for a series of biochemical and enzymatic events, often highly selective, which form the actual basis of neuronal activity.

1) Neuronal Cell Body

From a descriptive point of view, the neuron is surrounded by a very thin *membrane* (10-20 mμ) (YOUNG, 1956; FERNANDEZ-MORAN, 1957) that is believed to be formed by two parallel protein surfaces, separated from one another by a double layer of lipids (SCHMITT et al., 1935). This membrane becomes thick in the synaptic region. From a functional point of view, the neuronal membrane constitutes a barrier that permits, through an active process, probably of an enzymatic nature, the selective passage of only specific compounds; in this way, at the cellular level, there is some similarity to the selective mechanism observed for the penetration of compounds into the brain, a system that has been commonly referred to as the blood-brain barrier.

The neuronal cytoplasm contains a number of single elements present in granulated form, these are also enclosed by a thin membrane that constitutes a center of enzymatic processes (SJÖSTRAND, 1956); such elements, originally described by NISSL in 1894, have been defined and designated as *tigroid substance.* It is now believed that they are formed by liporibonucleoproteins (HYDÉN, 1960) and they represent a cytoplasmic ribonucleic acid (RNA) pool (FERNADEZ-MORAN, 1957). Other granules, present in the cell nucleus, but differing in size (around 1 mμ), contain nuclear deoxyribonucleic acid (DNA) (HYDÉN, 1960). At this point it is interesting to note that, in accord with hypotheses concerning the relationship between memory processes and brain RNA (see Chapter I), these latter granules appear to be quantitatively dependent upon the functional status of the neuron, so that neuronal RNA concentration can vary from 50 to 100 $\mu\mu$g (EDSTRÖM and EICHNER, 1958).

Another structure recognizable in the neuronal cytoplasm is that described by GOLGI in 1898; this has been designated as the *Golgi reticular apparatus.* With the use of electron microscopy it appears as a vacualized succession of filaments with a limiting membrane of 6-7 μ (SJÖSTRAND,

1956). From a functional point of view, the Golgi appartus has been interpretated as a lipoprotein chain which takes part in the formation of the granules; it therefore assumes an essential role in the biosynthesis of the cerebral amines (BAKER, 1954; NATH, 1957; VAN BREEMEN et al., 1958), which as potential synaptic mediators will be treated further and in more detail.

The *mitochondria* also have notable significance; they are numerous in the neuron and are provided with a particular structure. Their number can vary from neuron to neuron and can exceed more than 2,500 in a single cell (BLINKOV and GLEZER, 1968). In the same way as other subcellular organelles, the qualitative aspects of the mitochondria of the cell body are also extremely variable, depending on the maturational status of the neuron considered (GLEZER, 1963). Their basic morphology consists of a double outer membrane with ramifications into the core of the mitochondrial structure; these create the typical "crested" appearance of mitochondria.

The mitochondria are now considered as one of the most important elements of cellular metabolism, certainly constituting a center of essential and multiple enzymatic activities. These elements are composed of 65-70% protein, 25-30% lipid, mainly phosphatides, and about 0.5% RNA. As already mentioned, a series of metabolic processes, mainly of the oxidative type, occurs in the mitochondria, together with a release of energy utilized in the synthesis of adenosine triphosphate (ATP) which is accumulated in the mitochondrion itself (HYDEN, 1960). The functional importance of these biochemical processes is also reflected in the quantitative distribution of mitochondria in the neuron; the greatest density of mitochondria occurs along the axon, particularly at the synaptic ending (SCHARF and BLUME, 1964; GLEZER, 1966), where metabolic activity appears to be most intense, while in the cell body these organelles are relatively less numerous.

It remains now to briefly mention another series of microstructures, the so-called neurofibrils; these appear as very thin filaments with a diameter of approximately 10-20 mμ (SCHULTZ et al., 1957; GRAY, 1959). At present these structures have been interpreted as microtubular formations and have been designed as *neurotubules;* it is believed that the vesicles, possibly containing some of the cerebral amines, are transported along the axoplasm within these neural elements (DE ROBERTIS, 1964; SANDBORN, 1964; VAN BREEMEN et al., 1958).

2) The Nucleus

HERTWIG (1903) had demonstrated the existence of a definite ratio between nuclei and cytoplasms that was greater in the neuron than in the other cells of the organism; this ratio was further shown to be evolutionary and to increase as a function of neuronal maturation (HAMBURGER, 1955).

The nucleus is limited by a membrane with a thickness ranging from 26 to 39 mμ, formed by a double layer of laminar proteins (BLINKOV and GLEZER, 1968; CHINN, 1938; PORTER, 1955). Electron microscopic findings have indicated that the membrane possesses a series of invaginations, directed toward the nuclear center, forming pockets of a given depth. This morphological arrangement has been suggested as a means by which the surface area for metabolic exchanges that occur between nucleus and cytoplasm is increased; this process is very likely assisted by a series of pores, varying in size from 40 to 100 mμ (HARTMANN, 1953; DE ROBERTIS et al., 1960) (Fig. 9).

The nucleus of the neuron contains about 7.1% DNA, 20% RNA (HELLER and ELLIOTT, 1954), 20-30% lipids (BRATTGARD and HYDÉN, 1952; TYRRELL and RICHTER, 1951), and 20% protein (DEBUCH and STAMMLER, 1956). The ratio of DNA to RNA is completely reversed in the other endonuclear formation, the *nucleoles*, in which RNA content is only approximately 0.5% (HYDÉN, 1943). The nucleoles usually vary in number from one to five for each cell nucleus, with equally variable dimensions of from 2 μ^3 to 60 μ^3. They are formed by a foundation of basic proteins with a large quantity of free amino groups, and it is possible to classify them among those constituents having the greatest mass to volume values (HYDÉN and LARSSON, 1956).

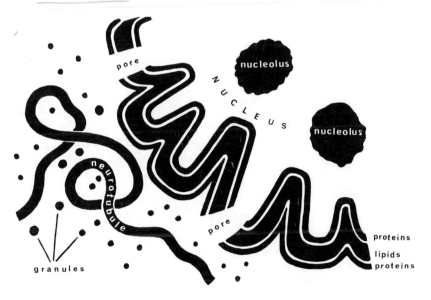

Fig. 9. Endo- and exonuclear structures.

3) The Dendrites

From a general point of view, the dendritic cytoplasm does not substantially differ from that of the neuronal cell body (HARTMANN, 1956; FERNANDEZ-MORAN, 1957; GRAY, 1959), so that it is possible to observe all of the structures present in the neuronal cell body in the dendrites as well; this includes all of those organelles from the mitochondria to the neurotubules. The only differences appear to be represented in the dendrites by an elongated appearance of the mitochondria and by the diameter of the neurotubules, which range from 18 to 20 $m\mu$ (GRAY, 1959).

4) The Axons

The axonal cytoplasm has been designated as axoplasm. The major characteristics of this intracellular medium are its high content of water, the longitudinal orientation of the fibrillar ultrastructures and neurotubules ranging in sizes from 40 to 90 $m\mu$ (DE ROBERTIS and SCHMITT, 1948). The fibrillar ultrastructures seem to be formed by filamentous proteins (HYDÉN, 1960), and at least one function to which these may be assigned is participation in the conduction of the nerve impulse or in the formation of a form of internal skeleton supporting the axonal structure. As far as neurotubules are concerned, it is now generally accepted that they contain vesicular formations (around 40 $m\mu$ in diameter; GRAY, 1961; PALAY, 1958), which are concentrated mainly in the synaptic region, and thus they have also been called *synaptic vesicles.* As previously indicated, these vesicles seem to be the carriers of those amines responsible for the transmission of the nervous impulse from neuron to neuron (SALMOIRAGHI et al., 1965; DAHLSTRÖM and FUXE, 1964).

Other elements such as the mitochondria, are present in the axoplasms, they do not possess any particular characterizations that allow them to be differentiated from those found in other portions of the neuron.

5) The Synapse

The synapse or the multiple sites for the functional interaction between synaptic zones present at interposed membrane surfaces in the neuron may be considered one of the most important and certainly essential regions of the entire neuronal structure. In fact, these regions of the nerve ending allow, through a series of biochemical mechanisms, for the transmission of the nerve impulse from one neuronal element to another and in this manner involve a vast complex of interrelated interactions involving considerable areas of cerebral activity and functions.

From a general point of view, the synapse consists of two distinct elements, the presynaptic terminal and the postsynaptic receptor, divided by a gap designed as the intersynaptic cleft. Descriptively, the presynaptic ending contains mitochondria, varying in number from one to ten, and is characterized by a membrane of greater thickness than that which surrounds the more distal segments of the nerve ending (Fig. 10).

Moreover, the synaptic vesicles, containing either acetylcholine (DE ROBERTIS, 1964; MICHAELSON et al., 1963; WHITTAKER, 1959), nor-epinephrine (DE ROBERTIS, 1964; MAYNERT et al., 1964; POTTER and AXELROD, 1963), serotonin (DE ROBERTIS, 1964; MAYNERT and KURIYAMA, 1964; MICHAELSON et al., 1963; RYALL, 1964), dopamine (LAVERTY et al., 1963), histamine (CARLINI and GREEN, 1963), or substance P (RYALL, 1964; WHITTAKER, 1964), are consistently observed as constitutents of presynaptic nerve endings. All the above-mentioned biologically active molecules are present in the synaptic vesicles in a granular form, probably bound to proteins and/or nucleotides that also require at least one divalent cation of a given ionic strength. It has been calculated that every single synaptic vesicle contains from several hundred to several thousand such molecules.

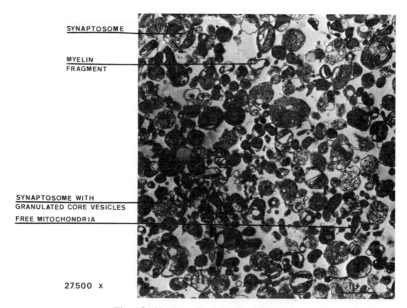

SYNAPTOSOME

MYELIN
FRAGMENT

SYNAPTOSOME WITH
GRANULATED CORE VESICLES
FREE MITOCHONDRIA

27.500 X

Fig. 10. Nerve ending constituents.

A space of about 10-20 mμ, the intersynaptic cleft, divides the pre-synaptic from the postsynaptic membrane (BLINKOV and GLEZER, 1968), the latter is thicker than that membrane covering the rest of the neuronal structure.

As previously mentioned, and to be treated in more detail later, a series of essential biochemical reactions and the operation of specialized mechanisms characterize the synaptic region when the nerve impulse is fired. It now seems possible to indicate that the mechanisms of action characteristic of synaptic events may be investigated, in one respect, through the use of selected psychotropic drugs believed to act upon one or more processes in the synaptic region. In this way functional studies of the synapse may be approached through pharmacological investigation.

The general description of the neuron and its ultrastructure up to this point should not be viewed in a static manner, since the neuron represents a substrate, the components of which integrate with each other continuously in a dynamic way to allow the multiple aspects of cerebral function to proceed, when such functions are considered to be due to the firing and the propagation of the nerve impulse within various pathways of the central nervous system.

B) THE NERVE IMPULSE

The substances which participate in constituting tissue excitability may be individually considered as possessing the same properties and characteristics that exist in any nonliving system, so that it may be assumed that such substances are transformed in a part of a living system by their capability to mutually interact in an organized manner; this condition places them within the context of other systems of the living structure (GABEL, 1965).

A peculiar characteristic of living systems is their excitability; this may be defined as that property of an organized group of particles which transfers environmental information along its constitutive elements while maintaining its structural integrity. This last condition is of essential importance since, if such information or stimuli are not transferred and utilized, the structural organization disintegrates; the stimulus itself may be viewed as initiating a "destructive" reaction, where the term, literally interpreted, connotes "capable of altering a structure". It may consequently be appropriate to consider that living systems become capable of expressing metastable and dynamic equilibria, show adaptation, and respond to various influences of environmental origin.

From this point of view, the nerve impulse and the expression of excitability and activity of the nervous system may be considered to be the main expression of a living system.

There are several highly specialized theories concerned with the phenomenon of electrogenesis, an analysis of which does not fall within the scope of this book. However, it is appropriate to consider that the electrochemical gradient characterizing the neuron is believed to be constituted by differences in potential that arise from differences in ionic concentration distributed selectively on the inner and on the outer surface of the poliphosphatide macromolecular complexes (GABEL, 1965). In this regard, the structure of excitable membranes has been described as a bimolecular layer of phospholipids, covered on both sides by a proteinic phase (ROBERTSON, 1960); this has been previously considered (see Fig. 9), and is typical of the neuronal membrane. With this type of membrane structure, the proteinic portion seems to be less important (STÄMPFLI, 1963) than the phospholipidic one. All of these considerations appropriately apply to the "membrane theory" of electrogenesis proposed by BERNSTEIN in 1902; this position integrates well with the equally classic ionic theory (HODKIN, 1964). In this context the exchanges between sodium and potassium, as well as the presence of calcium, become parts of a mechanism of dipole formation, fixed to the terminal groups of the membrane phosphatidic chains (GOLDMAN, 1962) so that the dipoles would determine the formation of differences in potential, which are responsible for the genesis of the nerve impulse which then spreads along the structure of the neuron.

The nerve impulse, when it reaches the synapses, excites the neurons which are in contact with them. This does not occur, however, in a direct way, since the discontinuity determined by the intersynaptic cleft, cannot be directly crossed by the small current that runs along the axon. In fact, nerve impulse transmission takes place only in a mediated way, through the release at the synaptic level of those biogenic substances which are functionally designated as *mediators of the nerve impulse.*

1) The Mediator Theory

The theory of biochemical mediation of the nerve impulse at the synapse developed in the past several years, beginning with biochemical studies concerning cerebral amines by AMIN et al. (1954), BRODIE and SHORE (1957), CARLSSON et al. (1958), FELDBERG (1945), VOGT (1954), VON EULER (1956), etc. The mechanisms for mediation of the nerve impulse generally have involved the initiation of the impulse, followed by a release, from the synaptic vesicles, of mediator molecules which spread, through the synaptic membrane into the intersynaptic cleft. Within the cleft these mediator molecules come in contact with a receptor membrane (BRODIE and BEAVEN, 1963).

This scheme, apparently simple, is supported, from an operational point of view, by a series of delicate regulatory mechanisms that moderate such mediatory function. For instance, it is known that transmitter substances are released in such quantity as to exceed the requirements of impulse mediation, so that at least two mechanisms exist by which excess quantities of transmitter substance may be inactivated. One of these is based upon the metabolic degradation of the transmitter molecules that are transformed into inactive derivatives; the other process consists of an active reuptake or retrieval of residual quantities of the transmitter that are reintroduced into the nerve ending by means of a membrane pump; in this way a system of transmitter storage pools is achieved. As may be seen later on, within the nerve ending, in accord with its specific transmitter molecule, there is a possibility for further partial metabolic degradation and vesicular reuptake which occur by means of an active transport mechanism similar to that previously indicated for the synaptic membrane.

It may be observed that most of these mechanisms which have been investigated empirically through the use of several psychotropic drugs as will be seen later, operate at the level schematically illustrated in Figure 11. In this figure they have been designated as COMT (catechol-0-methyltrans-ferase) and MAO (monoamine oxidase), respectively present in the synaptic cleft (outside the neuron) or in the mitochondria (inside the neuron), the

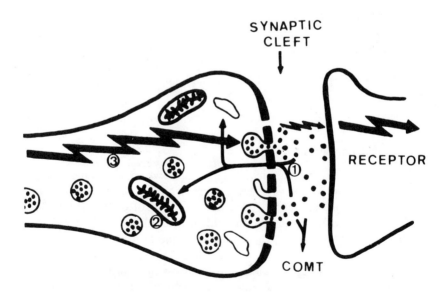

SYNAPTIC
CLEFT

RECEPTOR

COMT

Fig. 11. Schema of the synaptic mechanisms: (1) reuptake; (2) mitochondria; (3) nerve impulse. COMT: Catechol-oxydo-methyltransferase.

enzymes provided for the biochemical inactivation of at least three neurotransmitters (see Chapter III).

The foregoing proposal reintroduces the concept in which either brain functions or the behavior of living organism are related to the biochemistry of the neuron, and in particular to its biochemistry under both normal conditions and with pharmacological stimuli. At the same time such proposed relationships have provided bases upon which neurochemistry has been further developed to constitute a common denominator in the area of psychopharmacological research. In all likelihood, as usually occurs in the course of scientific evolution, the extension of the problem, generally coming through the refinement of experimental techniques, could provide bases for the consideration of new aspects or parameters of effect which at the present time still remain unclear.

2) The Glia

The attempt to better characterize the glial cells of the brain, and attribute a functional meaning to them has been a relatively recent effort.

The earliest descriptions of neuroglia (VIRCHOW, 1859) gave functional relevance to these cells as only cement (glia) binding adjacent neuronal elements together. Several other functional characteristics have been developed for glia, emerging largely from histological consideration of these cells themselves, or from their morphological relationship to adjacent neuronal structures. A common view, held for a considerable period of time, and serving as a convenient basis for excluding glia from further functional consideration, was that glial cells serve a nutritive function (BURNS, 1956) in supplying the neuron with its nutritive requirements, possibly by acting as channels between the neuron and proximal blood vessels (GOLGI, 1903). Repair or regenerative functions of glia have been suggested (WEIGERT, 1895; CAJAL, 1928, 1952) and their possible influence by neurons in a reciprocating relationship (CAJAL, 1928) has also been indicated. Additionally, secretory functions of these cells have been proposed (NAGEOTTE, 1910), and of course, these elements have also been cited as cellular loci constituting an anatomical basis for the blood-brain barrier.

Aside from some highly specific types of glia found in select areas of the central nervous system, there are, more generally, the fibrous and protoplasmic *astrocytes,* the former more prevalent in white matter and having some responsibility for myelin formation, are the *oligodendrocytes. Ependymal cells* have been frequently classed as a third general type of glia (Figs. 12 and 13).

Experimental consideration of the glia cells was reopened by two basic

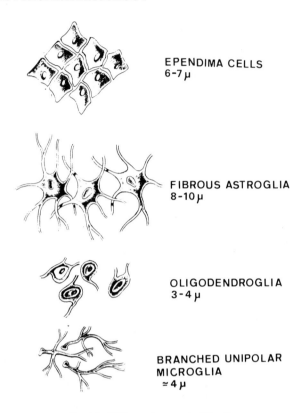

EPENDIMA CELLS
6-7 μ

FIBROUS ASTROGLIA
8-10 μ

OLIGODENDROGLIA
3-4 μ

BRANCHED UNIPOLAR
MICROGLIA
≈ 4 μ

Fig. 12. Different types of glial cells.

observations: one is concerned with the great quantity of these cells, in the brain the volume of which in man is equal to that of the neurons (BLINKOV and GLEZER, 1968); the other finding is that glia are also present even in the most elementary brains. It is interesting to note in this context that as early as 1886 NANSEN thought the glial population to be the seat of intelligence as "it increases in volume from the inferior animals to the superior ones."

In a brief consideration of glial function GALAMBOS (1961) advocated the hypothesis that the glia collaborate strictly with the neuron in determining animal behavior. In such a functional dualism, the glial cell assumes the function of "planning" activity for the neuron so that the latter acts only as a performer to instructions sent to it by the glia. Functional reevaluations of glial cells, particularly from a biochemical point of view, have been made by HYDÉN (1960) and GIACOBINI (1961); the observation that glial pro-

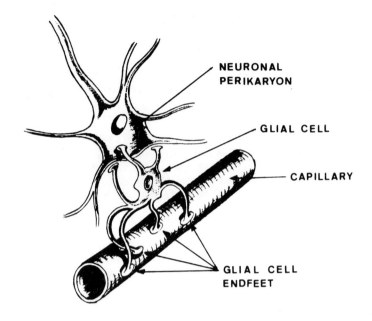

NEURONAL
PERIKARYON

GLIAL CELL

CAPILLARY

GLIAL CELL
ENDFEET

Fig. 13. Neuronal-circulatory glial connection.

cesses interpose themselves in the intersynaptic cleft (DE ROBERTIS, 1956;
DE ROBERTIS and BENETT, 1954; GRAY, 1959; PALADE and PALAY,
1956), could suggest the possibility that these cells could interfere in the
mediation of nerve impulse.

Several recent sources for a functionally dualistic role of glia have been
found in the application of new methodologies wherein glia have been either
morphologically, physiologically or metabolically distinguished from neurons.

Experimental studies of glial functions generally have been approached
using several possible techniques for the isolation of these cells from their
neuronal neighbors. Such methods have included (1) tissue culture of glia,
(2) use of gliomas, (3) microdissection of neurons and glia, and (4) tissue
fractionation to yield "enriched" fractions of these cells. These methodologies for isolating or purifying a population of glial cells, by which they may
be compared with the neuronal population with which they are associated,
have revealed several endogenous metabolic differences in macromolecules,
carbohydrates, and amino acids, as well as differences in response to
physiological and pharmacological stimulation (ROSE, 1969).

There are a number of cerebral functions for which glial participation
will, no doubt, ultimately be assigned a significant participatory role.

REFERENCES

Amin, A. H., Crawford, T. B. B., and Gaddum, J. H., (1954) J. Physiol., London **126**, 596.

Baker, J. R., (1954) J. R. Microsc. Soc. **74**, 217.

Blinkov, S. M. and Glezer, I. I., (1968) "The Human Brain in Figures and Tables," Basic Books Inc. Publ., Plenum Press, New York.

Bodian, D., (1962) Science **137**, 323.

Bodian, D., (1964) Bull. Johns Hopkins Hosp. **114**, 13.

Brattgard, S. O. and Hydén H., (1952) Acta Radiol (suppl.) **94**, 1.

Brodie, B. B. and Beaven, M. A., (1963) Med. Exper. **8**, 320.

Brodie, B. B. and Shore, P. A., (1957) Ann. N.Y. Acad. Sci. **66**, 631.

Burns, B. D., (1956) Can. J. Biochem. Physiol. **34**, 380.

Cajal, S. R. Y., (1928) in "Degeneration and Regeneration in the Nervous System," Milford, London.

Cajal, S. R. Y., (1952) in "Histologie du Systeme Nerveux de l'Homme et des Vertébres," Instituto Ramon y Cajal, Madrid.

Carlini, E. A. and Green, J. P., (1963) Biochem. Pharmacol. **12**, 1367.

Carlsson, A., Lindqvist, M., Magnusson, T., and Waldeck, B., (1958) Science **127**, 471.

Chinn, P., (1938) J. Cell. Comp. Physiol. **12**, 1.

Dahlström, A. and Fuxe, K., (1964) Acta Physiol. Scand. **60**, 293.

Debuch, H. and Stammler, A., (1956) Hoppe-Seyler's Z. Physiol. Chem. **305**, 111.

Deiters, O., (1865) "Untersuchungen über Gehirn und Rückenmark des Menschen und der Säugethiere," Hrsg. von M. Schutze, Vieweg, Braunschweig.

De Robertis, E., (1956) J. Biophys. Biochem. Cytol. **2**, 503.

De Robertis, E., (1959) Int. Rev. Cytol. **8**, 61.

De Robertis, E., (1962) in "Proceeding International Congress Neuropathology", Vol. 2, Munich, p. 35.

De Robertis, E., (1964) in "Progress in Brain Research," Vol. 8, "Biogenic Amines," Himwich, H. E. and Himwich, W. A., Eds., Elsevier Publ. Co., Amsterdam, p. 118.

De Robertis, E. (D. P.) and Benett, H. S., (1954) Fed. Proc. **13**, 35.

De Robertis, E. (D. P.), Nowinski, W. W., and Saez, F. A., (1960) "General Cytology," 3rd. ed., Saunders Co., Philadelphia.

De Robertis, E. and Schmitt, F. O., (1948) J. Cell. Comp. Physiol. **31**, 1.

Dutrochet, H., (1824) "Recherches Anatomiques et Physiologiques sur la Structure Intime des Animaux et des Végetaux et sur leur Motilité," Ballière, Paris.

Edström, J. and Eichner, D., (1958) Z. Zellforsch. Mikrosk. Anat. **48**, 187.

Ehrenberg, C. G., (1833) Poggendorf's Ann. Phys. Chem. **28**, 449.

Feldberg, W., (1945) Physiol. Rev. **25**, 596.

Fernandez-Moran, H., (1957) in "Metabolism of Nervous Tissue," Proc. Second International Symposium on Neurochemistry, Richter, D., Ed., Pergamon Press, London, p. 1.

Gabel, N. W., (1965) Life Sci. **4**, 2085.

Galambos, R., (1961) Proc. Nat. Acad. Sci. U.S. **47**, 129.

Giacobini, E., (1961) Science **134**, 1524.

Glezer, I. I., (1963) Zh. Nevropat. Psikhiat. **63**, 1189.

Glezer, I. I., (1966) in "Proceeding of the Symposium on Mitochondria: Structure and Function," Moscow, p. 24.

Goldman, D. E., (1962) in "Proceeding International Union Physiol. Sci., 22nd International Congress," Leiden, pt. II, Excerpta Medica Foundation, Amsterdam, p. 583.

Golgi, C., (1898) Arch. Ital. Biol. **30**, 60.
Golgi, C., (1903) "Opera Omnia," Vols. I & II, Hoepli, Milano.
Gray, E. G., (1959) J. Anat. **93**, 4.
Gray, E. G., (1961) J. Anat. **95**, 345.
Gray, E. G., (1962) Nature, London **193**, 82.
Hamburger, V., (1955) in "Biochemistry of the Developing Nervous System," Proc. 1st. Int. Neurochem. Symp., Waelsch, H., Ed., Academic Press, New York.
Hartmann, J. F., (1953) J. Comp. Neurol. **99**, 201.
Hartmann, J. F., (1956) J. Biophys. Biochem. Cytol. (Suppl.) **2**, 375.
Heller, J. H. and Elliott, K. A. C., (1954) Can. J. Biochem. Physiol. **32**, 584.
Hertwig, O., (1903) Biol. Zentbl. **23**, 49.
Hodkin, A. L. (1964) in "Les Prix Nobel en 1963", Nobel Foundation, Stockholm, p. 224.
Hydén, H., (1943) Acta Physiol. Scand. (suppl. 17) **6**, 136.
Hydén, H., (1960) in "The Cell", Brachet J. and Mirksky A. E., Eds., Vol. 4, Academic Press, New York p. 215.
Hydén, H. and Larsson, S., (1956) J. Neurochem. **1**, 134.
Inouye, A., Kataoka, K., and Shinagawa, J., (1963) Nature, London **198**, 291.
Laverty, R., Michaelson, I. A., Sharman, D. F., and Whittaker, V. P., (1963) Brit. J. Pharmacol. Chemother., **21**, 482.
Maynert, E. W. and Kuriyama, K., (1964) Life Sci. **3**, 1067.
Maynert, E. W., Levi, R., and De Lorenzo, A. J. D., (1964) J. Pharmol. Exper. Ther. **144**, 385.
McMahan, U. J., (1964) Anat. Rec. **148**, 310.
Michaelson, I. A., Whittaker, V. P., Laverty, R., and Sharman, D. F., (1963) Biochem. Pharm. **12**, 1450.
Nageotte, J. (1910) Comp. Rend. Soc. Biol. **68**, 1068.
Nansen, (1886) cited by Glees in "Neuroglia: Morphology and Function," Thomas C. C. Publ., Springfield, (1965), p. 9.
Nath, V., (1957) Nature, London, **180**, 967.
Nissl, F., (1894) Neurol. Zentbl. **13**, 676.
Palade, G. E. and Palay, S. L., (1956) J. Biophys. Biochem. Cytol. (Suppl.) **2**, 193.
Palay, S. L., (1958) Exper. Cell. Res. (Suppl.) **5**, 275.
Palay, S. L. and Palade, G. E., (1955) J. Biophys. Biochem. Cytol. **1**, 69.
Patterson, J. D. and Finean, J. B., (1961) J. Neurochem. **7**, 251.
Porter, K. R., (1955) Fed. Proc. **14**, 673.
Potter, L. T. and Axelrod, J., (1963) J. Pharmacol. Exper. Ther. **142**, 291.
Purkinje, J. E., (1838) in "Jan Ev. Purkiné, Opera Omnia," Purkyñova Společnost. T. 2, Prague (1937).
Remak, R. (1837) Froriep's neue Notizien aus dem Gebiete der Natur-und Heilkunde, pp. 36 & 216.
Robertson, J. D., (1960) Prog. Biophys. Biophys. Chem. **10**, 343.
Rose, S. P. R., (1969) in "Handbook of Neurochemistry," Lajtha, A., Ed., Vol. 2, Plenum Press, New York, p. 183.
Ryall, R. W., (1964) J. Neurochem. **11**, 131.
Salmoiraghi, G. C., Costa, E., and Bloom, F. E., (1965) Ann. Rev. Pharmol. **5**, 213.
Sandborn, E., (1964) Anat. Rec. **148**, 330.
Scharf, J. H. and Blume, R., (1964) J. Hirnforsch. **6**, 361.
Schmitt, F. O., Bear, R. S., and Clark, G. L., (1935) Radiology **15**, 131.
Schultz, R. L., Maynard, E. A., and Pease, D. C., (1957) Amer. J. Anat. **100**, 369.
Sjöstrand, F. S., (1956) Int. Rev. Cytol. **5**, 456.

Stämpfli, R., (1963) Ann. Rev. Physiol. **25,** 493.

Szentagothai, J., (1963) Acta Anat. **55,** 166.

Tyrrell, L. W. and Richter, D., (1951) Biochem. J. **49,** 4.

Van Breemen, V. L., Anderson, E., and Reger, J. F., (1958) Exper. Cell. Res. (suppl.) **5,** 153

Van der Loos, H. (1964) in "Progress in Brain Research," Vol. 6 "Topics in Basic Neurology," Bargmann, W. and Schadé J. P., Eds., Elsevier Publ. Co., Amsterdam, p. 43.

Van Leeuwenhoek, A., (1718) "Send-brieven, zoo aan de Hoog-edele Heeren van de koninklyke Societeit te Londen, als aan andere Aansienelyke en Geleerde Lieden," Beman, Delft.

Virchow, R., (1859) "Cellularpathologie," Hirchwald, Berlin.

Vogt, M., (1954) J. Physiol., London **123,** 451.

Von Euler, U. S., (1956) "Noradrenaline," Thomas, Springfield, Ill.

Whittaker, V. P., (1959) Biochem. J. **72,** 694.

Whittaker, V. P. (1964) in "Progress in Brain Research," Vol. 8 "Biogenic Amines," Himwich, H. E., and Himwich, W. A., Eds., Elsevier Publ. Co., Amsterdam, p. 90.

Young, J. L., (1956) in "Progress in Neurobiology," Ariens Kappers, J., Ed., Elsevier Publ. Co., Amsterdam, p. 3.

Chapter III

BRAIN NEUROTRANSMITTERS

As has been already mentioned in preceding chapters, the theory of biochemical mediation of the nervous impulse at the synaptic level is based on such extensive experimental evidence as to be generally well accepted. Those substances responsible for the mediation of synaptic transmission have been designated variously as neurohormones, neurotransmitters, nerve impulse modulators, brain mediators, etc. In the present context, not on the basis of any particular preference, but only in order to achieve uniformity of exposition, the term brain neurotransmitters, or more simply neurotransmitters will be used.

From the point of view of their chemical structure, neurotransmitters are mainly represented by several biogenic amines and, particularly, by some monoamines. Essentially, these are *serotonin* or *5-hydroxytryptamine* (5-HT), *norepinephrine* (NE), *dopamine* (DA), and *histamine* (Hia). While it does not directly fall within this particular class, *acetylcholine* (ACh), and several other molecules have also been strongly implicated as neurotransmitter agents (see Fig. 14).

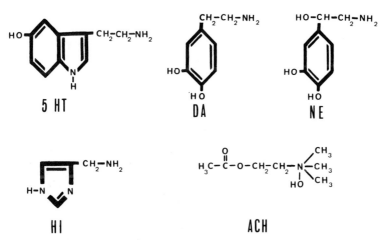

Fig. 14. Some neurotransmitter chemical structures.

It is believed in fact that certain other molecules such as substance P (RYALL, 1964; WHITTAKER, 1936, 1964) and γ - aminobuytyric acid (GABA: SALMOIRAGHI et al., 1965) may be given some significance as possible neurotransmitters at the central nervous system level. The former substance is believed to consist of a number of biologically active peptides, extractable from brain tissue, and inactivated by proteolytic enzymes. The latter, shown to act at crustacean synapses as an inhibitory transmitter and strongly indicated in a similar role for the mammalian central nervous system, is an amino acid apparently distributed generally as a cytoplasmic constituent rather than a specific nerve-ending component (WEINSTEIN et al., 1963; MANGAN and WHITTAKER, 1966). Studies concerning these molecules are still too fragmentary or inconclusive to permit them being more formally identified among other neurotransmitters.

A) NEUROTRANSMITTER CHARACTERIZATION

It becomes important to be able, within certain limits, to define as a neurotransmitter, such biologically active substances which take into account both the mechanisms of action of a variety of psychotropic drugs and also enter significantly into those cerebral changes associated with neuropathological conditions. It is immediately evident that several additional criteria, as well as definitive empirical studies, are required to more clearly define the nature of neurotransmitter molecules. In this context, some fundamental principles for the characterization of biogenic substances as neurotransmitters have been suggested (CURTIS, 1961; ECCLES, 1964; GADDUM, 1962; PATON, 1958).

At present these principles may be summarized as follows (SALMOIR-AGHI et al., 1965): a) the substance must be regionally localized together with a suitable series of enzyme systems responsible for either its formation or synthesis, and its metabolic inactivation; b) a substance hypothesized to be a neurotransmitter should show pharmacological activity at the postsynaptic cell that is typical for established transmitter molecules; and c) the neurotransmitter released at the nerve ending must, under all conditions, be identical with the substance stored in synaptic vesicles within the presynaptic nerve ending. The first principle of evaluation is probably the most important one, particularly since the localization of the transmitter molecule adheres to very strict limitations. This implies that for each of such substances there must be evidence for storage sites as well as specialized systems of transport at the synaptic level, while its presence in any major quantity should generally not occur in the synaptic axoplasm or

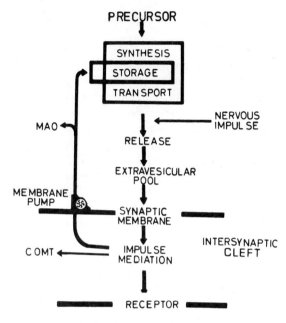

Fig. 15. Neuronal mechanisms.

cytoplasm. In other words, a putative transmitter substance has to limit itself within the context of those neuronal mechanisms, as have been schematically shown in Figure 15.

As generally considered up to this point, there may be a number of chemical substances the biological activity of which presents them as possible neurotransmitter candidates. Among these there are several that are highly prominent in terms of their meeting both the aforementioned criteria, as well as exerting behavioral effects when their metabolism or content is altered through the action of psychotropic drugs.

1) Serotonin (5-Hydroxytryptamine (5-HT))

Serotonin, so called by REID and RAND (1952) because of its peripheral vasoconstrictor activity, is identical with enteramine, an active substance derived from peripheral tissue by ERSPAMER in a series of studies begun in 1933 (ERSPAMER, 1954; VIALLI and ERSPAMER, 1933).

The significance of this substance as a neurotransmitter in the central nervous system had been postulated by BRODIE and SHORE (1957) and further confirmed by other authors (ROTHBALLER, 1959; CROSSLAND, 1960), initially on the basis of its selective distribution in different and functionally important areas of the brain (AMIN et al., 1954; BOGDANSKI et al., 1957).

From a chemical point of view, 5-HT is an indole-amine (Fig. 14) deriving from tryptophan, an essential amino acid, which is initially hydroxylated in the 5-position of the indole ring by a specific enzyme, *tryptophan-5-hydroxylase*, to form 5-hydroxytryptophan; this is further decarboxylated by another enzyme, *5-hydroxytryptophan-decarboxylase* which, in turn, leads to 5-HT formation. Under normal conditions it has been calculated that no more than 1 or 2% of an animal's body supply of tryptophan follows this metabolic route (UDENFRIEND et al., 1956). Therefore, this percentage can vary to a great extent, mainly in such pathological conditions as carcinoidosis, leading to profound alterations of serotonin metabolism (BEAN et al., 1955; FEIN and KNUDTSON, 1956; PAGE et al., 1955; VALZELLI, 1960; ZEITLIN and SMITH, 1966). In the body periphery serotonin is further metabolized through a number of different metabolic pathways, beginning with the oxidation by monoamine oxidase, to sulfatation, glycuronization, methylation, and various other routes (GARATTINI and VALZELLI, 1965). In the brain, however, the only pathway for inactivation is represented by monoamine oxidase, a mitochondrial enzyme which leads, through the intermediate formation of 5-hydroxyindolaldehyde (KEGLEVIĆ et al., 1968), to a final inactive product which is 5-hydroxyindoleacetic acid (PLETSCHER et al., 1961; ZELLER, 1961). This fact is of great importance, from a biochemical point of view, since it permits determination of the dynamic aspects of the 5-HT synthesis rate in the brain by means of the simple device of completely blocking the metabolic activity of monoamine oxidase; this will be further considered.

The conditions necessary for the definition of 5-HT as a neurotransmitter are partially satisfied by the fact that all of the metabolic steps required for its formation and inactivation are present in the brain. In this context it was initially believed that 5-HT was formed from the 5-hydroxytryptophan carried from areas in which tryptophan was hydroxylated by the peripheral blood to the brain. This source of the amine formation was mainly dependent upon the assumption that the amino acid crossed the blood-brain barrier with difficulty; hydroxylated homologues of the amino acid, however crossed the barrier easily, and in vitro experiments did not provide sufficient evidence to confirm any active hydroxylation of tryptophan by the brain tissue. Recently, however, it was shown, in vivo, that brain tissue can utilize available tryptophan, being able to hydroxylate it directly into 5-hydrotryptophan (CONSOLO et al., 1965; GAL et al., 1963; GRAHAME-SMITH, 1964; AIRAKSINEN et al., 1968).

Moreover, the technique of fluorescence in microscopy (Fig. 16) has indicated that 5-HT is stored in a granular form in vesicles which can travel

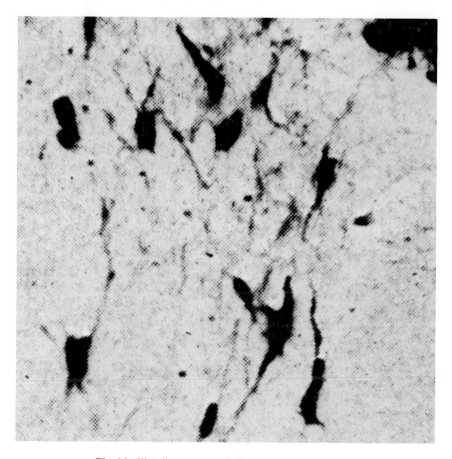

Fig. 16. Histofluorescence of 5HT containing cells.

along the axon at a speed of 5 mm/hr (LIVETT et al., 1968). When these
have reached the synapse, 5-HT is realeased from storage by nerve impulses
(DAHLSTRÖM and FUXE, 1964, 1965; FALCK, 1962; FUXE, 1965), as
indicated in the schemes shown in Figures 11 and 15. The metabolic
pathways for 5-HT and for brain norepinephrine and dopamine have been
summarized in Figure 17.

2) Norepinephrine (NE)

In a preliminary series of studies, VON EULER (1947, 1948) developed
the hypothesis that norepinephrine was the transmitter for mediation of the
nerve impulse within the sympathetic nervous system. Further studies (VON
EULER, 1961; VON EULER and HILLARP, 1956; VON EULER and

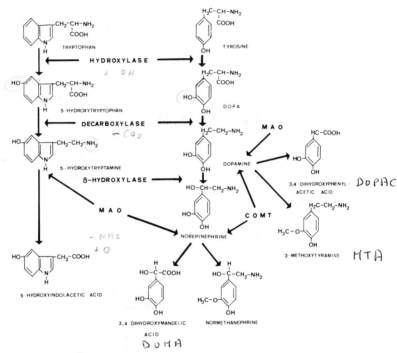

Fig. 17. Metabolic pathways of serotonin (5HT), dopamine (DA), and norepinephrine (NE).

LISHAJKO, 1960; STJÄRNE, 1966; THAEMERT, 1966) confirmed this initial postulate, also showing that NE was stored in granules within the synaptic vesicles. Also in the case of NE, it was shown that the technique of fluorescence microscopy could be applied to allow for either the direct visualization of the neurotransmitter within the synaptic structures (FALCK et al., 1962; FALK, 1962; DAHLSTRÖM and FUXE, 1964, 1965), or for verification of findings of related pharmacological interest (Fig. 18).

It was thus possible to observe that NE concentration was selectively elevated in those synapses where its concentration was higher that that found in other parts of the neuron. Furthermore, this amine is synthesized within the pericarya of the cell body, stored, as already indicated in the synaptic vesicles, and released from the granules by the nerve impulse (DAHLSTRÖM, 1967; DAHLSTRÖM and HÄGGENDAL, 1966).

As far as its metabolism is concerned, brain norepinephrine derives tyrosine which is initially hydroxylated to dihydroxyphenylalanine (DOPA) by a hydroxylating enzyme, which in some respects appears identical with the enzyme that hydroxylates tryptophan (GAL et al., 1966; ICHIYAMA et

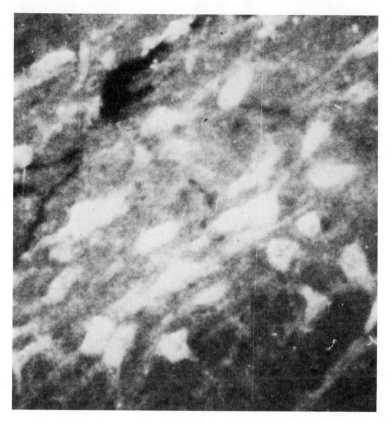

Fig. 18. Histofluorescence of norepinephrine containing cells (hypothalamus).

al., 1968). DOPA is then decarboxylated to dopamine (DA) and then, as a result of another enzyme, *dopamine-β-hydroxylase,* NE is formed. Neurotransmitter inactivation is accomplished through a dual mechanism, so that NE is partially inactivated in the synaptic cleft, and thereupon, extraneuronally by catechol-oxy-methyltransferases (COMT), which gives rise to the so-called basic metabolites (normetanephrine from NE, and 3-methoxytyramine from dopamine); that portion of the transmitter that is contributed to synaptic reuptake is inactivated by mitochondrial monoamine oxidases (MAO), as was noted for 5-HT, degrading the amine into the acid metabolites (3, 4-dyhydroxymandelic acid from NE and 3, 4-dyhydroxyphenylacetic acid from dopamine; see Fig. 13). However, after their removal from the synaptic terminal, the acid metabolites, which are individually inactive metabolically, are further modified by the extraneuronal COMT, which transforms them, respectively, into vanililmandelic acid and homovanillic acid.

3) Dopamine (DA)

Dopamine is the second of the suggested adrenergic transmitters of the catecholamine-type present in the central nervous system. As has previously been described for NE, DA derives from the same metabolic pathway and it is the precursor of NE (Fig. 17). It has all the necessary characteristics to merit its consideration as a neurotransmitter, and its neurobiological activity is particularly specific to certain specialized brain structures, such as the extrapyramidal system and the corpora striata (SOURKES and POIRIER, 1968). The identification and direct visualization of DA, by means of the techniques of histochemical fluorescence and fluorescence microscopy, has been extensively described by IVERSEN (1967).

4) Acetylcholine (ACh)

Surprisingly and somewhat paradoxically, acetylcholine, which has been known for many years as a transmitter for the peripheral parasympathetic nervous system, is at the brain level, less well understood, although it certainly is characterized among the neurotransmitters.

The explanation for this apparent conceptual gap is mainly accounted for by differences in techniques for tissue extraction and determination of this substance which, because of its physico-chemical characteristics, is not easily nor precisely measurable.

One of the earliest hypotheses concerning the importance of ACh in the brain was advanced by DALE in 1937; this was further considered by other authors (WHITTAKER, 1959; CURTIS and ANDERSEN, 1962; DE ROBERTIS et al., 1962; LAVERTY et al., 1963; RENTSCH, 1966) with suggestive evidence in support of its activity as neurotransmitter. From a metabolic point of view, ACh derives from the reaction of choline with acetylic radicals, in the presence of coenzyme A and of acetylkinase, and is then inactivated by acetylcholinesterase, leading to the formation of choline and acetate. Regarding the specificity of ACh at the neuronal level, GIA-COBINI and HOLMSTEDT (1958) showed that isolated nerve cells had the ability to hydrolyze esters of choline; these findings were also confirmed by other investigators by means of histochemical techniques (HÄRKÖNEN, 1964; SÖDERHOLM, 1965, ZELENA and LUBINSKA, 1962). Moreover, at the neuronal level, the presence of high cholineacetylase activity was demonstrated (McCAMAN, 1963; McCAMAN and HUNT, 1965), and thought to be mainly confined to the neuronal membrane structures (HEBB and WHITTAKER, 1958; DE ROBERTIS et al., 1963). Other studies confirmed the presence of ACh and cholineacetylase in the synaptic vesicles (WHITTAKER et al., 1963; DE ROBERTIS et al., 1963), in this way meeting the criteria outlined for qualification as a possible neurotransmitter.

5) Histamine (Hia)

The possibility that histamine is a neurotransmitter, is based upon findings of its presence and localization in brain structures (CARLINI and GREEN, 1963; MICHAELSON and DOWE, 1963). KWIATOWSKI (1943) had observed a difference in the distribution of histamine in different brain structures, and subsequent studies (NAITO and KURIAKI, 1957) indicated the presence of a selective distribution of histidinedecarboxylase. From a metabolic point of view histamine is simply formed from the decarboxylation of histidine and is then inactivated by diamineoxidase of histaminase (ZELLER, 1965); it also appears that histamine can also be metabolized to a certain extent by monoamine oxidases (ZELLER et al., 1956).

Data is too incomplete to permit an accurate representation of the role of histamine in the central nervous system.

B) DISTRIBUTION AT THE BRAIN LEVEL

Generally, the presence of a specific biologically active molecule in a particular tissue, in this case the brain, is considered the first clue to possible functional participation of that substance in the tissue considered. Further and more definite, support for this premise derives from findings of a selective distribution of such active substances in structures or specialized areas of the brain. Of those neurotransmitters previously considered, and particularly for 5-HT, NE, and DA, a considerable number of experimental studies have demonstrated differences in concentration that vary for specific brain areas; this has been observed in experimental animals and in man.

A brief overview of this differential distribution is shown in Tables I, II, and III.

Obviously, the data reported represent only a very small segment of those existing in the literature and have been intended only as an example. In fact, it is possible to find variations among absolute concentration levels of brain amines reported by different authors; this is probably due either to differences in the animal species or strain studied, to the method of tissue extraction employed to determine the concentration of the substance under examination, or possibly due to the sampling reliability, depending upon the size and number of tissue samples. However, these facts do not diminish the value of the differential distribution concept for neurotransmitter localization in different brain regions. In the case of DA, for example, its maximal concentration is evident in striated nuelei, both in man and in animals; it is now well known that this substance serves to mediate neurological changes characterizing the extrapyramidal syndromes, particularly, in Parkinson's disease (BARBEAU, 1969; BIRKMAYER and HORNIKIEVICZ, 1961;

TABLE I

5HT Distribution (γ/g of tissue) in Various Brain Areas of Different Animal Species

Brain Areas	Mouse[a]	Rat[b]	Dog[c]	Man[c]
Whole brain	0.65 ± 0.03	0.37 ± 0.01	–	–
Hemispheres	0.36 ± 0.03	0.25 ± 0.01	0.01	–
Hypothalamus	–	0.65 ± 0.01	0.99	0.81
Thalamus	–	0.36 ± 0.01	0.47	0.62
Corpora quadrigemina	1.10 ± 0.07	0.63 ± 0.04	–	0.76
Medulla oblongata	–	0.55 ± 0.01	–	0.34
Corpora striata	–	0.30 ± 0.04	–	–
Cerebellum	n.m.[d]	n.m.	0.02	0.03
Olfactory bulbs	0.39 ± 0.01	0.21 ± 0.03	0.08	0.39
Mesencephalon	0.62 ± 0.03	–	0.72	–
Diencephalon	0.94 ± 0.02	–	–	–

[a]Valzelli, 1967.

[b]Valzelli and Garattini, 1968.

[c]Garattini and Valzelli, 1965 (Appendix V).

[d]n.m. denotes quantities not measurable.

TABLE II

NE Distribution (γ/g of tissue) in Various Brain Areas of Different Animal Species

Brain Areas	Mouse[a]	Rat[b]	Dog[c]	Man[c]
Whole brain	0.45 ± 0.02	0.28 ± 0.01	0.14	–
Hemispheres	0.36 ± 0.03	0.17 ± 0.03	–	–
Hypothalamus	–	0.73 ± 0.03	1.03	1.11
Thalamus	–	0.35 ± 0.01	–	0.04
Corpora quadrigemina	0.60 ± 0.05	0.28 ± 0.03	–	0.15
Medulla oblongata	–	0.32 ± 0.03	–	0.14
Corpora striata	–	0.71 ± 0.01	–	–
Cerebellum	0.10 ± 0.02	0.10 ± 0.01	–	0.01
Olfactory bulbs	0.11 ± 0.02	0.26 ± 0.01	0.05	–
Mesencephalon	0.39 ± 0.05	–	0.37	'–
Diencephalon	0.55 ± 0.05	–	–	–

[a]Valzelli, 1967.

[b]Valzelli and Garattini, 1968.

[c]Garattini and Valzelli, 1965 (Appendix V).

COTZIAS et al., 1969; EHRINGER and HORNIKIEVICZ, 1960). On the other hand, the maximal concentrations of NE are found in the hypothalamus, as is the case for 5-HT, which however is also particularly concentrated in the corpora quadrigemina.

At this time only scattered data concerning acetylcholine concentration

TABLE III

DA Distribution (γ/g of tissue) in Various Brain Areas of Different Animal Species

Brain Areas	Mouse[a]	Rat[b]	Dog[c]	Man[c]
Whole brain	1.09 ± 0.05	0.49 ± 0.02	0.22	–
Hemispheres	1.77 ± 0.01	0.50 ± 0.04	–	–
Hypothalamus	–	0.52 ± 0.05	0.26	1.12
Thalamus	–	0.22 ± 0.03	–	0.29
Corpora quadrigemina	0.71 ± 0.02	0.15 ± 0.01	–	0.07
Medulla oblongata	–	0.09 ± 0.01	–	0.17
Corpora striata	4.21 ± 0.03[d]	5.25 ± 0.15	–	–
Caudate nucleus	–	–	6.5	–
Putamen	–	–	–	8.25
Cerebellum	n.m.[e]	n.m.	0.03	0.02
Olfactory bulbs	0.63 ± 0.02	0.19 ± 0.01	–	–
Mesencephalon	0.06 ± 0.01	–	0.20	–
Diencephalon	0.29 ± 0.01	–	–	–

[a]Valzelli, 1967.

[b]Valzelli and Garattini, 1968.

[c]Garattini and Valzelli, 1965 (Appendix V).

[d]Valzelli and Ramirez del Angel, unpublished data.

[e]n.m. denotes quantities not measurable.

in the different brain areas are available. As previously mentioned, this is partially a consequence of the lack of a direct and suitable method for the determination of this neurotransmitter. Consequently, most of the data concerning ACh have been expressed in terms of cholinacetylase activity (BEANI et al., 1964; McCAMAN and HUNT, 1965) or as the quantity of acetylcholine-like activity emerging from a biological test which responds proportionally to the different concentrations of neurotransmitter; this has been so, even when employing new methods of purification and tissue extraction and the increasing reliability of results (TAKAHASHI and APRISON, 1964; TORU and APRISON, 1966; TORU et al., 1966).

More recently (FELLMAN, 1969) the problem concerning brain distribution of this transmitter has been considerably revised. In Table IV, the ACh content of different areas of rat brain, have been summarized according to TAKAHASHI and APRISON (1964). Recent developments combining separation techniques involving gas chromatography and analysis with mass spectrometry (JENDEN, 1970; JENDEN et al., 1970; JENDEN and CAMPBELL, 1971) have made microdetermination of brain ACh much more feasible. From the use of such a methodological approach several interesting descriptive and functional observations have been made possible; these have included, for example, the regional distribution of ACh in the rat

TABLE IV

ACh Contents (mμ moles/g of tissue) in
Different Brain Areas of the Rat

Brain Areas	ACh Contents
Diencephalon	22.3 ± 1.84
Mesencephalon	16.7 ± 2.68
Pons and medulla	12.3 ± 2.39
Cerebellum	2.3 ± 0.74
Caudate nucleus	37.5 ± 2.69
Olfactory bulbs	16.4 ± 4.07
White matter	7.9 ± 1.87
Gray matter	3.3 ± 0.80

brain, a description of the effects of cholinergic and anticholinergic drugs, and their interaction, upon brain ACh levels, and measurement of circadian variations in brain ACh content in the rat (HANIN et al., 1969). Certainly more functional studies of brain ACh may be anticipated with the availability of such recent methodologies.

As has already been described for DA, ACh is maximally concentrated in striated formations (caudate nucleus) and this localization has found some functional significance in that the ester has been associated with motor activity.

The data concerning histamine and its determination in the brain are also somewhat in question; in this case, this is perhaps due to the analytic methods employed for localization; the problem might be overcome by the spectrofluorometric techniques now available (SHORE et al., 1959; KREMZNER and PFEIFFER, 1966; MEDINA and SHORE, 1966). However even these techniques are not completely free from sources of interference with fluorescence measurements by other substances, and it must be emphasized that a certain degree of caution must be exercised in accepting suggested correlations between variations in brain amine level and the activity of psychotropic drugs. In fact, a number of behaviorally active substances exist which, both in animals and man, modify brain neurotransmitter content; these include reserpine and monoamine oxidase inhibitors and their analogs. There are also a considerable number of other psychotropic drugs, of equipotent pharmacological activity, which do not produce appreciable variations in brain neurotransmitter levels.

A possible interpretation of this fact is that drugs, such as the latter, selectively influence very specialized brain areas, so that, possible neurotransmitter variations that may actually occur can be overlooked in a quantitative, global determination, the differences being too small and too selectively localized. Another possible explanation may be provided in the fact that the concentration of a particular transmitter substance at a particular time following the administration of a drug that does not act directly or strongly upon normal levels of such a transmitter molecule may still be extremely significant when possible variations in the dynamic aspects of this molecule, as represented by its synthesis and inactivation, are considered.

On the basis of present evidence, the level of a specific neurotransmitter at a given time is the result of its synthesis rate, which is balanced against a given inactivation rate. As a consequence, it is possible to have a transmitter, which although unchanged in concentration under given conditions, is sustained by different synthesis and inactivation rates. This has been noted in different strains of rats and mice under normal conditions (Table V).

TABLE V

Brain 5HT Contents and Turnover in Different Mouse and Rat Strains

(male = M; female = F)[a]

			Turnover	
Strain	Sex	Brain 5HT μg/g $\pm$ SE	rate (μg/g/hr)	Time (min)
Mice				
Albino Swiss	M	0.69 ± 0.03	0.58	67
Albino Swiss	F	0.64 ± 0.05	0.64	59
CFW/Sel	M	1.01 ± 0.08	0.95	57
CBA/J	M	1.07 ± 0.08	0.53	86
BALB/C	M	0.95 ± 0.04	0.55	96
DBA/2J	F	0.96 ± 0.07	0.69	77
Rats				
Sprague-Dawley	M	0.48 ± 0.03	0.38	70
Buffalo	M	0.35 ± 0.01	0.37	85
Wistar	M	0.40 ± 0.02	0.21	108
ACI	M	0.49 ± 0.02	0.35	76

[a]Valzelli, Giacalone, and Consolo, unpublished data.

Considering the dynamic evolution of neurotransmitter synthesis and inactivation (*turnover process*) as a self-regulating mechanism (*feedback mechanism*), it is easily seen how, within limits, decreases or increases in neurotransmitter inactivation rate will correspond respectively to an increase or a decrease in its rate of synthesis (Figs. 19 and 20).

Hence, the concept of neurotransmitter turnover must be considered as being somewhat more important than the simple concentration of the neurotransmitter itself. It is possible, therefore, that several psychotropic drugs, which do not appreciably alter neurotransmitter concentration, may however, act upon its turnover, providing consequently, a different orienta-

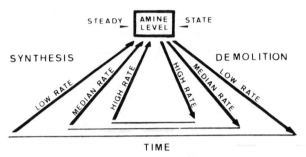

Fig. 19. Schema of different kinds of turnover.

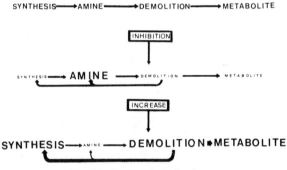

Fig. 20. Feedback mechanism.

tion to the functional and biochemical aspects of synaptic transmission in the brain.

It should be further pointed out that an error of formulation frequently encountered is the development of a hypothesis based upon concentration changes in single neurotransmitter, without taking account of a mutual integration of different concentrations of multiple transmitters; such considerations could well encompass further bases for explanation of the experimental results.

It is within this context that consideration may be given to the functional integration of the "trophotropic" and "ergotropic" centers hypothesized by HESS (1954): the first concept referred to mastery of "recovering" activities and was held to be responsible for sedation in general, the other center was believed to be of the "activating" type and responsible for excitation. Later, this hypothesis was given biochemical significance by BRODIE (BRODIE and SHORE, 1957; BRODIE and COSTA, 1961) who indicated that 5-HT could represent the mediator for "trophotropic" centers and NE and DA, the neurotransmitters of "ergotropic" centers. This theory has led to many fascinating areas of research

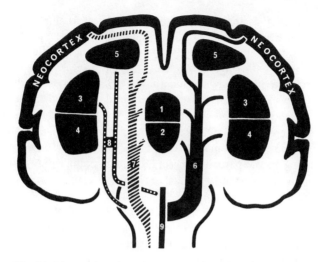

Fig. 21. Monoaminergic pathways: (1) thalamus; (2) hypothalamus; (3) neostriatum; (4) paleostriatum; (5) anterior
limbic formation; (6) serotoninergic pathways; (7)
noradrenergic pathways; (8) dopaminergic pathways;
(9) mesencephalic raphe.

involving both neurochemical and neuropharmacological studies for several
years, and considerable experimental effort is still being devoted to testing
hypotheses concerned with initial formulation.

C) MONOAMINERGIC NERVE FIBERS

According to SALMOIRAGHI and BLOOM (1964), it is possible to
consider the present period of experimental effort in the neurochemical and
psychopharmacological areas, as a strongly evolutionary one. It has been
previously seen that experimental approaches considering brain neurotransmitter concentration changes were extended to include the turnover concept; this has opened the way for more molecular levels of neurotransmitter
analysis—turning to the application of techniques of cell biology to treat
neurotransmitter variations at the cellular and subcellular levels as a consequence of a pharmacological stimulation (HÖKFELT, 1966; VAN ORDEN
et al., 1966; FUXE, 1965). All these approaches have been directed toward
the possibility of evolving a series of neural routes comprised of serotoninergic, noradrenergic, and dopaminergic pathways (ANDÉN et al., 1966a, b;
see Fig. 21).

Such experimental study was facilitated by the use of histochemical
fluorescence and fluorescence microscopy methods combined with other

methodologies such as anatomical lesions or electrical stimulation of several localized brain regions; these were designed to provide variations at a "distance" in monoamine contents for some brain specific nuclei and regions (ANDÉN et al., 1964, 1966a, b).

Through the use of such methods it was possible to establish that an ascending nigro-striatal system depended upon dopaminergic mediation, as did other projections of this type innervating the olfactory tubercules and the acumbens septi nucleus. Other ascending pathways having noradrenergic mediation originate from some neuronal aggregates localized in the pons and medulla oblongata and partially project into the hypothalamus (paraventricular and periventricular dorsomedial nucleus), preoptic and septal area, amygdaloid complex, hippocampus, and cingulate gyrus and, to some extent the neocortex. It may be of interest to note that several of these structures are part of the limbic circuit already described (see Chapter I, B and Fig. 2).

Another series of pathways operating essentially on the basis of serotoninergic mediation, originates in neurons of the median and dorsal nuclei of the mesencephalic raphé and project directly to the telencephalon and diencephalon, particularly to globus pallidus, septal area, amygdaloid complex, hypothalamus, and cingulate gyrus as well as to the neocortex.

It appears from these findings that for those brain areas believed to be responsible for emotional and affective states and also the elaboration of such conditions on a behavioral level, a balancing system may be considered wherein appropriate anatomo-functional circuits are integrated to encompass both HESS' hypothesis and the biochemical theory formulated by BRODIE.

REFERENCES

Airaksinen, M., Giacalone, E., and Valzelli, L., (1968) J. Neurochem. 15, 55.

Amin, A. H., Crawford, T. B. B., and Gaddum, J. H., (1954) J. Physiol., London, 126, 596.

Andén, N. E., Carlsson, A., Dahlström, A., Fuxe, K., Hillarp, N.-Å., and Larsson K., (1964) Life Sci. 3, 523.

Andén, N. E., Dahlström, A., Fuxe, K., Larsson, K., Oslon, L., and Ungerstedt, U., (1966a) Acta Physiol. Scand. 37, 313.

Andén, N. E., Dahlström, A., Fuxe, K., Olson, L., and Ungerstedt, U., (1966b) Experientia 22, 44.

Barbeau, A., (1969) Union Med. Con. 98, 183.

Bean, W. B., Olch, D., and Weinberg, H. B., (1955) Circulation 12, 1.

Beani, L., Bianchi, C., and Megazzini, P., (1964) Experientia 20, 677.

Birkmayer, W. and Hornikiewicz, O., (1961) Wien Klin. Wschr. 73, 787.

Bogdanski, D. F., Weissbach, H., and Undenfriend, S., (1957) J. Neurochem. 1, 272.

Brodie, B. B. and Costa, E., (1961) in "Monoamines et Système Nerveux Central," Proc. Symposium Bel-Air, Genève, Georg & C.ie S.A., Genève, p. 13.

Brodie, B. B. and Shore, P. A., (1957) Ann. N.Y. Acad. Sci. 66, 631.

Carlini, E. A. and Green, J. P. (1963) Biochem. Pharmacol. **12**, 1367.

Consolo, S., Garattini, S., Ghielmetti, R., Morselli, P., and Valzelli, L., (1965) Life Sci. **4**, 625.

Cotzias, G., Papavasiliou, P. S., and Gellenf, R., (1969) N. Eng. J. Med. **280**, 337.

Crossland, J., (1960) J. Pharm. Pharmacol. **12**, 1.

Curtis, D. R., (1961) in "Nervous Inhibition", Florey, E., Ed., Pergamon Press, Oxford.

Curtis, D. R. and Andersen, P., (1962) Nature, London **195**, 1105.

Dahlström, A., (1967) Arch. Pharmak. Exper. Pathol. **257**, 93.

Dahlström, A. and Fuxe, K., (1964) Acta Physiol. Scand. (Suppl. 232) **62**, 1.

Dahlström, A. and Fuxe, K., (1965) Acta Physiol. Scand. (Suppl. 247) **64**, 1.

Dahlström, A. and Häggendal, J., (1966) Acta Physiol. Scand. **67**, 271.

Dale, H. H., (1937) Harvey Lect. **32**, 229.

De Robertis, E., Pellegrino de Iraldi, A., Rodriguez de Lores Arnaiz, G., and Salganicoff L., (1962) J. Neurochem. **9**, 23.

De Robertis, E., Rodriguez de Lores Arnaiz, G., Salganicoff, L., Pellegrino de Iraldi, A., and Zieher L. M., (1963) J. Neurochem **70**, 225.

Eccles, J. C., (1964) "The Physiology of Synapses," Academic Press, New York.

Ehringer, H. and Hornikiewicz, O., (1960) Klin. Wschr. **38**, 1236.

Erspamer, V., (1954) Rendiconti Scientifici Farmitalia **1**, 1.

Falck, B., (1962) Acta Physiol. Scand. (Suppl. 197) **56**, 1.

Falck, B. Hillarp, N.-Å., Thieme, G., and Torp, A., (1962) J. Histochem. Cytochem. **10**, 348.

Fein, S. B. and Knudtson, K. P., (1956) Cancer, Philadelphia **9**, 148.

Fellman, J. H., (1969) J. Neurochem. **16**, 135.

Fuxe, K., (1965) Acta Physiol. Scand. (Suppl. 247) **64**, 39.

Gaddum, J. H., (1962) in "Proc. 1st. International Pharmacological Meeting," Vol. 8 "Pharmacological Analysis of Central Nervous Action," Paton W. D. M. and Lindgren P., Eds., Pergamon Press., Oxford, p. 1.

Gal, E. M., Armstrong, J. C., and Ginsberg, B., (1966) J. Neurochem. **13**, 643.

Gal, E. M., Poczik, M., and Marshall, F. D., Jr., (1963) Biochem. Biophys. Res. Commun. **12**, 39.

Garattini, S. and Valzelli, L., (1965) "Serotonin," Elsevier Publ. Co., Amsterdam.

Giacobini, E. and Holmstedt, B., (1958) Acta Physiol. Scand. **42**, 12.

Grahame-Smith, D. G., (1964) Biochem. Biophys. Res. Commun. **16**, 586.

Hanin, I., Massarelli, R., and Costa, E., (1969) Physiologist **12**, 246.

Härkönen, M., (1964) Acta Physiol. Scand. (Suppl. 237) **63**, 1.

Hebb, C. O. and Whittaker, V. P., (1958) J. Physiol., London **142**, 187.

Hess, W. R., (1954) "Diencephalon: Autonomic and Extra Pyramidal Function," Grune and Stratton, New York.

Hökfelt, T., (1966) Experientia **22**, 56.

Ichiyama, A., Nakamura, S., Nishizuka, Y., and Hayaishi, O., (1968) in "Advances in Pharmacology," Vol. 6A, Garattini, S. and Shore, P. A., Eds., Academic Press, New York, p. 5.

Iversen, L. L., (1967) Nature, London **214**, 8.

Jenden, D. J., (1970) in "Drugs and Cholinergic Mechanisms in the CNS," Heilbronn, E. and Winter, A., Eds., Res. Inst. Nat. Defense, Stockholm, p. 3.

Jenden, D. J. and Campbell, L. B., (1971) in "Methods of Biochemical Analysis," Vol. 19, Glick D., Ed., Wiley, New York, p. 183.

Keglević, D., Kveder, S., and Iskrić (1968) in "Advances in Pharmacology," Vol. 6A, Garattini, S. and Shore, P. A., Eds., Academic Press, New York, p. 79.

Kremzner, L. T. and Pfeiffer, C. C., (1966) Biochem. Pharmacol. **15**, 197.

Kwiatowski, H., (1943) J. Physiol., London **102**, 32.

Laverty, R., Michaelson, I. A., Sharman, D. F., and Whittaker, V. P., (1963) Brit. J. Pharmacol. **21**, 482.

Livett, B. G., Geffen, L. B., and Austin, L., (1968) Nature, London **217**, 278.

Mangan, J. L. and Whittaker, V. P., (1966) Biochem. J. **98**, 128.

McCaman, R. E. (1963) Fed. Proc. Fed. Amer. Soc. Exper. Biol. **22**, 170.

McCaman, R. E. and Hunt, J. M., (1965) J. Neurochem. **12**, 253.

Medina, M. and Shore, P. A., (1966) Biochem. Pharmacol. **15**, 1627.

Michaelson, I. A. and Dowe, G., (1963) Biochem. Pharmacol. **12**, 949.

Naito, T. and Kuriaki, K., (1957) Arch. Exper. Pathol. Pharmak. **232**, 481.

Page, I. H., Corcoran, A. C., Undenfriend, S., Szoedsma, A., and Weissbach, H., (1955) Lancet **1**, 198.

Paton, W. D. M., (1958) Ann. Rev. Physiol. **20**, 431.

Pletscher, A., Gey, K. F., and Zeller, P., (1961) Progr. Drug Res. **2**, 417.

Reid, G. and Rand, M., (1952) Aust. J. Exper. Biol. Med. Sci. **29**, 401.

Rentsch, G., (1966) Med. Welt, Berlin. **7**, 321.

Rothballer, A. B., (1959) Pharmacol. Rev. **11**, 494.

Ryall, R. W., (1964) J. Neurochem. **11**, 131.

Salmoiraghi, G. C. and Bloom, F. E., (1964) Science **144**, 493.

Salmoiraghi, G. C., Costa, E., and Bloom, F. E. (1965) Ann. Rev. Pharmacol. **5**, 213.

Shore, P. A., Burkhalter, A., and Chon, V. H., Jr., (1959) J. Pharmacol. Exper. Ther. **127**, 182.

Söderholm, U., (1965) Acta Physiol. Scand. (Suppl. 256) **65**, 3.

Sourkes, T. L. and Poirier, L. J., (1968) in "Advances in Pharmacology," Vol. 6A, Garattini, S. and Shore, P. A., Eds., Academic Press, New York, p. 335.

Stjärne L. (1966) Acta Physiol. Scand. **67**, 441.

Takahashi, R. and Aprison, M. H., (1964) J. Neurochem. **11**, 887.

Thaemert, J. C., (1966) J. Cell. Biol. **28**, 37.

Toru, M, and Aprison, M. H., (1966) J. Neurochem. **13**, 1533.

Toru, M., Hingtgen, J. N., and Aprison, M. H., (1966) Life Sci. **5**, 181.

Udenfriend, S., Weissbach, H., and Sjöerdsma, A. (1956) Science **123**, 669.

Valzelli, L., (1960) Recenti Progr. Med. **29**, 426.

Valzelli, L., (1967) in "Neuropsychopharmacology" (Proc. V. Int. CINP Symp., Washington,D.C. 1966), Excerpta Medica Foundation, Amsterdam, p. 781.

Valzelli, L. and Garattini, S., (1968) J. Neurochem. **15**, 259.

Van Orden, L. S. III, Bloom, F. E., Barnett, R. J., and Giarman, N. J., (1966) J. Pharmacol. Exper. Ther. **154**, 185.

Vialli, M. and Erspamer, V., (1933) Zellforschung **19**, 321.

Von Euler, U. S., (1947) Acta Physiol. Scand. **12**, 73.

Von Euler, U. S., (1948) Acta Physiol. Scand. **16**, 63.

Von Euler, U. S., (1961) Harvey Lect. **55**, 43.

Von Euler, U. S. and Hillarp, N.-A., (1956) Nature, London **177**, 44.

Von Euler, U. S. and Lishajko, F., (1960) Science **132**, 351.

Weinstein, H., Roberts, E., and Kakefuda, T., (1963) Biochem. Pharmacol. **12**, 503.

Whittaker, V. P., (1959) Biochem. J. **72**, 694.

Whittaker, V. P., (1963) in "Proc. 1st International Pharmacological Meeting," Vol. 5 "Methods for the Study of Pharmacological Effects at Cellular and Sub-Cellular Levels," Lowry, O. H. and Lindgren, P.,Eds., Pergamon Press, Oxford, p. 61.

Whittaker, V. P., (1964) in "Progress in Brain Research," Vol. 8 "Biogenic Amines," Himwich, H. E. and Himwich, W. A., Eds., Elsevier Publ. Co., Amsterdam, p. 90.

Whittaker, V. P., Michaelson, I. A., and Kirkland, R. J., (1963) Biochem. Pharmacol. **12**, 300.

Zeitlin, I. J. and Smith, A. N., (1966) Lancet **2**, 986.

Zelena, J. and Lubinska, L., (1962) Physiol. Bohemoslov. **11**, 261.

Zeller, E. A., (1961) in "Monoamines et Système Nerveux Central" (Proc. Symposium Bel-Air Genève), Georg & C.ie S. A., Genève, p. 51.

Zeller, E. A., (1965) Fed. Proc. Fed. Amer. Soc. Exper. Biol. **24**, 766.

Zeller, E. A., Stern, P., and Blanksma, L. A., (1956) Naturwissenschaften **43**, 157.

Chapter IV

METHODS IN PSYCHOPHARMACOLOGY

There appears to be some indication that a gap exists between experimental and clinical psychopharmacology; this potential dichotomy has been essentially based upon a relatively philosophical interpretation of the term "psychopharmacology", much more than upon a practical or operational definition. In other words, the concept of drugs acting upon "psychic" processes, implied by the term, is the main idea requiring additional interpretation. It may be stated that, even if the term itself is applied exclusively to experimental investigation at the human level, this denotation cannot be taken as a sufficiently valid reason to exclude, on the basis of such a species-specific definition, all of the extremely important data derived from experimental psychopharmacology with animals.

Moreover, there is a critical position held by some clinicians, which tends to further minimize the utility of experimental animal research in this field; this view basically argues that experimental studies in animals have no meaningful significance for man, lacking validity and mutual grounds for generalization (SHEPHERD et al., 1968). Also, in this context, such an attitude derives much more from a polemic position, rather than from an unbiased one. It may be considered, for instance, that the general formulations of brain mechanisms, ranging from the biochemical concommitants of nerve impulses mediation and the mapping of brain monoaminergic pathways, the concept of functional circuits, illustrate one way in which methodologically significant contributions of psychopharmacology are made to the growing body of information concerning the functional properties of the central nervous system. These derive mainly from those data obtained experimentally from animals.

Another relevant consideration is that several experimental approaches to the brain and its functions, particularly biochemical investigation, become possible only through animal investigation.

On the other hand, it is noteworthy that some psychopharmacological research approaches tend to focus mainly upon the pharmacology of psychotropic drugs, and moreover, that the development of psychopharmacology has been so rapid, and is still progressing at such a rapid rate, so as to make difficult the unification and reciprocal integration of the multiple experimental techniques, the interdisciplinary methodologies, and the emerging results thereof.

From an experimental point of view, it is noteworthy that the human brain consists of a series of extremely important functional circuits which are to a considerable extent similar to those described in animals (Chapter I; Fig. 3); in conjunction with this, most of the emotional substrates regulating several behavioral patterns are shared in common among species. Beginning with this fundamental consideration, a series of experimental investigations have recently been carried out in order to derive models of altered animal behavior which may approximate several features of human psychopathology; it has been through the medium of such analogs that biochemical studies related to altered functional brain states have emerged, and extended investigation of neurochemical individuality and variation may be further explored.

A) GENERAL BEHAVIOR

By the term "general behavior" we include all of those different activities that a given animal shows within a familiar environment, both from the point of view of inserting itself into the social context of its group and in terms of the stimulation provided by the mean level of existing environmental inputs. When confined within these limits, the various steps that shape and drive general behavior derive essentially from previously rewarding or frustrating experiences as well as from those environmental emotional cues providing for species- and self-preservation.

Obviously, it is possible to observe a number of behavioral differences between wild animals and animals of the same species bred under highly standardized laboratory conditions. In this regard, BARNETT (1963) has reported a highly experimentally derived and comparative study of the rat.

The animals' general behavior may be considered to result from the integration of imputs deriving from the environment impinging upon the central nervous system and thus upon the peripheral capacity of an organism to deliver a response or a coordinated sequence of responses. This fact necessarily implies a certain amount of caution to be exercised in the accurate evaluation of a drug's central activity which may be masked by a series of peripheral effects. Thus, for instance, a muscle-relaxant drug can conceal central sedation or can mimic antiaggressive activity simply by impairing the muscular capacity required to initiate or maintain fighting behavior.

The evaluation of general behavior is mainly based upon direct observation and, then, on the observer's discriminative ability; only in part does it take advantage of a certain more specific evaluative technique, the more common of which are measurements of the spontaneous motor activity and of peripheral muscle tonus.

1) Evaluation of Spontaneous Motor Activity

In the experimental literature several techniques for the measurement of spontaneous motor activity or, more briefly, the spontaneous locomotor activity of small mammals have been described. Some of these methods, developed several years ago, are still employed, largely because of their simplicity, as in the case of the *revolving drum,* or *activity wheel,* first described and employed by STEWART in 1898. This method essentially consists of a centrally pivoted drum-shaped cage in which the animal is placed so that its gross movements are transformed by the drum into revolving motions that are counted within a specified interval of time.

Some modifications of this basic method were proposed and later described (SKINNER, 1933; SIEGEL, 1946) but have not substantially changed the characteristics and performance of this apparatus which is more suitable for the measurement of drug-induced decreases rather than increases of motor activity. In particular, very minimal animal movements cannot be recorded using this type of apparatus, so that RICHTER (1927) has described and employed another method, designated as the *swinging cage*; this consists of a cage resting upon pneumatic sockets connected by tubes to a pen writing on smoked paper. WILBUR (1936) and HUNT and SCHLOSBERG (1939) proposed some minor variations of this apparatus, mainly consisting of a spring system on which a cage was suspended to allow for swinging to be initiated by movement within the cage.

In contrast to the rotating drum, the swinging cage is very efficient for recording and measuring small animal movements and tremors but it is quite unsuitable for the careful measurement of extensive gross movements.

DEWS (1953) employed a cage with transparent walls, across which a thin luminous or infrared beam, invisible to the animals, was directed; deviations in the constancy of this beam were recorded by a photocell, so that an interruption of the circuit passing through the beam, caused by an animal's movement, may be recorded on a counter which summarizes the movements within a fixed period of time (*Dews' Test*). With this technique, as well, small animal movements are not counted while a source of error may derive from a long-lasting interruption of the beam when an animal happens to stop in front of the light source.

Recently a new apparatus has become available which is based essentially upon a series of electromagnetic fields which are modified by the animal's passage within them. This system, completed by a counter and a timer, is quite sensitive and contains no "dead-ground"; however, it cannot record tremor in small animals, which is often an important aspect of locomotor capacity, particularly as initiated by psychotropic drugs. Other similar types of apparatus have been based upon the use of a piezoelectric head (FROMMEL, 1965).

From a general point of view, the ideal apparatus for the measurement of spontaneous locomotor activity must be (a) sensitive to every type of animal movement, (b) sensitive to the slightest changes in the animal's activity, (c) without any dead-ground in its functioning, and (d) constant in its function. It may be reasonably concluded that an apparatus which functions to include the first two measurement requirements is still not available.

It should be emphasized that there are a number of variables that are capable of contributing significantly to differences and variations in loco-motor activity measurements in experimental animals. While several of these variables are readily subject to experimental control their potential effect upon activity measurement, individually or in interaction with psychoactive drugs, should not be overlooked. It has long been observed that periodic episodes of increased locomotor activity occur in animals that have been deprived of food. This relationship between a "hunger drive" and increased activity is also superimposed upon another characteristic of animal activa-tion—namely, its cyclical nature. RICHTER (1927) has shown that periodic episodes of increased activity in a food-deprived rat were correlated with periodic stomach contractions, and that given the opportunity to gain access to food, the rat took this opportunity during peak periods of activity. Aside from the hunger-periodicity interaction contributing to activity differ-ences in the animals, there is also a hunger-illumination interaction that has been investigated (JEROME et al., 1957). The effects of illumination, per se, upon locomotor activity are probably closely related to or interact with cyclical variations in locomotion. Greater activity levels for rats housed in darkness, with increases every few hours (HUNT and SCHLOSBERG, 1939) are probably related to the primarily nocturnal nature of these animals.

Other factors such as temperature (BROWMAN, 1942, 1943), age (RICH-TER, 1922), sex hormone level (HOSKINS, 1941), estrous (RICHTER, 1932), genetic factors (BRODY, 1942), and, of course, physiological, ana-tomical, or biochemical intervention in the central nervous system can contribute significantly to the level of locomotor activity in experimental animals. It may be of further interest to observe that body weight, upon which drug dosage in laboratory animals is primarily based, has been found to be positively and significantly correlated ($r = 0.60; p < 0.001$) with activity level in the rat, measured over a 24 hour interval (TURNBULL, cited by CROSSLAND, 1970). These findings indicated that 36 percent of the locomotor activity variation found for a group of rats could be attributed to weight differences.

2) Evaluation of Muscle Strength

In the evaluation of the effects of a psychotropic drug, an important issue is represented by possible muscle relaxant effects; these may reflect either the central activity of the drug under examination or, simply an effect secondary to other underlying activities.

One of the simplest methods for recording a muscle relaxant effect consists of placing rats or mice in a position whereby they are supported by their forelimbs with the paws grasping a small bar approximately 30 cm above the laboratory bench; in this situation the duration of clinging by the animal may be noted. Obviously, it is necessary to obtain basal grasping time indices from appropriate control animals before evaluating a possible drug effect.

Another method, which combines both the aspects of muscle strength and coordinated movements, has been called the *rotating bar* or *rota-rod*; this consists of a rod, the diameter of which is varied depending upon its use with mice (1.5 cm) or with rats (3 cm). The rod is rotated on its axis by a motor at a velocity of 5 rpm and is elevated above a surface by about 20 cm. Using this test, the time during which drug-treated animals are able to maintain themselves on the rota-rod, may be compared with those times comparably obtained for control animals.

One methodological variation on this general theme consists of putting the animal into a tube, 50 cm in length with a diameter suitable to the size of the experimental animal; the tube is then lifted up at one end so that it becomes oblique and, by its angle, causes the animal to slide back into the tube; the difference in angles required to displace the control animals and those treated with the specific drug under study, provides a measure of the general strength of the muscular apparatus.

There are, however, some conditions in which the animal's general overt posture may immediately suggest a general involvement of muscular tonus, and preclude the necessity of any more precise functional test. This is typical of the *muscular hypertonus* of the extrapyramidal rigidity type, which may be observed in reserpinized animals, which may develop cataleptic-like states characterized by plasticity, postural flexibility, and the maintenance of abnormal positions of rigidity (Fig. 22).

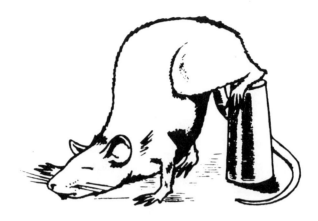

Fig. 22. Catalepsia (by reserpine).

Of a similar overt nature, the opposite situation may also be observed, where there is a development of deep *muscle relaxation,* causing an impairment of maintenance of normal posture; moreover, when an animal is placed in nonphysiological positions such as on its back, it may be barely able or completely unable to return to an upright position (reduction or abolition of the *righting reflex*).

Another overt sign of muscle involvement is *ataxia,* which may be measured by a method in which the animal's paws are inked and then it is allowed to walk on a surface where its paw prints will be imprinted; measurement of such prints from some reference point may thereby provide a precise evaluation of the possible anomalies of gait that have developed (KHAÏRY, 1961).

At this point it seems useful to note that the two essentially contrasting situations represented by muscular hypertonus and by muscular relaxation, when measured by means of one of those techniques previously described for the evaluation of motor activity (Section 1), both yield the common result of an apparent decrease in the measure obtained. In fact, a strongly excitatory drug which may induce tremors, muscular hypertonus, and ataxia in animals can lead to impaired performance as measured by these techniques in much a similar manner to the attenuated performance that may be brought about by sedatives or muscle-relaxants.

3) Behavioral Profile

Analysis of a certain specific number of components of the behavioral repertoire of a given laboratory animal, may provide a means of developing a satisfactory behavioral profile. IRWIN (1959) has listed a series of patterns divided into three categories, respectively concerned with behavioral, neurological, and autonomic activities, which yield a profile reasonably indicative of the animal's general functional status and capacity (Tables VI, VII, VIII).

TABLE VI

Behavioral Profile

Consciousness	Motor Activity	Affective Reactions
Spatial orientation	spontaneous activity	grooming
Arousal	reactivity to environment	vocalization
Stupor	response to touch	restlessness
Visual discrimination	response to pain	irritability
Catalepsy		aggressivity
Stereotypsy		fear

TABLE VII

Neurological Profile

Central Excitation	Motor Incoordination	Muscular Tonus	Reflexes
Starts	body position	limb tonus	corneal
Tail "Straub's reaction"	limb position	grasping strength	pineal
Tremors	waving gait	bodily tonus	scratching
Dysmetria	abnormal gait	abdominal tonus	righting
Muscle twitching			torsion
Opystotomes			
Convulsions			

TABLE VIII

Autonomic System Profile

Eyes	Secretions and Excretions	General	Lethality
Pupillary size	lacrimatin	piloerection	late
Eyelid opening	urination	hypothermia	acute
Exophtalmus	salivation	cyanosis	
Eye opacity	diarrhoea	heart rate	
		respiratory rate	
		respiratory or heart arhythmia	

The items listed in the tables are scored utilizing arbitrary units as referred to normal animal patterns.

Generally, this test, known as *Irwin's Test*, even if functionally complete, must be integrated through observation and measurement of other aspects of behavior which provide access to those animal responses which may be taken as the expression of higher nervous activities and which are revealed by specialized behavior.

B) SPECIALIZED BEHAVIOR

The problem of animal intelligence is still a *vexata quaestio* having as many supporters as it has deniers.

The fundamental characteristics of human nature, according to psychologists, are essentially of two kinds. One series of such characteristics concerns consciousness—the thoughts and feelings of inner life, mainly described as "self-consciousness" and "awareness", while the second series pertains to behavior as an expression of those living activities which, lying beyond access by physical, chemical, anatomical, and physiological analysis, are brought together under the general terms of "intelligence" and "character" (THORNDIKE, 1965).

Without exceeding the limits of simple experimental commentary, it is possible to assert that animal psychology possesses the same double content, so that such terms as perception, attention, memory, learning, etc. are appropriately employed by both animal and human behaviorists. Moreover, in many animal species it is possible to demonstrate the presence of discriminative as well as associative processes, which are investigated in man with several experimental conditioning techniques.

What seems peculiar to man is his ability to elaborate and integrate information of varied origin and to accumulate a logical, speculative, or applied capacity that is identified with reasoning skill. It is however interesting to note that the learning abilities, as shown by most different animals, and by vertebrates in particular (BITTERMAN, 1960, 1965), may be considered as the foundation of a theory concerning the potential development of intelligent behavior (STENHOUSE, 1965), the main components of which are curiosity and exploratory behavior (BERLYNE, 1966).

It then becomes evident that it is important to carefully evaluate those experimental parameters which actively reflect the animal's higher nervous functions (SOKOLOV, 1963) and wherein several psychoactive drugs can induce a series of complex modifications.

1) Exploratory Behavior

One of the first pieces of basic evidence that derived from the PAVLOV experiences in the study of higher nervous functions (1927), concerned the exploratory or orienting reflex; this essentially consists of a response made by an animal to novel or unanticipated stimulus; the response involves cessation of ongoing activity with an attentional shift to the stimulus source. Such a reflex is characterized by the fact that, if the frequency of the stimulus presentation is increased within a brief interval, the orienting response gradually disappears. The response may reappear if the stimulus is represented, for instance, on the following day but, after a series of subsequent reinforcements and extinctions, the response permanently fades (BERLYNE, 1960) as it gradually loses its properties of uniqueness or novelty.

On the same basis, a rat is more inclined to maintain interest in an object or situation that has not previously been experienced in the experimental situation than in some conditions just explored within the previous ten minutes (BERYLNE, 1950); similarly, an animal maintained in a new environment develops a mode of behavior orientation toward exploration of the characteristics of such an environment. Also in this case, the exploratory or orienting reflex diminishes and tends to disappear when the experimental situation is repeated in time (BERLYNE, 1955; MONTGOMERY, 1953).

Apart from the influence of novelty, the intensity of the drive underlying exploratory behavior depends, both in man and animal, upon the level of stimulus complexity, so that exploratory behavior becomes more active and prolonged as the object or environment provides an increased number of novel and unpredictable stimuli (WILLIAMS and KUTCHA, 1957; WEL-KER, 1956).

Without further detailing this issue, it seems clear that exploratory behavior is based upon a series of central activities, among which emotion-ality plays a prominent role. In fact, all of those factors capable of leading to increases in the arousal level, such as painful sensations, fear, range, noise, distraction from an exploratory task, etc. tend to render both animal and man less inclined to become aware of the novelty or complexity of the stimulus (CHAPMAN and LEVY, 1957; HAYWARD, 1962; THOMPSON and HIGGINS, 1958).

FISKE and MADDI (1961) have developed a behavioral theory based upon the assumption that, in the absence of a specific task to perform, the behavior of a given organism tends to maintain that inner activation level which is normal or characteristic for it; so that, those animals, whose activation level is more elevated than normal, do not show exploratory behavior. Moreover, deprived animals will explore less than others whose environment has been provided with stimulus variety. Obviously, such factors as hunger and thirst (FOSTER, 1959; GLICKMAN and JENSEN, 1961; RICHARDS and LESLIE, 1962), sex (LESTER, 1967a,b), and differ-ences in basic level of emotionality (VALZELLI, 1966; GREGORY, 1968; GUPTA and HOLLAND, 1969) can induce variations in exploratory behavior. Those methods probably most appropriately employed to study animal exploratory behavior, are mainly represented by open-field tests, the maze, and the hole-board. As generally used the *open-field* test is essentially represented by a square or round surface of about one square meter, with walls 40 cm high, painted in quenched and opaque colors to avoid light reflections that might serve as a source of distraction for the animal (MEAD, 1960; VALLE, 1970). The apparatus is uniformly illuminated and its floor is divided into a series of squares. Some investigators (HENDERSON, 1967) have used such an apparatus provided with two photoelectric circuits with the beams orthogonally arranged to register the animal's spontaneous activity. The scoring of open-field activity is generally performed within a five minute interval, taking account of how the animal traverses the subdivisions designated on the floor of the open-field. The floor subdivisions are usually kept within predetermined scoring values, such that the peripheral sector adjoining the walls of the area are of a smaller value than the central sectors, which are most traversed as a function of a more intense exploratory drive.

The intensity and number of defecations have also been used as a measure reflecting the emotional level of the animal (BRUELL, 1963; HENDERSON, 1967). The frequency with which an animal shows the typical exploratory posture of standing on its hindlegs (Fig. 23) has also been employed as a potential measure of emotionality.

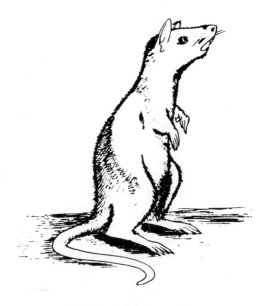

Fig. 23. Orienting reaction.

This test, simple in its conception, even if more difficult in its interpretation, remains a reliable index of the emotional status of the animal (DENENBERG et al., 1964; IVINSKINS, 1966).

Regarding *mazes,* their type, pattern, dimensions, and complexity have been widely varied in accordance with their use by different investigators, so that it has been extremely difficult to standardize both the methodology as well as the results obtained. However, from the historical point of view, the maze is perhaps the first setup employed for studies of animal psychology (LASHLEY, 1929; SMALL, 1899; WATSON, 1907, 1914).

Aside from the "map" differences and complexity (Fig. 24), some common and important maze characteristics are represented by the diffuse and undazzling illumination and by the quenched color coating of the apparatus. Indeed the extensive variability in experimental design construction allows, according to some authors, the inclusion of a series of motivated drives, such as hunger or thirst, so that an animal at the end of a positive trial, is rewarded with some food or water (SMALL, 1899; WATSON, 1907; TSANG, 1934; HUNTER, 1940) while others add a conditioning component such as a soft electric shock (KUO, 1922; MÜNZIGER, 1934; VALENTINE, 1930) or a bell sounded (MÜNZIGER, 1936) when the animal takes the wrong way, so that the maze is transformed into a complex learning situation. It has to be considered that animal performances in a maze are the results of a series of sensorial interactions which imply the integration of the visual, olfactive, acoustic, and tactile controls (MUNN, 1950) with the participation of the learning processes, all of which are based

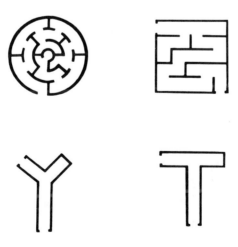

Fig. 24. Different types of mazes.

upon the common ground of the emotional shape of the experimental animal.

Recently, BOISSIER and SIMON (1962, 1964), described and successfully employed the *hole-board test,* an extremely simple and most useful setup to study animal behavior in a free environment. The hole-board consists merely of a board, kept some 20 cm from the desk, with a series of holes which appear endless to the exploring animal.

The surface dimension is of about one-half square meter on which sixteen holes, 3 cm in diameter, are uniformly distributed. The method is somewhat related to the open-field situation but presents the animal with a stronger stimulus for exploratory behavior, represented by the holes which the animal explores by inserting its head into them. The measure of exploratory activity is represented by the number of holes explored within a predetermined period of time, usually varying between three and five minutes. Recently there have been some commercially available automated devices offered* (BOISSIER and SIMON, 1967; VALZELLI, 1971) which automatically register the number of holes explored by the animal during a period of time that can be varied by the investigator (Fig. 25).

The hole-board test is particularly useful for the measurement of differences in exploratory behavior after drug treatment (BOISSIER et al.,

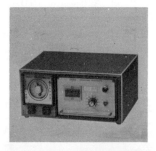

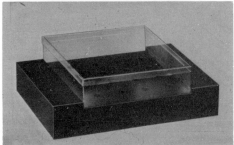

Fig. 25. Automatized hole-board apparatus.

*LP Italiana, Via Lepanto 6, Milano, Italy; Apelab, Bagneaux, France.

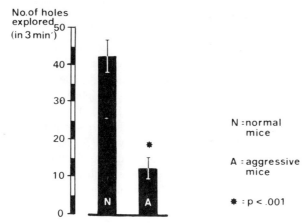

Fig. 26. Exploratory behavior of normal (N) and aggressive (A) mice.

1964), and also for describing differences in emotional level between animals, for example, variances of normal and aggressive mice derived from the same strain following a suitable period of differential housing. According to the FISKE and MADDI postulate (1961; see page 67) aggressive animals, that are in a situation of social deprivation as a consequence of isolation, explore much less than normal animals living together and interacting with one another (Fig. 26).

Moreover, it can be observed that with differential housing (grouping or isolation) providing for differences in emotional status, some psychoactive drugs show a differential activity (VALZELLI, 1969a, 1971, 1973).

However, as previously indicated for the maze, the use of the hole-board test with too brief an intertrial interval leads to a decrease of exploratory behavior due to stimulus satiation, the attenuation of task novelty, and a presumed reduction of the exploratory drive.

The hole-board test is particularly suitable for studies with mice, and a variation of this method that is quite effective with rats consists of a board with a series of tunnels which can be explored by the animals (SHILLITO, 1969).

Aside from exploratory behavior, there are several other parameters which should be included in the analytical study of specialized animal behavior, such as sexual and social patterns. These are both extremely important to the comprehensive study of animal behavior but, at the same time, they are not too easily utilized, or quantified as potential measures of psychotropic drug activity; this is due, in part, to the complexity and variability of those factors that may be involved in measurement, such as the degree of specialization required for an observer to correctly evaluate the results.

2) Conditioning Techniques

During the past several years, the use of conditioning techniques has become so elaborate and complicated as to become a highly specialized area endowed with its own characteristic terminology, placing this branch of methodology into an almost independent discipline within the general framework of psychopharmacology (DEWS, 1953).

Conditioning studies find their origin in the earlier experimental observations of PAVLOV (1927); these studies were, in part, concerned with stimulus continuity, where the repeated coupling of a nonspecific stimulus, or conditional stimulus (CS), with another stimulus (unconditioned stimulus: US) capable of consistently evoking an unconditioned response (UCR), resulted in a conditioned response (CR)—i.e., eliciting a response, similar to or identical with the UCR—to the presentation of the CS alone.

From a practical point of view, in accordance with PAVLOV's classical observations, the presentation of food (US) to a hungry dog induces an intense salivary response (UCR) and when a bell is sounded (CS) immediately prior to the food presentation the ringing of the bell alone becomes capable, after a number of CS-US pairings, of inducing salivation (CR). Moreover, other stimuli, different from the bell, are capable of eliciting the conditioned response, so that both the discriminative and selective properties of the animal can be studied; this suggests one avenue through which the investigation of drug activity on the acquisition or extinction of the conditioned reflex may be carried out.

From this initial framework, two major classes of conditioning techniques originated—avoidance conditioning and free-operant conditioning.

In *avoidance conditioning*, there is a visual or auditory stimulus utilized to signal the subsequent onset of a noxious stimulus, so that the animal must provide responses capable of mediating the avoidance or postponement of the noxious stimulus; this stimulus usually consists of a mild electric shock. The earliest types of apparatus for conditioning this type of response in the rat, which is the species most frequently employed in this situation, were described by WARNER (1932a,b), HUNTER (1935), MOTE (1940), and GELLHORN et al., (1942, 1943). The basic operational mode of these methods is that, following a visual or auditory warning stimulus, the animal must: (a) climb a pole or on a rope to avoid foot-shock delivered through the cage floor, (b) press a lever to postpone the shock for a certain time, (c) pass through a small door in order to reach a nonelectrified portion of the cage where shock may be avoided. In a modified version of this latter method, the cage floor is balanced so that the weight of the moving animal alternatively activates and deactivates an electric circuit in each one of the two halfs of the cage. This type of apparatus is called a "shuttle box" and several further variations of this basic design have been utilized to take into account such parameters as time before shock onset, shock intensity and duration, and the complexity of the exit response.

A typical form of shuttle box avoidance conditioning consists in placing a rodent in one side of a double compartment box with a grid floor which can be alternatively electrified on either side. A light is usually fixed to the wall of each compartment, which, when illuminated, signals the subsequent onset of foot-shock, usually delayed by some interval of seconds. The animal can avoid foot-shock by crossing to the opposite compartment, where, after an appropriate time delay, the light cue again warns of a forthcoming shock that can be avoided by shuttling back to the other compartment.

The conditioning process has been considered to be the basic element of learning (WATSON, 1916; PAVLOV, 1927; HULL, 1943) and it therefore seems appropriate to study the activity of drugs upon avoidance behavior, especially with regard to the differences induced in the animal's response to the conditional stimulus and to shock (HERZ, 1960).

A higher degree of associative complexity is required by the animal for the numerous types of *free-operant conditioning* that have been utilized in several ways to assess different aspects of behavior already presumably within the organism's response capacity. Here the animal is not always punished by shock when it commits an error or fails to emit a required response, but it may be rewarded (positively) when it, for example, correctly presses a lever, for food, water, or some other positive consequence, being completely free to repeat that response.

The techniques for this type of conditioned behavior have been elaborated from a relatively simple mechanical bar-press apparatus (SKINNER, 1938) to very sophisticated relay- and transistor-operated switching, counting, and timing circuits that can be regulated to provide for various schedules of reinforcement (FERSTER and SKINNER, 1957). By such a procedure, the animal may be (a) rewarded every time it presses the lever (*continuous reinforcement*), (b) rewarded only after a fixed or variable period of time (*fixed and variable interval reinforcement*), (c) rewarded after a fixed variable number of correct responses (*fixed and variable ratio reinforcement*), and (d) rewarded only when the lever is pressed at a low-rate frequency (*differential reinforcement of low rates*). Obviously these different operative possibilities correspond to an equal number of learning situation that, moreover, can be further elaborated by the combination of different schedules. Thus, it is possible to combine a visual stimulus signaling a fixed-interval reinforcement to another different stimulus, associated with a fixed-ratio reinforcement; in such a way that it is possible to test and analyze the perceptive and the discriminatory abilities of the animal under experimental conditions (STEBBINS, 1966). It is also possible to combine a free-operant conditioning with an avoidance situation (SIDMAN, 1963).

It still remains open to question whether punishment of an incorrect response or rewarding of a correct one is the more effective means of contributing to the learning process.

Some investigators (HOGE and STOCKING, 1912; WARDEN and AYLESWORTH, 1927) demonstrated experimentally that shock increases the rate of discriminatory learning more than food reinforcement does; THORNDIKE (1932a,b) has emphasized that reward reinforces the connection with the expected response, while punishment is ineffective or even exerts a slightly negative effect upon this behavior.

It is then more appropriate to consider the importance of the implications deriving from observations made in the study of animal behavior, and at the same time, how a drug can lead to differences in response depending upon the experimental situation adopted, as a function of those different mechanisms developed by the animal under examination to perform a requested task. As a consequence, in order to derive a profile accurate enough to assess the activity of a drug on learning processes, such a behavioral description must be derived through the use of the techniques described (BRADY, 1959; BRADY and ROSS, 1960).

C) FACTORS INFLUENCING BEHAVIOR

Apart from basic drives such as hunger, thirst, sexual stimuli, etc. there are several factors that can influence animal behavioral patterns and which, to a great extent, even operate to shape behaviors in man. Such factors are of importance in the field of psychopharmacology because they can differentially modulate, from time to time, the activity of a drug on the central nervous system (FISHER, 1970).

One of the most important of these elements, especially because of its potential interaction with the developmental process in animals or man, is represented by the _mean level of environmental stimulation_ (WELCH, 1964). This concept refers to the effect of the reciprocal interaction between a living organism and its environment, so that the animal responds continuously to the influences of its typical environment and to a certain extent modifies and transforms in accordance with its own needs. In turn, the environment provides stimulation to the animal which lives therein where it utilizes personal behaviors derived from physical and social interaction; these become more complex as the number of animals present in the same environment is increased. As a consequence, by varying environmental complexity, it is possible to induce changes in brain biochemistry and morphology as well as in behavioral patterns (KRECH et al., 1960, 1965; ROSENZWEIG et al., 1962; ROSENZWEIG, 1966; QUAY et al., 1969; BENNETT and ROSENZWEIG, 1968). In fact, animals living in a deprived environment, lacking the opportunity for social interaction, show a reduced brain weight, a reduced cerebral cortical thickness, and a decrease in cholinesterase activity both in the whole brain and in visual and somesthesic cortex in particular (KRECH et al., 1965). In contrast, animals raised in an environment enriched with a variety of sources of stimulation and social interaction, show an increase in the cerebral cortical depth and an increased number of cortical glial cells (DIAMOND et al., 1966) which, in connection with the increased level of behavioral adaptability observed, possibly bears upon GALAMBOS' suggestion of a binomial entity, the neuron-glial inter-action (GALAMBOS, 1961), and its significance for behavior (Chapter II).

The *effect of previous experiences* with frustrating or rewarding events is notably important in the shaping of behavioral patterns (SCOTT, 1958a,b), so that, particularly in laboratory animals, *handling* and *gentling* during early life represents an important positive factor both for their growth (WEININGER, et al., 1954; RUEGAMER and SILVERMAN, 1956; LEVINE, 1957; LEVINE and OTIS, 1958) and subsequent behavior (COWLEY and WID-DOWSON, 1965). Similar observations concerning the influence of the level of environmental stimulation upon child development have been made by WIDDOWSON (1951). Moreover, the significant influence of an enriched or deprived environment has been demonstrated for the behavioral perfor-mance of retarded children (SAYEGH and DENNIS, 1965; SHEPPS and ZIGLER, 1962; SPITZ, 1949; ZIGLER, 1963; VOGEL et al., 1967).

The contribution of rewarding experiences and handling to variations in emotional behavior of rats has been considered (ADER, 1965; 1968); such variations can be measurably converted into better performance in open-field tests as a consequence of a higher level of emotional stability than that characteristic of control animals never exposed to social contact or handling during their period of infancy (DENENBERG et al., 1964). Incidentally, if these latter animals are considered to have experienced a deprived situation, this could represent a confirmation of the FISKE and MADDI hypothesis.

Animals of the same species but of a different *strain,* can also show differences in emotional behavior which, in some strains, is correlated with brain 5-HT levels; more emotional strains show elevated brain levels of this amine (MAAS, 1962, 1963; SUDAK and MAAS, 1964a). Moreover, negative and significant correlations were found between the 5-HT content of the limbic system and levels of motor activity in different rat strains (SUDAK and MAAS, 1964b). Different strain-dependent emotional levels also result in measurable differences on learning abilities (OLIVERIO et al., 1968; OLIVERIO, 1969).

In conclusion, it seems apparent that several genetic and/or environmen-tal effects may profoundly influence the behavioral patterns of the experi-mental animal as well as its response to drugs (GUPTA and HOLLAND, 1969; GREGORY, 1968; KATZ and STEINBERG, 1970; PORSOLT et al.,

1970; VALZELLI, 1969a, 1971, 1973; VALZELLI and BERNASCONI, 1971). Moreover this general schema for animals, parallels the drug-personality-milieu interactions which have also been considered operative in man (FISHER, 1970; McNAIR et al., 1970a,b; HEIMANN, 1969; FORREST et al., 1967).

D) EXPERIMENTAL MODEL OF BEHAVIORAL ALTERATIONS

A very important issue in psychopharmacological research concerns the use of animals presenting specific behavioral alterations as potential "models" of some aspects of human psychopathology. This possibility allows for the analysis of the anatomical, physiological, and biochemical parameters of brain function which participate in behavioral alterations; in this way gaining a better understanding of the grounds upon which both behavioral abnormalities and differences in drug activity may be sought.

Some of these models introduce the danger of excessive anthropomorphic interpretation of the results but are, however, of notable interest as they represent an area that psychopharmacology must amplify and further develop in order to reach the transitional point that exists between the behaviorally altered animals and the psychologically impaired man; this should allow a more immediate and complete application of experimental results to clinical and therapeutic use.

1) Experimental Neurosis

This experimental approach finds origin in studies carried out by PAVLOV (1927) on conditioned reflexes. He conditioned a dog to salivate upon presentation of a circle and to stop salivating when an ellipse was presented, in order to study the discriminative ability of the animal. Subsequently the dog was presented with a series of ellipses which were gradually transformed into a circular shape until the point was reached at which the animal lost its discriminatory ability. At this point the animal showed a symptomatology similar to that of a human neurosis. In fact, mydriasis, tachycardia, tic-like movements, altered respiration, disregard for learned tasks, phobias, and deviations of social and sexual behavior became evident and persisted for a prolonged time after the experimental situation (RUSSEL, 1950).

The common principle upon which the techniques for obtaining experimental neurosis are based is that of producing a conflict between a previously learned pattern for obtaining a reward and the introduction of an unexpected experience, capable of becoming traumatically disruptive and fear-inducing, which is substituted for the expected reward (MASSERMAN, 1960). To bring about such a behavioral situation it is possible to modify the conditioning paradigm in such a way that an animal, previously conditioned to obtain food as a reward for its performance is given an electric shock instead of the anticipated reward.

Obviously these methods are suitable for studying those drugs that may prevent, limit, or change the behavioral abnormalities that derive from such an induced "neurosis".

2) Sleep Deprivation

As outlined in Chapter I, sleep deprivation in man induces a series of alterations in behavioral capacity as well as accounting for the appearance of psychotic-like syndromes. In laboratory animals it is also possible to obtain a forced state of sleep deprivation which, when sufficiently prolonged, induces a typical behavioral picture, characterized by hyperirritability, tremors, piloerection, and vocalization. Some preliminary studies have indicated that such symptomatology is accompanied by variations in brain amine turnover.

3) Brain Stimulation and Lesions

For some time methods for the localization of nuclei and specific brain structures in different animal species, have employed suitable neurosurgical techniques and stereotaxic devices in such a way as to provide for the delivery of an electrode-delivered current, such that coagulation of tissue and lesions could be induced; or the delivery of such a current could be used as an extraphysiological source of stimulation to the cells comprising these brain areas. Behavioral modification have been observed with both of these effects, suggesting possible functional links in structure-function relationships. In a similar way, such methods may also be employed as tools for the investigation of drugs capable of initiating behavioral modification, particularly with respect to their possible target areas in the brain.

Another experimental method is represented by the microinjection of minute amounts of psychoactive drugs directly into brain nuclei or structures.

Obviously, based upon the enormous number of lesions that can be placed, or points in the brain to which stimulation may be applied, it becomes virtually impossible to systematically summarize all of the experimental work accomplished in this area which is currently still actively developing.

A very interesting experimental technique that has found a wide range of applications is brain self-stimulation (OLDS, 1958), in which a rat, permanently implanted with brain electrodes, is trained to press a lever which can either initiate stimulation through the implanted electrodes or terminate ongoing stimulation through the same implanted device. When such stimulating electrodes are implanted into the median forebrain bundle (MFB), an animal responds by increasing its rate of bar-pressing to continue such stimulation, suggesting that the stimulus serves to mediate positive reinforcement; the magnitude of the positive reinforcing properties of MFB self-stimulation by the rat is indicated by the observation that the course of responding at such a high rate is not interrupted, even in a hungry animal presented with the option of a food reward. In contrast the mesodiencephalic periventricular system (MPS) when electrically stimulated in the rat, leads to bar-pressing for the termination of such stimulation; this suggests that electrical stimulation of the MPS may be negatively reinforcing (OLDS, 1962; STEIN, 1968). Both the MFB and MPS are a part of the *limbic mesencephalic area* (NAUTA, 1964) and the use of experimental paradigms in which anatomical loci mediating apparently rewarding or punishing effects are utilized, seem to provide appropriate bases of emotional behavior upon which the effects of psychoactive drugs may be investigated.

A variation of this basic technique consists in animals self-injecting minute amounts of drugs (GOLDBERG et al., 1971) into the brain (OLDS, 1959) or bloodstream (MILLER, 1964) through an implanted cannula; in this way when a fear-producing stimulus is presented, the animal, by pressing a lever, can self-inject a drug that is capable of restoring a preferred level of affective experience.

Similar, but somewhat more complex experiments have been performed by DELGADO (1967, 1969, 1973) in monkeys using radio frequency telestimulator or self-stimulator devices. These monkeys, living in colonies and moving freely, are permanently implanted with over 40 microelectrodes in different brain structures, and respond to a telemetered control with a series of responses and emotional reactions, ranging from rage to aggressiveness, dominance, subordination, fear, excitation, quiescence, sedation, and several others. Permanent implantation of brain electrodes has also been performed in some human volunteers suffering from intractable schizophrenic reactions or psychotic symptomatology with homicidal impulses (DELGADO, 1969, 1973). Experimental use of brain lesion or stimulation techniques has also been made in the study of sleep mechanisms and the anatomical structures involved therein (HERNÁNDEZ-PÉON and CHÁVEZ-IBARRA, 1963; JOUVET, 1962, 1965, 1968). Recently it was shown that a lesion of the medial raphe nucleus of the mesencephalon produced extreme excitation and restlessness in rats and induced a pronounced decrease in the forebrain content of 5-HT and 5-HIAA (KOSTOWSKI et al., 1968);

whereas, electrical stimulation of the same nucleus produced quiescence, sedation, and sleep, as well as a slight decrease in forebrain 5-HT content and an increase in 5-HIAA level, indicating an increased brain 5-HT turnover (KOSTOWSKI et al., 1969; GUMULKA et al., 1969). Even more pronounced are the changes in forebrain 5-HT following electrical stimulation of the dorsal raphe nucleus (GUMULKA et al., 1971). These experimental findings support JOUVET's hypothesis (1968) that 5-HT plays an important role in the neurohumoral mediation of the state of sleep.

4) Induced Aggressiveness

In wild animals, aggressiveness may be considered as a normal behavioral component that has been developed for the survival, elimination, or removal of those objects or stimuli that threaten the physical or psychological integrity of an organism. Aggressive responses are to some extent genetically determined and consequently apparent to varying degrees among different animal species, including man (LORENZ, 1963; SCOTT, 1958b). Aggressive behavior is, in part, learning-dependent to the extent that it can occur as a function of previous defeats or victories with frustrating or rewarding associations, respectively (KAHN, 1951; SEWARD, 1945, 1946). The basic drives of aggression are represented by competition for food (FREDERIC-SON and BIRNBAUM, 1954), social rank (KAHN, 1954; KING, 1957), reproduction (KAHN, 1961), and territory (SCOTT, 1958b, 1962). The term territoriality is used to indicate that area within which the animal establishes its living space and concomitantly the levels and limits of interchange developed therein with other animals; it may, moreover, be noted that territoriality plays a double role in aggressive behavior, since all violations of habitual territory trigger aggressive reactions and, at the same time, a well organized system of territories acts as a control of aggressive activity (CLARK, 1962; FREDERICSON, 1950; KING and GURNEY, 1954; SCOTT, 1958b, 1962).

It is well known that animals that show aggressive behavior in their natural habitat will lose this characteristic to a considerable extent when they are domesticated or bred in standard conditions; such animals react defensively only when improperly handled or painfully stimulated.

In fact, laboratory rats and mice are usually bred under such highly standardized conditions that most of their drives for aggression are essentially inoperative; this is due to the absence of competitive drives for food, which is usually abundantly and uniformly distributed, for females, which are singly put in contact with a single male for reproductive purposes at a predetermined time, for territory, which is generally represented by the living cage, and is uniformly and constantly distributed among a fixed number of animals. As a consequence, the experimental means by which aggressive behavior can be induced in laboratory animals becomes quite important, as it raises the possibility of inducing a new, or at least unusual, behavioral component (VALZELLI, 1966; 1967a). The techniques adopted to achieve this result are mainly represented by cerebral lesions, painful stimulation, and isolation.

The rationale for the use of the *brain lesion* technique to induce aggressive behavior in animals has been based upon the demonstrated relationship between several anatomical structures comprising the limbic system and the behavioral components which are regulated by them (KARLI, 1968; Chapter I). For example, the septal nuclei and amygdala (Fig. 2) are important in the mediation of the diencephalic and hypothalamic activities which govern emotional vegetative and motor impulses (KING, 1962); so that, lesions of the septal nuclei can induce an extreme degree of hyperirritability in rats (BRADY and NAUTA, 1953, 1955). Such lesioned animals, however, do not directly manifest aggressive behavior; truly aggressive behavior is shown by rats lesioned in one of the structures comprising the olfactory pathways such as the olfactory bulbs, the lateral olfactory bandelets, or the prepyriform cortex; lesions of the amygdala or of the lateral hypothalamus can abolish the aggressiveness induced in the same animal by the previously described lesions (KARLI, 1956; KARLI and VERGNES, 1963; VERGNES and KARLI, 1963, 1965).

It is interesting to note, however, that ablation of the olfactory bulbs blocks the aggressive tendencies of animals that are spontaneously aggressive (MOYER, 1968; MURPHY, 1970), thus this observation may suggest that one type of neural intervention can lead to opposite results, as a function of the previous behavioral status of the animal.

With regard to laboratory rats and to the aggressiveness induced by the previously cited lesions, such animals may also be characterized behaviorally by the term "muricide", as they will consistently and repetitively kill a mouse that is put into their cage. The use of lesion-induced aggressiveness is a very useful technique for the study of anatomo-physiological correlates of aggressive behavior, but it raises some doubt concerning its use in the pharmacological evaluation of possible antiaggressive drugs; since there is substantial evidence that every lesion made in brain tissue can alter the permeability of the blood-brain barrier (ADLER, 1961) there is some question as to the resulting influence of such intervention upon the pharmacological response.

The technique of *painful stimulation* for the initiation of aggressive behavior is based upon the exasperation of the normal reactive response of an animal to pain (SCOTT, 1958a,b) and, in fact, it is well known that wounded or sick animals are more inclined to respond aggressively to stimuli than normal ones. In this way, a painful stimulus, as for example, an electric shock applied to the paws of rats through the cage floor (foot-shock), is capable of enhancing a reciprocal aggressive response (O'KELLY and STECKLE, 1939; MILLER, 1948; LEVINE, 1959). Similar results have also been obtained in mice (TEDESCHI et al., 1959); several other species such as snakes, monkeys, birds, and felines also show both intraspecific and interspecific aggressive behavior (AZRIN et al., 1963; ULRICH and AZRIN, 1962) as well as aggressive responses toward inanimate objects (AZRIN et al., 1964). This technique seems to be more suitable for behavioral studies than for pharmacological evaluation of the antiaggressive properties of drugs, mainly because the aggressive response obtained is short-lasting and transient and, moreover, the response of the animal to drugs can possibly be misinterpreted due to any possible analgesic or anesthetic properties of the compound under investigation.

The simplest method for inducing prolonged aggressive behavior, which holds several sources of conceptual as well as methodological implication for behavior, is represented by *isolation.* This technique has been developed from indications of YEN et al. (1959), SEWARD (1946), ALLEE (1942), and SCOTT (1947). The method essentially consists in isolating standard albino mice for approximately four weeks in an individual cage with *ad libitum* water and food. The animals show an initial stage of general hyperreactivity to usual environmental stimuli and then develop aggressiveness, which is shown consistently whenever another mouse, previously isolated or not, is put into the same area. Fighting occurs almost immediately after contact; there are some interesting social-aggressive interactions that may be developed in such a situation, specifically when three previously isolated mice are exposed to one another (VALZELLI, 1969b) (Fig. 27).

Prolonged isolation represents a drastic variation of the social environment within which the animal has previously lived, and there is a profound reduction in stimulus level, which would normally derive from grouped animals; a new concept of territory is thereby established for isolated animals such that an alteration of emotional stability and the capacity to sustain aggressive reactions occur. The observation of an isolated animal showing an "emotional explosion" without any apparently motivating stimulus, is somewhat similar, observationally, to outbursts that occur in human neurotic reactions wherein a conflict situation is insoluble by the subject. In this context, it may be of interest to mention that profound isolation as obtained in man by means of complete sensory deprivation (tactile, visual, auditory, and kinesthetic deprivation for several hours) results in schizophrenic-like symptoms (LEFF, 1968; MILLER, 1962; POLLARD et al., 1963; ROSENZWEIG and GARDNER, 1966), even more

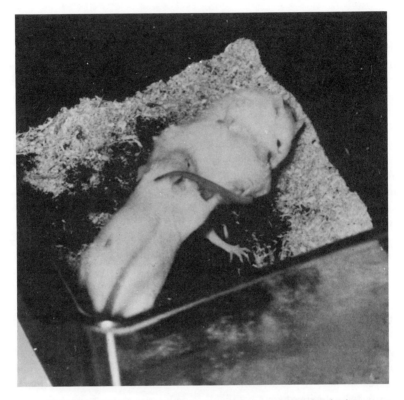

Fig. 27. Fighting behavior among previously long-time isolated mice.

intense than the "model psychoses" that have been induced by psycho-
tominetic agents such as mescaline or LSD (ROSENZWEIG, 1959). This
fact seems to further support the hypothesis that aggressive behavior developed in animals by isolation is the result of a complex interaction of social,
behavioral, sensory, and neurological variables and may bear certain similarities to certain components of human psychopathology.

    Aggressiveness produced by isolation in mice is long-lasting and tempo-
rally stable and may be usefully employed to study the activity of psychoactive drugs (SOFIA, 1969; VALZELLI, 1969a,b, 1971, 1972, 1973; VAL-
ZELLI et al., 1967; YEN et al., 1959), although there are variations in
the extent to which animals may become aggressive after isolation; this may
be dependent upon the strain, sex, age, and several other environmental
factors (VALZELLI, 1967a,b, 1969b, 1972). Aggressive mice show a differential sensitivity to drugs as compared with nonaggressive animals, so that, for
instance, amphetamine is much more toxic in aggressive than in normal mice

(CONSOLO et al., 1965a), while some sedative drugs are less active in the former than in the latter (CONSOLO et al., 1965b). Many other drug effects are modulated by different emotional responses typical for differences in the expression of aggressive behavior (VALZELLI, 1969a, 1971; VALZELLI et al., 1971).

Isolation is also an effective means of inducing aggressive behavior in some strains of rat, providing some basis for muricide behavior in which rats repetitively kill every mouse put into their cage (SOFIA, 1969; VALZELLI, 1969c; VALZELLI and BERNASCONI, 1971; VALZELLI and GARATTINI, 1972). Isolation can also lead to other behavioral alterations (VALZELLI, 1969c; VALZELLI and GARATTINI, 1972) which are affected differently by psychotropic drug administration; these may be potentially considered additional animal models for various psychopathological conditions in man.

E) PHARMACOLOGICAL TECHNIQUES

There are a considerable number of techniques, derived from classical pharmacology, that may be employed to characterize the more traditionally pharmacological aspects of psychotropic drugs; these are generally discussed in current pharmacology textbooks (GOODMAN and GILMAN, 1970; WILSON and SCHILD, 1968; AIAZZI-MANCINI and DONATELLI, 1957; CROSSLAND, 1970). In this context the study of the activity of such drugs upon the cardiovascular system, autonomic nervous system, gastrointestinal system, renal or respiratory apparatus, and endocrine axis are considered; the synergistic or antagonistic effects of psychotropic drugs toward acetylcholine, histamine, serotonin, and other biologically active substances and on isolated organs and tissues have also been viewed and their possible actions on in vitro enzymatic activities have been summarized.

Other pharmacological tests are based upon the potentiating or antagonizing effects of psychotropic drugs on other compounds acting on the central nervous system. The potentiation of ether, or barbiturate narcosis, is a standard test (WINTER, 1948) in which the test drug is given to experimental animals 30 minutes before a subnarcotic dose of a barbiturate, so that the possible potentiation can be measured by the time course of narcosis and by the percentage of narcotized animals as compared with saline-barbiturate control animals. Anticonvulsant drugs can be tested by their ability to prevent convulsions induced by electroshock, pentylenetetrazol, strychnine or amphetamine. The antireserpine effects of a given drug may be evaluated in terms of its ability to counteract or to invert the typical reserpine-induced symptomatology and, in particular, the sedation, hypothermia, and ptosis induced by this drug.

Also, the antiamphetamine effect is commonly adopted employing amphetamine in a dose capable of inducing only hyperthermic and hyperexcitant effects without any convulsions; in this test the extent to which other psychoactive drugs can modify the effects of amphetamine are measured.

All of these techniques, as well as several others, are important for obtaining a preliminary profile of the general properties of a drug, but are insufficient to elucidate its intrinsic properties. Moreover, some questions concerning the correct interpretation of results obtained may arise from possible interactions, or molecular and metabolic competition between drugs employed; in this way, possible direct effects of a psychotropic drug under examination upon specific brain structures or functions may be obscured.

F) HUMAN TECHNIQUES

Some authors believe that a review of those methods employed in experimental psychopharmacology would demonstrate a lack of satisfactory animal models which can elucidate the mode of action of psychotropic drugs in man and evaluate their efficacy; as a consequence, "the evaluation of drugs has to be carried out on humans, both healthy and diseased" (SHEPHERD et al., 1968).

Apart from the ethical considerations which necessarily strongly limit certain types and extension of experimental studies in humans, the quoted affirmation appears somewhat arbitrary, when it may be considered, for example, that responses to drugs are incomparably much more variable in humans than in animals, due to the absence, of highly standardized genetic and environmental parameters. It is widely known that these parameters allow for reproducibility and statistical evaluation of results. Moreover, it may be considered that a uniform nomenclature system for different mental illnesses has not yet been adopted, primarily because the same psychiatric syndrome can be "personalized" and modulated by an individual patient in different ways, in accord with his own behavioral characteristics. It seems appropriate, in this context, to recall, as an example, the various subdivisions of the depressive disorders; the array of functional and phasic labeling indicates quite plainly that there is little hope for a systematization from which the clinical psychopharmacology may work, and that it seems more useful and productive to attempt the integration of animal and human psychopharmacological experiences than to keep these two fields independent from one another.

It is certainly not an easy task to briefly summarize the wide range of techniques that have been proposed to study the effect of psychotropic drugs in man. However, many pertinent examples can be found in a recent book by SHEPHERD et al., (1968). Generally speaking, there are *pharmacological techniques* which are based upon the evaluation of the changes in heart rate, salivary secretion, pupil size, and skin resistance, as indications of the peripheral influence of drugs. Also the study of the muscular apparatus is suggested as an indirect indicator of central drug action, so that surface electromyography has been employed in the evaluation of both the anxiety level and of the antianxiety drug effects of drugs in psychiatric patients (SAINSBURY, 1959).

More appropriate *neuropharmacological techniques,* so comprehensively utilized in animal studies, are necessarily limited in human investigation wherein electroencephalographic measurement, and variations therein produced by the administration of psychotropic drugs, have been utilized both in healthy and psychiatric subjects (BRAZIER, 1964). Although it is considered relatively nonspecific, this technique has been retained as an index of the pharmacological activity of a drug (PFEIFFER et al., 1963; 1964).

There are also several *behavioral techniques* which BURDOCK et al., (1959) have designated as physiological, sensory, perceptual, psychomotor, and conceptual, or pertaining to the higher nervous activities. These methods refer to a large extent, to several tasks associated with manual dexterity, fine movement coordination, reaction time, problem-solving skill, speed of learning and memorization, associative productivity, etc., while other behavioral components are assessed with a series of psychological tests, such as the Rorschach test, the Clyde Mood Scale (CLYDE, 1960), the Taylor Manifest Anxiety Scale (TAYLOR, 1953), the Minnesota Multiphasic Personality Inventory (HATHAWAY and MEEHL, 1951), the Impatient Multidimensional Psychiatric Scale (LORR, 1962), and several others of a similar format.

In the evaluation of behaviorally active drugs two sets of factors which can, to various degrees, modify the drug efficacy must be taken into account. The elements of one group pertain mainly to the pharmacodynamics of the compound, indicated by the differences in rate of absorption, distribution, and metabolism, to the dosage, route of administration, individual tolerance or sensitization, undesired side effects, etc; the second group includes variables of a more strict psychological type, such as the placebo effect, the personality characteristics of the physician, the characteristics of the familial, social, and ward milieu or environment, as well as the personality traits of the normal subject or patient receiving the drug

(RINKEL, 1963; RICKELS, 1963; LINDEMANN and VON FELSINGER, 1961; HONIGFELD, 1964; McNAIR et al., 1970a,b; FISHER, 1970).

Other sources of variation in the response of man to psychoactive drugs are represented by age and sex, the presence of other peripheral pathological conditions that can interfere, to varying degrees, with the absorption and utilization of a psychoactive drug. At the same time, it may be considered that any drug can be assessed as efficacious if it is administered for a suitable period of time at a correct dosage, in patients screened for some select aspect of the clinical pattern. Available methods of evaluation should, furthermore, be sensitive enough to measure the level and the degree of possible amelioration of the behavior disorder characterizing the patient.

Due to the large number of variables which can interfere with both the experimental and clinical evaluation of psychopharmacological results, it was recently suggested that computers be given the task of analyzing the collected data (BUHLER, 1968; CLYDE, 1968). A very effective review of the different aspects and problems inherent in the clinical evaluation of psychopharmacological therapy has been recently made by LEHMANN (1968).

REFERENCES

Ader, R., (1965) J. Comp. Physiol. Psychol. 60, 233.

Ader, R., (1968) J. Comp. Physiol. Psychol. 66, 264.

Adler, M. W., (1961) J. Pharmacol. Exper. Ther. 134, 214.

Aiazzi-Mancini, M. and Donatelli, L., (1957) "Trattato di Farmacologia", F. Vallardi Publ., Milano.

Allee, W. C., (1942) Science 95, 289.

Azrin, N. H., Hutchinson, R. R., and Hake, D. F., (1963) J. Exp. Anal. Behav. 6, 620.

Azrin, N. H., Hutchinson, R. R., and Sallery, R. D., (1964) J. Exp. Anal. Behav. 7, 223.

Barnett, S. A., (1963) "The Rat: A Study in Behaviour," Aldine Publ. Co., Chicago.

Bennett, E. L., and Rosenzweig, M. K., (1968) in "Mind as a Tissue," Rupp C., Ed., Harper and Row, New York, p. 63.

Berlyne, D. E., (1950) Brit. J. Psychol. 41, 68.

Berlyne, D. E., (1955) J. Comp. Physiol. Psychol. 48, 238.

Berlyne, D. E., (1960) "Conflict, Arousal and Curiosity," McGraw-Hill, New York.

Berlyne, D. E., (1966) Science 153, 25.

Bitterman, M. E., (1960) Amer. Psychol. 15, 704.

Bitterman, M. E., (1965) Sci. Amer. 212, 92.

Boissier, J. R. and Simon, P., (1962) Thérapie 17, 1226.

Boissier, J. R. and Simon, P., (1964) Arch. Int. Pharmacodyn. Ther. 147, 372.

Boissier, J. R. and Simon, P., (1967) Physiol. Behav. 2, 447.

Boissier, J. R., Simon, P., and Lwoff, T.-M., (1964) Thérapie 19, 571.

Brady, J. V., (1959) in "Psychopharmacology: Problems in Evaluation," Nat. Acad. Sci., Nat. Res. Council, Washington, D.C., p. 46.

Brady, J. V. and Nauta, W. J. H., (1953) J. Comp. Physiol. Psychol. **46**, 339.
Brady, J. V. and Nauta, W. J. H., (1955) J. Comp. Physiol. Psychol. **48**, 412.
Brady, J. V. and Ross, S., (1960) in "Drugs and Behavior," Uhr, L. and Miller, J. G., Eds., Wiley, New York.
Brazier, M. A. B., (1964) Clin. Pharmacol. Ther. **5**, 102.
Brody, E. G., (1942) Comp. Psychol. Monogr. **17**, 24.
Browman, L. G., (1942) J. Exp. Zool. **91**, 331.
Browman, L. G., (1943) J. Comp. Psychol. **36**, 33.
Bruell, J. H., (1963) American Psychological Association Meeting, Philadelphia.
Buhler, R., (1968) in "Psychopharmacology," Proc. 6th Ann. Meeting of Amer. College of Neuropsychopharmacol., Public Health Service Publ. no. 1836, p. 1013.
Burdock, E. J., Sutton, S., and Zubin, J., (1959) J. Abnorm. Soc. Psychol. **56**, 18.
Chapman, R. M. and Levy, N., (1957) J. Comp. Physiol. Psychol. **50**, 233.
Clark, L. D., (1962) in "The Roots of Behavior," Harper and Row, New York, p. 179.
Clyde, D. J., (1960) in "Drugs and Behavior," Uhr., L. and Miller, J. G., Eds., Wiley, New York.
Clyde, D. J., (1968) in "Psychopharmacology," Proc. 6th Ann. Meeting of Amer. College of Neuropsychopharmacol., Public Health Service Publ. no. 1836, p. 1019.
Consolo, S., Garattini, S., and Valzelli, L., (1965a) J. Pharm. Pharmacol. **17**, 53.
Consolo, S., Garattini, S., and Valzelli, L., (1965b) J. Pharm. Pharmacol. **17**, 594.
Cowley, J. J. and Widdowson, E. M., (1965) Brit. J. Nutr. **19**, 397.
Crossland, J., (1970) "Lewis's Pharmacology," 4th ed., Williams & Wilkins, Baltimore.
Delgado, J. M. R., (1967) Endeavour **26**, 149.
Delgado, J. M. R., (1969) in "The Present Status of Psychotropic Drugs," Cerletti, A. and Bové, F. J., Eds., Excerpta Medica Foundation, Amsterdam, p. 36.
Delgado, J. M. R., (1973) in "The Benzodiazepines," Garrattini, S. and Randall, L. O., Eds., Raven Press, New York.
Denenberg, V. H., Morton, J. R. C., and Haltmeyer, G. C., (1964) Anim. Behav. **12**, 205.
Dews, P. B., (1953) Brit. J. Pharmacol. **8**, 46.
Diamond, M. C., Law, F., Rhodes, H., Lindner, B., Rosenzweig, M. R., Krech, D., and Bennett, E. L., (1966) J. Comp. Neurol. **128**, 117.
Ferster, C. B. and Skinner, B. F., (1957) "Schedules of Reinforcement," Appleton Century, New York.
Fisher, S., (1970) in "Clinical Handbook of Psychopharmacology," Di Mascio, A. and Shader, R. I., Eds., Science House, New York, p. 17.
Fiske, D. W. and Maddi, S. R., (1961) "Functions of varied Experience," Dorsey, Homewood, Ill.
Forrest, G. L., Bortner, T. W., and Bakker, C. B., (1967) J. Psychiat. Res. **5**, 281.
Foster, S. G., (1959) Diss. Abstr. **19**, 2656.
Fredericson, E., (1950) J. Psychol. **29**, 89.
Fredericson, E. and Birnbaum, E. A., (1954) J. Genet. Psychol. **85**, 271.
Frommel, E., (1965) Arch. Int. Pharmacodyn. Ther. **154**, 231.
Galambos, R., (1961) Proc. Nat. Acad. Sci. U.S.A. **47**, 129.
Gellhorn, E., Kessler, M., and Minatoya, H., (1942) Proc. Soc. Exper. Biol. Med. **50**, 260.
Gellhorn, E. and Minatoya, H., (1943) Fed. Proc. Fed. Amer. Soc. Exper. Biol. **2**, 15.
Glickman, S. E. and Jensen, G. D., (1961) J. Comp. Physiol. Psychol. **54**, 83.
Goldberg, S. R., Hoffmeister, F., Schlichting, U. U., and Wuttke, W., (1971) J. Pharmacol. Exper. Ther. **179**, 277.

Goodman, L. S. and Gilman, A., Eds., (1970) "The Pharmacological Basis of Therapeutics," 4th ed., MacMillan, New York.

Gregory, K., (1968) Psychopharmacologia (Berl.) 13, 29.

Gumulka, W., Samanin, R., Garattini, S., and Valzelli, L., (1969) Europ. J. Pharmacol. 8, 380.

Gumulka, W., Samanin, R., Valzelli, L., and Consolo, S., (1971) J. Neurochem. 18, 533.

Gupta, B. D. and Holland, H. C., (1969) Psychopharmacologia (Berl.) 14, 95.

Hathaway, S. R. and Meehl, P. E., (1951) "An Atlas for the Clinical Use of the Minnesota Multiphasic Personality Inventory," University Press, Minnesota.

Hayward, H. C., (1962) J. Personality 30, 63.

Heimann, H., (1969) Confin. Psychiat. 12, 205.

Henderson, N. D., (1967) Anim. Behav. 15, 364.

Hernández-Peón, R. and Chávez Ibarra, G., (1963) Electroenceph. Clin. Neurophysiol. (Suppl.) 24, 188.

Herz, A., (1960) Int. Rev. Neurobiol. 2, 229.

Hoge, M. A. and Stocking, R. J., (1912) J. Anim. Behav. 2, 43.

Honigfeld, G., (1964) Dis. Nerv. Syst. 25, 145.

Hoskins, R. G., (1941) "Endocrinology; the Glands and their Functions," Norton, New York, p. 388.

Hull, C. L., (1943) "Principles of Behavior," Appleton Century, New York.

Hunt, J. McV. and Schlosberg, H., (1939) J. Comp. Psychol. 28, 23.

Hunter, W. S., (1935) Brit. J. Psychol. 26, 135.

Hunter, W. S., (1940) Science 91, 267.

Irwin, S., (1959) "General philosophy and methodology of screening: A multidimensional approach," Communication held at Gordon Res. Conf. on Medicinal Chemistry, Colby Junior College, New London, New Hampshire, August 3-7.

Ivinskins, A., (1966) Aust. J. Psychol. 18, 276.

Jerome, E. A., Moody, J. A., Connor, T. J., and Fernandez, M. B., (1957) J. Comp. Physiol. Psychol. 50, 588.

Jouvet, M., (1962) Arch. Ital. Biol. 100, 125.

Jouvet, M., (1965) in "Progress in Brain Research," vol. 18 "Sleep Mechanisms," Akert, K., Bally, C., and Schadé, J. P., Eds., Elsevier, Amsterdam, p. 20.

Jouvet, M., (1968) in "Advances in Pharmacology," vol. 6B, Garattini, S. and Shore, P. A., Eds., Academic Press, New York, p. 265.

Kahn, M. W., (1951) J. Genet. Psychol. 79, 117.

Kahn, M. W., (1954) J. Genet. Psychol. 84, 65.

Kahn, M. W., (1961) J. Genet. Psychol. 98, 211.

Karli, P., (1956) Behaviour 10, 81.

Karli, P., (1968) J. Physiol., London (Suppl. 1), 60, 3.

Karli, P. and Vergnes, M., (1963) C.R. Soc. Biol. 157, 372.

Katz, D. M. and Steinberg, H., (1970) Nature, London, 228, 469.

Khaïry, M., (1961) in "Neuropsychopharmacology," Proc. 2nd CINP International Congress, vol. 2, Rothlin E., Ed., Elsevier, Amsterdam, p. 159.

King, J. A., (1957) J. Genet. Psychol. 90, 151.

King, J. A., (1962) IX Riunione Monotematica di Psichiatria, Milano.

King, J. A. and Gurney, F., (1954) J. Comp. Physiol. Psychol. 47, 325.

Kostowski, W., Giacalone, E., Garattini, S., and Valzelli, L. (1968) Europ. J. Pharmacol. 4, 371.

Kostowski, W., Giacalone, E., Garattini, S., and Valzelli, L., (1969) Eruop. J. Pharmacol. 7, 170.

Krech, D., Rosenzweig, M. R., and Bennett, E. L., (1960) J. Comp. Physiol. Psychol. 53, 509.
Krech, D., Rosenzweig, M. R., and Bennett, E. L., (1965) Physiol. Behav. 1, 99.
Kuo, Z. Y., (1922) J. Comp. Psychol. 2, 1.
Lashley, K. S., (1929) "Brain Mechanism and Intelligence," Chicago University Press, Chicago, Ill.
Leff, J. P., (1968) Brit. J. Psychiat. 114, 1499.
Lehmann, H. E., (1968) in "Psychopharmacology," Proc. 6th Ann. Meeting of Amer. College of Neuropsychopharmacol., Public Health Service Publ. no. 1836, p. 949.
Lester, D., (1967a) Psychol. Rec. 17, 55.
Lester, D., (1967b) Psychol. Rec. 17, 63.
Levine, S., (1957) Science 126, 405.
Levine, S., (1959) J. Genet. Psychol. 94, 77.
Levine, S. and Otis, L. S., (1958) Can. J. Psychol. 12, 103.
Lindemann, E. and Von Felsinger, J. M., (1961) Psychopharmacologia (Berl.) 2, 69.
Lorenz, K., (1963) "Das sogenannte Böse; Zur Naturgeschichte der Aggression," Dr. G. Borotha-Schöler Verlag, Wien.
Lorr, M., (1962) Ann. N.Y. Acad. Sci. 93, 851.
Maas, J. W., (1962) Science 137, 621.
Maas, J. W., (1963) Nature, London, 197, 255.
Masserman, J. H., (1960) in "Drugs and Behavior," Uhr, L. and Miller, J. G., Eds., Wiley, New York.
McNair, D. M., Fisher, S., Kahn, R. J., and Droppleman, L. F., (1970a) Arch. Gen. Psychiat. 22, 128.
McNair, D. M., Fisher, S., Sussman, C., Droppleman, L. F., and Kahn, R. J., (1970b) J. Psychiat. Res. 7, 299.
Mead, A. P., (1960) Anim. Behav. 8, 19.
Miller, N. E., (1948) J. Abnorm. Psychol. 43, 155.
Miller, N. E., (1964) in "Animal Behavior and Drug Action," Ciba Foundation Symp., Churchill Ltd., London, p. 1.
Miller, S. C., (1962) Int. J. Psycho-Analysis 43, 1.
Montgomery, K. C., (1953) J. Comp. Physiol. Psychol. 46, 129.
Mote, F. A., Jr., (1940) J. Comp. Psychol. 30, 197.
Moyer, K. E., (1968) Commun. Behav. Biol. 2 pt A, 65.
Munn, N. L., (1950) "Handbook of Psychological Research on the Rat," Houghton Mifflin, Boston, Mass.
Münziger, K. F., (1934) J. Comp. Psychol. 17, 267.
Münziger, K. F., (1936) J. Exper. Psychol. 19, 116.
Murphy, M. R., (1970) 41st Ann. Meeting of Eastern Psychological Assoc., April 2-4.
Nauta, W. J. H., (1964) in "The Frontal Cortex and Behavior," Warren, J. M. and Akert, K., Eds., McGraw-Hill, New York, p. 397.
O'Kelly, L. J. and Steckle, L. C., (1939) J. Psychol. 8, 125.
Olds, J., (1958) Science 127, 315.
Olds, J., (1959) in "Neuropsychopharmacology," Vol. 1, Bradley, B. B., Deniker, P., and Radouco-Thomas, C., Eds., Elsevier, Amsterdam, p. 20 and 386.
Olds, J., (1962) Physiol. Rev. 42, 554.
Oliverio, A., (1969) Commun. Behav. Biol. 4, 7.
Oliverio, A., Satta, M., and Bovet, D., (1968) Life Sci. 7, 799.
Pavlov, J. P., (1927) "Conditioned Reflexes," Oxford University Press, Oxford.
Pfeiffer, C. C., Goldstein, L., Munoz, C., Murphree, H. B., and Jenney, E. H., (1963) Clin. Pharmacol. Ther. 4, 441.

Pfeiffer, C. C., Goldstein, L., Murphree, H. B., and Jenney, E. H., (1964) Arch. Gen. Psychiat. **10**, 446.
Pollard, J. C., Uhr, L., and Jackson, C., (1963) Arch. Gen. Psychiat. **8**, 435.
Porsolt, R. D., Toyce, D., and Summerfield, A., (1970) Nature, London **227**, 286.
Quay, W. B., Bennett, E. L., Rosenzweig, M. R., and Krech, D., (1969) Physiol. Behav. **4**, 489.
Richards, W. J. and Leslie, G. R., (1962). J. Comp. Physiol. Psychol. **55**, 834.
Richter, C. P., (1922) Comp. Psychol. Monogr. **1**, 2.
Richter, C. P., (1927) Rev. Biol. **2**, 307.
Richter, C. P., (1932) Amer. J. Orthopsychiat., **2**, 345.
Rickels, K., (1963) J. Nerv. Ment. Dis. **136**, 540.
Rinkel, M., (1963) "Specific and Non-Specific Factors in Psychopharmacology," Philosophical Library, New York.
Rosenzweig, M. R., (1966) Amer. Psychol. **21**, 321.
Rosenzweig, M. R., Krech, D., Bennett, E. L., and Diamond, M. C., (1962) J. Comp. Physiol. Psychol. **55**, 429.
Rosenzweig, N., (1959) Amer. J. Psychiat. **116**, 326.
Rosenzweig, N. and Gardner, L. M., (1966) Amer. J. Psychol. **122**, 920.
Ruegamer, W. R. and Silverman, F. R., (1956) Proc. Soc. Exper. Biol. Med. **92**, 170.
Russel, R. W., (1950) Brit. J. Psychol. **41**, 95.
Sainsbury, P., (1959) in "Quantitative Methods in Human Pharmacology and Therapeutics," Laurence, D. R., Ed., Pergamon Press, Oxford.
Sayegh, Y. and Dennis, W., (1965) Child Develop. **36**, 81.
Scott, J. P., (1947) J. Comp. Physiol. Psychol. **40**, 275.
Scott, J. P., (1958a) "Animal Behavior," Chicago University Press, Chicago, Ill.
Scott, J. P., (1958b) "Aggression," Chicago University Press, Chicago, Ill.
Scott, J. P., (1962) in "The Root of Behavior," Harper and Row, New York, p. 167.
Seward, J. P., (1945) J. Comp. Psychol. **38**, 213.
Seward, J. P., (1946) J. Comp. Psychol. **39**, 51.
Shepherd, M., Lader, M., and Rodnight, R., (1968) "Clinical Psychopharmacology," English University Press, London.
Shepps, R. and Zigler, E., (1962) Amer. J. Ment. Defic. **67**, 262.
Shillito, E. E., (1969) J. Physiol., London **200**, 35P.
Sidman, M., (1963) in "Psychopharmacological Methods," Votava Z., Ed., Pergamon Press, Oxford, p. 162.
Siegel, P. S., (1946) J. Psychol. **21**, 227.
Skinner, B. F., (1933) J. Genet. Psychol. **12**, 313.
Skinner, B. F., (1938) "The Behavior of Organisms," Appleton Century, New York.
Small, W. S., (1899) Amer. J. Psychol. **11**, 80.
Sofia, R. D., (1969) Life Sci. **8** pt 1, 705.
Sokolov, E. N., (1963) Ann. Rev. Physiol. **25**, 545.
Spitz, R. A., (1949) Child Develop. **20**, 145.
Stebbins, W. C., (1966) in "Methods in Medical Research," vol. 11, Year Book, Chicago, Ill.
Stein, L., (1968) in "Review of Psychopharmacology," Efron, D. E., Ed., U.S. Government Printing Office, Washington D.C., p. 105.
Stenhouse, D., (1965) Nature, London **208**, 815.
Stewart, C. C., (1898) Amer. J. Physiol. **1**, 40.
Sudak, H. S. and Maas, J. W., (1964a) Nature, London, **203**, 1254.
Sudak, H. S. and Maas, J. W., (1964b) Science **146**, 418.

Taylor, J. A., (1953) J. Abnorm. Soc. Psychol. **48**, 285.

Tedeschi, R. E., Tedeschi, D. H., Mucha, A., Wook, L., Mattis, P., and Fellows, E. J., (1959) J. Pharmacol. Exper. Ther. **125**, 28.

Thompson, W. R. and Higgins, W. H., (1958) Can. J. Psychol. **12**, 61.

Thorndike, E. L., (1932a) Comp. Psychol. Monogr. **8**, 65.

Thorndike, E. L., (1932b) "Fundamentals of Learning," Teachers College Ed., New York.

Thorndike, E. L., (1965) "Animal Intelligence: Experimental Studies," Hafner Publ. Co., New York.

Tsang, Y. C., (1934) Comp. Psychol. Monogr. **10**, 56.

Turnbull, M. J., cited in: Crossland, J., (1970) "Lewis's Pharmacology," Edinburgh, Livingstone, p. 112.

Ulrich, R. E. and Azrin, N. H., (1962) J. Exper. Anal. Behav. **5**, 511.

Valle, F. P., (1970) Amer. J. Psychol. **83**, 103.

Valentine, W. L., (1930) J. Comp. Psychol. **10**, 421.

Valzelli, L., (1966) Med. Clin. Sper. **16**, 404.

Valzelli, L., (1967a) in "Advances in Pharmacology," vol. 5, Garattini, S. and Shore, P. A., Eds., Academic Press, New York, p. 79.

Valzelli, L., (1967b) in "Neuropsychopharmacology," Proc. Vth CINP Int. Congr., Excerpta Medica Foundation, Amsterdam, p. 781.

Valzelli, L., (1969a) Psychopharmacologia (Berl.) **15**, 232.

Valzelli, L., (1969b) in "Aggressive Behavior," Proc. 1st Int. Congress, Milan, 1968, Garattini, S. and Sigg, E. B., Eds., Excerpta Medica Foundation, Amsterdam, p. 70.

Valzelli, L., (1969c) "Proc. II Riunione Nazionale Società Italiana di Neuropsicofarmacologia," Pacini-Mariotti, Pisa, p. 20.

Valzelli, L., (1971) Psychopharmacologia (Berl.) **19**, 91.

Valzelli, L., (1972) in "1st C.I.A.N.S. Congress," Pacini-Mariotti, Pisa, p. 396.

Valzelli, L., (1973) in "The Benzodiazepines," Garattini, S. and Randall, L. O., Eds., Raven Press, New York.

Valzelli, L. and Bernasconi, S., (1971) Psychopharmacologia (Berl.) **20**, 91.

Valzelli, L. and Garattini S., (1972) Neuropsychopharmacology **11**, 17.

Valzelli, L., Giacalone, E., and Garattini, S., (1967) Europ. J. Pharmacol. **2**, 144.

Valzelli, L., Ghezzi, D., and Bernasconi, S., (1971) Totus Homo, **3**, 73.

Vergnes, M. and Karli, P., (1963) C.R. Soc. Biol. **157**, 1061.

Vergnes, M. and Karli, P., (1965) C.R. Soc. Biol. **159**, 972.

Vogel, W., Kun, K. J., and Meshorer, E., (1967) J. Consulting Psychol. **31**, 570.

Warden, C. J. and Aylesworth, M., (1927) J. Comp. Psychol. **7**, 117.

Warner, L. H., (1932a) J. Genet, Psychol. **41**, 57.

Warner, L. H., (1932b) J. Genet, Psychol. **41**, 91.

Watson, J. B., (1907) Psychol. Rev. Monogr. **8**, 2.

Watson, J. B., (1914) J. Anim. Behav. **4**, 56.

Watson, J. B., (1916) Psychol. Rev. **23**, 89.

Weininger, O., McClelland, W. J., and Arima, R. K., (1954) Can. J. Psychol. **8**, 147.

Welch, B. L., (1964) in "Symposium on Medical Aspects of Stress in the Military Climate," Walter Reed Army Medical Center, Washington, D.C., p. 39.

Welker, W. I., (1956) J. Comp. Physiol. Psychol. **49**, 181.

Widdowson, E. M., (1951) Lancet **1**, 1316.

Wilbur, K. M., (1936) Science **84**, 274.

Williams, C. D. and Kutcha, J. C., (1957) J. Comp. Physiol. Psychol. **50**, 509.

Wilson, A. and Schild, H. O., (1968) "Applied Pharmacology," 10th ed., Churchill Ltd., London.

Winter, C. A., (1948) J. Pharmacol. Exper. Ther. **94**, 7.
Yen, C. Y., Stanger, L., and Millman, N., (1959) Arch. Int. Pharmacodyn. Ther. **123**, 179.
Zigler, E., (1963) J. Personality **31**, 258.

Chapter V

NEUROCHEMICAL CORRELATES
OF BEHAVIOR

It has been generally accepted that different patterns of animal behavior depend upon the activation and mutual integration of a series of neural circuits, the development and complexity of which vary as a function of the elaboration and disposition of an organism's response to a specific stimulus, Consistent with this view is the notion that the activity of such neural circuits can occur, not only through the action of putative neurotransmitters, but must also be regulated by the availability of such molecules at receptor sites; such regulation would appear to be flexibly regulated and dependent upon functional needs. As a consequence of such an emerging schema, different behavioral responses can be tentatively related to different biochemical situations at the central nervous system level.

This basic formulation originates in a speculative framework, which has been developing for over a century; the centrally stimulating effects of exercise (SPURZHEIM, 1815), and of environmental factors (DARWIN, 1874), upon brain organization and its specialized functions have been observed, as well as the perhaps more impressive finding that such effects can lead to increases in cell number and in a possible reorganization and development of cortical interconnections (RAMON y CAJAL, 1895). In another respect the concept is related to KÖHLER's hypothesis (1938) which emphasizes that the prime effect of the nerve impulse consists of a series of chemical events; it has recently been demonstrated, for example, in the findings of ROSENZWEIG et al. (1962: see Chapter IV), that environmental characteristics can affect several anatomical and biochemical parameters of the brain. These considerations have led to the concept of a neural plasticity in biochemical and anatomical brain systems for certain environmental experiences and influences (BENNETT et al., 1964). It may, therefore, become possible to consider the correlation of behavioral differences with specific changes in brain biochemistry, or to relate the effects of psychotropic drugs to their possible biochemical correlates, as RUSSELL (1958, 1964) has proposed. In this manner it becomes possible to formulate hypotheses in terms of a relationship between behavioral responses and biochemical events, rather than between drugs and behavior.

The practical problems and difficulties in the application of such an experimental approach essentially consist in having sufficiently selective methods available for the extraction of biologically significant molecules from tissue, as well as methods for the quantitative determination of the highly specific substances that are isolated by such tissue extraction procedures. Moreover, it may be considered that some changes in spontaneous or pharmacologically induced behavior can be sustained by very selective central biochemical variations and limited to a few anatomical sites, or even to some specific neuronal pathway; these restricted changes may not register any obvious influence upon monoamine levels as determined for the whole brain. As already mentioned in Chapter III, a lack of change in brain neurotransmitter level does not exclude the possibility that there has been a turnover change; these changes may even more significantly reflect some new and different operative mechanisms in the central nervous system.

The extension of studies concerned with interrelations between neurochemical substrates and behavioral components, will provide a better understanding of brain mechanisms as well as of the mode of action of psychotropic drugs; such defined interrelationships may serve as a basis for the synthesis of new drugs more and more selective and effective in mediating their therapeutic effect.

A) ASSAY METHODS

Obviously, it is not possible to list and analyze the advantages and limitations of the numerous qualitative and quantitative assay methods described in the scientific literature, which have been employed to derive all of the possible biologically active constituents present in the brain. Therefore, it seems more appropriate to outline only those most frequently used, while leaving the more detailed technical description for the references cited.

A significant contribution to a methodological facility in the investigation, particularly of biogenic amines—and their likely role as neurotransmitters—was made by the introduction into biological research of the *spectrofluorometer* (BOWMAN et al., 1955); several commercially available models of such instruments are currently available. This optical method is emphasized because of its extensive use in the analysis of biogenic amines and its high level of sensitivity, as compared with other standard photometric techniques.

The basic principle of this technique is that a molecule, after the absorption of radiation, will emit light because of a change in its excited state. Specifically, the working principle of these devices is essentially based on an *activating monochromatic ray* of sufficient intensity, provided either through a prism or grating machromotor, which reaches a cell containing the dissolved molecule under examination. When a molecular structure possesses some particular physicol-chemical characteristics, the activating ray, which has to be powerful enough to shift out from their normal orbital level one or more electrons of the atomic groups typical of the molecule, provides the molecule to give back a part of the energy employed for the activation as a photon emission that gives origin to a new luminous ray (*emission ray*), the wavelength of which is always greater than that of the activating ray, typical of the molecular structure of the substance under examination.

There are several practical and theoretical considerations which must be taken into account when this technique is employed (UDENFRIEND, 1962, 1969; HERCULES, 1966), however, spectrofluorometric methods are generally considered as one of the most selective and sensitive techniques available for experimental purposes.

As far as neurotransmitter determination, particularly serotonin, dopamine, and norepinephrine is concerned, the first spectrofluorometric method was described for serotonin assay by BOGDANSKI et al. (1956), and was further modified by several investigations (SHORE and OLIN, 1958; MEAD and FINGER, 1961; CALLINGHAM and CASS, 1963) in such a way as to allow for the simultaneous determination of both serotonin and norepinephrine content in the same tissue sample. More recently, the method described by ANSELL and BEESON (1968) provided for the possibility of a simultaneous determination of all three monoamines. There are also methods for the determination of 5-hydroxyindoleacetic acid concentration in the brain (QUAY, 1963; ROOS et al., 1963; GIACALONE and VALZELLI, 1966); these latter procedures are important when brain serotonin turnover has to be estimated, using an inhibitor of monoamine oxidase activity and then mathematically integrating the linearity of the increase in serotonin and the corresponding decrease of 5-hydroxyindoleacetic acid within a fixed period of time (TOZER et al., 1966). Recently, a method has been described that allows for the simultaneous determination of serotonin and its metabolite in the same brain tissue sample, so that both rate constants are simultaneously provided (GIACALONE and VALZELLI, 1969). A more recently described method is that of WELCH and WELCH (1969) in which serotonin, norepinephrine, dopamine, and 5-hydroxyindoleacetic acid are simultaneously extracted from the same tissue sample. Obviously, the possibility of obtaining simultaneous determinations of all the major monoamines and one of their important metabolites from the same brain tissue of a single animal is notably advantageous, and particularly appropriate when information concerning the absolute levels of such bio-

genic molecules and their mutual interrelationships at a given function point
is sought.

Recently methods for improved spectrofluorometric detection of serotonin have been described; these are based upon a reaction of this molecule
with orthophtaldialdehyde (OPT) (MAICKEL and MILLER, 1966; CUR-
ZON and GREEN, 1970; THOMPSON et al., 1970) and permits detection
of serotonin levels as low as 2.7 ng/ml in comparison with 56 ng/ml detecta-
ble by the traditional procedures.

The estimation of brain catecholamine turnover presents a somewhat
different problem since these compounds are partially metabolized by
monoamine oxidase (MAO) and partially by catechol-oxydo-methyltransferase (COMT) (see Fig. 13).

A steady state method for turnover estimation would require the use of
two different types of metabolic inhibitors which, because of the possibility
of a mutual pharmacodynamic interaction, leading to confounding results
and interpretative difficulties, would not be practical. The turnover estimate
is therefore based upon the linear decrease in brain norepinephrine and
dopamine, following inhibition of synthesis at the hydroxylating step,
which is common to both of these amines, following the administration of
alpha-methyl-p-tyrosine (BRODIE et al., 1966).

As mentioned in Chapter III, there are histochemical methods, based
upon fluorescence microscopy, with which one may identify and localize
specific monoamines in cellular populations and subcellular sites within the
central nervous system (FUXE et al., 1967, 1968).

This method basically consists of exposing thin slices of brain tissue to
formaldehyde vapors, following which tetrahydroisoquinolines develop,
which in the presence of protein, are transformed into dihydroisoquinolines,
in the case of catecholamines, and into dihydronorharmane derivatives in
the case of indoles. The former derivatives have a green or yellow-green
fluorescence that differs from a typical yellow fluorescence of the latter.
Obviously, such techniques are extremely valuable for qualitative experimental use, but are not ideally suited to quantitative applications, such as
where tissue amine levels are required. An example of this method has been
given in Chapter III (Figs. 16,18). An enzymatic method (SAELENS et al.,
1967) has been recently introduced for the determination of norepinephrine
in tissue samples of as little as 10 μg. Moreover, there are methods for the
spectrofluorometric determination of monoamines oxidase activity (SNY-
DER and HENDLEY, 1968), as well as radioisotopic methods, utilizing
labeled molecules, both for the determination of such enzymes as well as for
5-hydroxytryptophan decarboxylase activity (McCAMAN et al., 1965).
These methods are also appropriate for the identification and distribution of
serotonin (AGHAJANIAN and BLOOM, 1967; PALAIC et al., 1967) and

norepinephrine (GLOWINSKI et al., 1965). There is also the possibility of determining the concentration of catecholamine metabolites, both directly in brain tissue and in the cerebrospinal fluid (ANDÉN et al., 1963a).

The quantitative determination of tissue acetylcholine concentration has represented a difficult technical and methodological problem for some time. The assay of this amine has usually been accomplished through the use of classical bioassay procedures, such as measuring its effect upon the contractile properties of either the guinea pig ileum, clam heart, or leech dorsal muscle; such responses have usually been titrated against those produced by known concentrations of acetylcholine.

More recently, radioisotopic (KRAMER et al., 1968), gas chromatographic (CRANMER, 1968), and spectrofluorometric (FELLMAN, 1969) methods for estimation of tissue acetylcholine levels have been described. Techniques for the determination of choline acetylase activity (McCAMAN and HUNT, 1965) and acetylcholinesterases (HANIN et al., 1968; POTTER, 1967) have also been developed.

Methods for the detection of histamine content have been less prevalent; however, like previously described assays, this amine has also been assayed on isolated organs, and subsequently a spectrofluorometric assay technique for its determination has been developed (KREMZNER and PFEIFFER, 1966; MEDINA and SHORE, 1966).

Obviously, those methods cited for the study of brain biochemistry are not the only ones which are available. Beyond those experimental paradigms in which neurotransmitters and their various metabolic pathways are considered, there are a considerable number of additional experimental procedures which provide for the identification and quantitative determination of a continuously increasing number of biologically active molecules present in brain tissue; there are, further methodological means by which the functional significance of such molecules may be explored, but all such approaches require more space than has herein been allotted for their complete description.

It must also be considered that, for the present, the correlations between behavioral variations and neurochemical substrates are still primarily intended as general relationships with putative neurotransmitters, particularly serotonin, norepinephrine, and dopamine, so that this general area is still one that is being actively developed.

Obviously, the possibility of such biochemical investigations as have been described are extremely limited in man because of the impossibility of determining such potential neurotransmitters directly in brain tissue (unless obtained from autopsy material), so that assays are more commonly performed with biological fluids such as urine, blood, or cerebrospinal fluid. In urine it is possible to determine serotonin content using a method described

by SHORE and OLIN (1958) and by BOGDANSKI et al. (1956), recogniz-
ing the fact that this monoamine is present in only negligible quantities
under normal conditions. Urinary 5-hydroxyindoleacetic acid concentration
can also be determined utilizing an unmodified application of a method
described by GIACALONE and VALZELLI (1966). Methods for the determination of urinary catecholamine content are less simple; the most classical
of these methods is that of CROUT (1961), following which another was
described by ANTON and SAYRE (1962), which was recently modified by
SPANO et al. (1967).

A method by MATTOK et al. (1967a) allows for the urinary assay of
epinephrine, norepinephrine, dopamine, and several catecholamine metabolites such as metanephrine and normetanephrine. For other catecholamine
metabolites there is a spectrofluorometric method described by SATO
(1965) which provides for the assay of other metabolites such as homovanillic acid, while vanililmandelic acid can be spectrofluorometrically determined with a method described by MAHLER and HUMOLLER (1962).

 There are a series of technical problems involved with the assay of
catecholamines and indole amines in blood and urine; these are due both to
the small quantities of these substances normally present in the blood
stream, and to numerous sources of possible nonspecific fluorescence which
may interfere with a correct spectrofluorometric determination.

The methods available for the measurement of serotonin concentration
in blood and urine are still substantially the same as were developed several
years ago by WAALKES (1959) and by DAVIS (1959) and more recently
technically modified by MATRAY and MOREAU (1964). For the determination of blood and urinary catecholamine content there are other
methods by HÄGGENDAL (1963), and LINDSTEDT (1964), aside from
those already mentioned (SPANO et al., 1967).

From a general point of view, it should be considered that biochemical
studies in man that yield results which derive from the analysis of body
fluids are probably poor indices of the cerebral situation. In fact, monoamines, under normal conditions, do not cross the hematoencephalic barrier;
moreover such constituents undergo extensive and quantitatively significant
peripheral metabolism. These conditions can, to a great extent, obscure the
biochemical variations which can take place not only in the whole brain, but
also in limited cell populations, structures, or area. Such considerations
should necessarily provide cautionary limits for the interpretation of possible monoamine variations in human blood and urine as correlates for some
particular aspect of behavior.

A more direct approach to the assessment of amine content, as potentially more relevant to brain function in man, has been in the analysis of
human cerebrospinal fluid (CSF). Although the concentrations of such

substances in the CSF are lower than found either in brain tissue or peripheral fluids, these levels are still perhaps more relevant to the functional disposition of the brain, and certainly, in the case of neuropathology, reflect aminergic changes that are consistent with those observed in brain. Serotonin has been assayed in CSF (AKCASU et al., 1960), as has its major metabolite, 5-HIAA (ASHCROFT and SHARMAN, 1962). Norepinephrine has been detected in CSF (CIPLEA et al., 1964) as well as catecholamine metabolites, such as homovanillic acid and 3-methoxy-4-hydroxymandelic acid (ANDÉN et al., 1963b). Histamine has also been measured in human CSF (JACKSON and ROSE, 1949). Because of a plasma-CSF barrier and the fluid mechanics necessary to accommodate the diffusion of amines from the brain into CSF, it seems likely that this more accessible source of indices for central nervous system change may provide a more appropriate medium from which such change may be assessed.

B) BEHAVIORAL ASPECTS AND BIOCHEMICAL VARIATIONS IN ANIMALS

In 1915 CANNON suggested that rage and fear reactions in animals could have a biochemical substrate consisting in the release of a biologically active amine, epinephrine. With the development of research, particularly in recent years, a series of experimental data have accrued which reinforce the premise that a number of biologically active substances exert a regulating effect on the behavior of living organisms; such an influence occurs either directly or through a series of mutual interactions with central nervous system activity (APRISON et al., 1962).

Within the general area of biochemistry-behavior interrelationships experimental approaches have essentially consisted in administering either metabolic precursors of biogenic amines which, upon easily reaching the brain, can substantially modify the normal levels of a neurotransmitter, or such drugs, which by acting on the enzyme systems regulating the synthesis or inactivation of a putative transmitter can alter its concentration. A third experimental approach is represented by the administration of psychotropic drugs and investigating the possible modifications in neurotransmitter content that can take place. Obviously, the common denominator of these experimental approaches consists in the possibility of establishing correlations between biochemical variations and specific aspects of behavior in laboratory animals.

For example, 5-hydroxytryptophan administered to animals trained in a specific conditioning paradigm induces a decrease in acquired responses and results in the appearance of atypical behavior that is temporally correlated with the increase in brain serotonin content (APRISON et al., 1962). It has also been shown that dopamine level varies in diencephalic and pontomesencephalic structures in such a way as to correlate with the behavioral variations, while norepinephrine concentration does not significantly change (APRISON and HINGTGEN, 1965). The concentration changes of these last two amines has been explained on the basis that 5-hydroxytryptophan decarboxylase, which mediates the synthesis of serotonin, and DOPA-decarboxylase, which mediates the synthesis of dopamine (see Fig. 13, Chapter II), are probably a unique enzymatic substrate (YUWILER et al., 1959; KUNTZMAN et al., 1961), so that, the administrations of large doses of 5-hydroxytryptophan would tend to engage that enzymatic step involving indoles, resulting in both a catecholamine decrease (YUWILER et al., 1959) and a serotonin increase. This would occur, not only in those neurons wherein it is normally stored, but also in those which generally contain only dopamine and/or norepinephrine (HIMWICH and COSTA, 1960; COSTA et al., 1962). In the experimental paradigm previously described, the administration of alpha-methyl-p-tyrosine, an inhibitor of catecholamine-decarboxylating enzymes (HESS et al., 1961; COSTA et al., 1962; ANDÉN, 1964), to laboratory animals brought about a series of behavioral modifications which were not correlated in magnitude or time with brain norepinephrine and dopamine decreases, whereas they corresponded very well with the relative modification in brain serotonin level (APRISON and HINGTGEN, 1966). This observation tends to suggest that, within certain limits, increased levels of brain serotonin may provide for behavioral deficits or performance decrements that can be operative upon the learning process. However, WOOLLEY and VAN DER HOEVEN (1963, 1965) had previously observed that, in mice, learning ability was inversely related to brain serotonin content. More recently, it has been observed that inhibition of serotonin synthesis, as provided by the administration of p-chlorophenylalanine, a drug which does not influence catecholamine synthesis (KOE and WEISSMAN, 1966), induces an obvious increase in the discriminative learning ability of rats (STEVENS et al., 1967); such responses were not enhanced by an increase in brain catecholamines.

Experiments performed with alpha-methyl-m-tyrosine indicated that several behavioral indices, such as avoidance behavior, motor activity, and rota-rod performances, are dramatically impaired by a decrease in brain catecholamines (RECH et al., 1968a,b). An increase in brain dopamine produced by the combined administration of dihydroxyphenylalanine (DOPA), the precursor common to both the brain catecholamines and of diethyldithiocarbammate, which blocks beta-hydroxylase activity (Fig. 13), results in the appearance of stereotyped behavior (RANDRUP and MUNKVAD, 1966; SCHEEL-KRÜGER and RANDRUP, 1967).

This series of experiments is certainly suggestive of several bases of potential relationships that may be developed between putative neurotransmitters and a series of behavioral components. However, it remains to be emphasized that such results, for the present, must be considered as only indicative of a series of more complex functional biochemical relationships, which could be clarified and extended when methodological approaches permit data acquisition more selectively referable to specific brain pathways, nuclei, or regions.

Over the past several years, other experimental approaches have attempted to develop relationships between environmentally induced behavioral alterations and specific neurochemical parameters; this approach has avoided the direct effects of drugs, precursors, or metabolic inhibitors previously relied upon.

This general area of research includes the experiments of KRECH et al. (1960, 1965) and of ROSENZWEIG (1966), previously mentioned, and is concerned with the influence of different controlled environments upon several aspects of animal behavior and some brain parameters (Chapter IV). Also relevant in this area of research are the experiments of MAAS (1962, 1963), which demonstrated that mouse strains that show a high level of emotionality have higher brain serotonin levels than other strains of mice that were less emotional. The same type of general correlation has also been developed in rats, particularly with serotonin concentrations in the limbic area (SUDAK and MAAS, 1964a,b), an area well known as an essential structure in the control and manifestation of emotional behavior. Stress situations and stress or stimuli can bring about modifications of the content of presumed neurotransmitters (THIERRY et al., 1968a,b; PUJOL et al., 1968; GORDON et al., 1966). In this context, it becomes fundamentally important to provide experimental evidences that purely psychological stimulations are capable of inducing specific neurochemical changes, in order to comprehend etiological factors of mental diseases where, almost certainly, social and emotionally relevant influences from the environment exert physiological effects, modify biochemical events, and alter the influence of psychotropic drugs.

WELCH and WELCH (1968) have demonstrated that a mouse given the opportunity to observe fighting episodes between other mice, will show a statistically significant decrement in pontine and medullary norepinephrine levels; the emotional stimulus apparently accounting for the central catecholamine change did not involve physical participation in the fighting behavior.

In aggressiveness induced in mice by isolation (Chapter IV) it has been possible to describe brain biochemical variations which do not mainly consist in significant modification of brain amine levels between aggressive

TABLE IX

Brain Serotonin (5HT), Norepinephrine (NE), and
Dopamine (DA) Contents in Normal (N) and Aggressive (A) Mice

	Brain Contents γ/g ± Standard Error					
	N			A		
Brain Areas	5HT	NE	DA	5HT	NE	DA
Cerebellum	–	0.10 ± 0.02	–	–	0.10 ± 0.02	–
Olfactory bulbs	0.39 ± 0.01	0.11 ± 0.02	0.63 ± 0.02	0.40 ± 0.06	0.12 ± 0.04	0.73 ± 0.08
Corpora quadrigemina	1.10 ± 0.07	0.60 ± 0.05	0.71 ± 0.02	1.01 ± 0.04	0.49 ± 0.03	0.61 ± 0.03
Mesencephalon	0.62 ± 0.03	0.39 ± 0.05	0.06 ± 0.005	0.56 ± 0.04	0.36 ± 0.03	0.04 ± 0.002
Diencephalon	0.94 ± 0.02	0.55 ± 0.05	0.29 ± 0.01	0.94 ± 0.02	0.50 ± 0.04	0.28 ± 0.02
Remainder of the brain	0.36 ± 0.06	0.36 ± 0.03	1.77 ± 0.01	0.47 ± 0.02	0.29 ± 0.04	1.60 ± 0.02
Whole brain	0.65 ± 0.03	0.45 ± 0.02	1.09 ± 0.05	0.65 ± 0.03	0.42 ± 0.03	1.04 ± 0.04

and normal mice (DA VANZO et al., 1966; VALZELLI, 1967a; VALZELLI and GARATTINI, 1968; Table IX), but rather in changes in the turnover of brain amines VALZELLI, 1967a, 1971a, ESSMAN, 1968, 1969, 1971; ESSMAN and FRISONE, 1966).

Depending upon the strain of mouse employed, and the age at which they were subjected to isolation, there is a decrease of brain serotonin turnover in aggressive mice (VALZELLI, 1967a; GARATTINI et al., 1967; VALZELLI and GARATTINI, 1972), a minor decrease of norepinephrine turnover, and an increase of dopamine turnover (VALZELLI, 1971a), while other strains show an increased brain serotonin turnover (ESSMAN, 1971). Changes in brain neurotransmitter turnover can be observed also in rats made aggressive by isolation (VALZELLI and GARATTINI, 1972; GOLDBERG and SALAMA, 1969). Another series of experiments has been concerned with another functionally significant component of brain biochemistry, N-acetylaspartic acid; this free amino acid, which appears well correlated with brain serotonin level and changes, has been shown to decrease in concentration in the brain of the aggressive mouse (MARCUCCI et al., 1968), while there are no variations that occur in either brain aspartic acid or glutammic acid (GIACALONE and VALZELLI, 1972). Moreover, isolation housing in mice induces a decreased liver microsomal ATPase activity and an increased rate of microsomal protein synthesis. There are similar, although smaller, changes in equivalent measurements occurring in the brain following isolation (ESSMAN et al., 1972). A particularly interesting observation is that these brain biochemical changes do not occur in those animals which, even after isolation for a sufficient period of time, do not become aggressive (Table X).

The experimental data deriving from this behavioral model, emphasize that alterations in the normal social context, as represented by isolation, are capable of inducing at least two major effects in laboratory animals. The first of these consists of a series of changes in brain biochemistry, while the second involves drastic effects upon emotional behavior and responsivity; at least for the present there is no single obvious direct cause-and-effect relationship between the biochemical changes and aggressive behavior.

The previously mentioned effects of isolation in man (Chapter IV), seem to clearly demonstrate that there are several factors which serve to abnormally influence emotional behavior, and are of sufficient duration to induce a series of different behavioral changes; knowledge of such isolation-induced aberrant perceptual behavior, together with some of the biochemical modifications that have been described in pathologic states in man, is still limited by technical difficulties inherent in the assessment of biochemical changes in man and the significance of such changes for brain function.

TABLE X

Physiological, Neurochemical, Pharmacological, and Behavioral
Changes Observed in Isolation-Housed Male Albino Mouse

Observation	References
Initial increase of locomotor activity	VALZELLI (1969a)
Increased general reactivity	VALZELLI (1969a)
Increased response to painful stimulation	VALZELLI (1969a)
Induction of gastric pathology	ESSMAN and FRISONE (1966); ESSMAN (1966)
Hyperirritability	VALZELLI (1969a)
Increased vocalization	VALZELLI (1969a)
Tremor	VALZELLI (1969a)
Piloerection	VALZELLI (1969a)
Compulsive aggression	VALZELLI (1967b); ESSMAN and SMITH (1967)
Decreased brain 5HIAA	VALZELLI and GARATTINI (1968)
Decreased brain 5HT turnover	VALZELLI and GARATTINI (1968)
Decreased 5HT turnover in diencephalon	GARATTINI et al. (1969)
Minor decrease in brain NE turnover	VALZELLI (1971a)
Increased DA turnover	VALZELLI (1971a)
Cerebellar neuronal RNA decrement with increased duration of isolation	ESSMAN (1970a)
Cerebellar glial RNA increment with increased duration of isolation	ESSMAN (1970a)
Decrease in brain N-acetyl-L-aspartic acid	MARCUCCI et al. (1968)
Unchanged brain MAO activity	CONSOLO and VALZELLI (1970)
Unchanged brain choline acetylase activity	CONSOLO and VALZELLI (1970)
Increased AChE activity associated with external synaptic membrane of nerve endings from cerebral cortex	ESSMAN (1970b)
Unchanged brain aspartic acid	MARCUCCI and GIACALONE (1969)
Unchanged brain glutamic acid	MARCUCCI and GIACALONE (1969)
Faster release of brain amines by low doses of reserpine	VALZELLI (1967a)
Decreased exploratory behavior	VALZELLI (1969b)
Reduced avoidance response acquisition	VALZELLI (1971a)
Decreased barbiturate-induced sleeping time	CONSOLO et al. (1965a)
Decreased potentiation of chlorpromazine on barbiturate-sleeping time	CONSOLO et al. (1965a)
Increased amphetamine toxicity	CONSOLO et al. (1965b)
Increased fencamfamine toxicity	CONSOLO et al. (1965a)
Different response to various psychotropic drugs on exploratory behavior	VALZELLI (1969b, 1971b)
Different response to muscular-relaxant activity of various benzodiazepines	VALZELLI (1973)

104

C) BEHAVIORAL ASPECTS AND BIOCHEMICAL VARIATIONS IN MAN

Over the past several years data from hundreds of experimental studies have accumulated in clinical psychiatry in which the approach has been based upon the investigation of biochemical parameters measured in the blood and/or urine of patients in an attempt to evolve possible correlations between such measures and differences in behavior. This general area of research can be divided into three major categories; the first deals with the analysis of relationships between biochemical variations and emotional situation; the second searches for possible comparisons between biochemical constants of behaviorally healthy subjects with those of psychiatric patients, particularly in schizophrenia; the third approach concerns the activity of psychotropic drugs upon the biochemistry of normal subjects and those manifesting behavior disorders.

Only the first two categories will be considered further, since they are more strictly related to the general theme of this chapter. It is currently a generally accepted premise that life events and emotional situations associated with them, influence the central nervous system in such a way that its function varies, reflecting upon the status of the living organism (RAHE and ARTHUR, 1968).

In particular, aside from the well known variations in corticosteroids that characterize normal or emotionally stressful conditions (FOX et al., 1961; FISHMAN et al., 1962; WADESON et al., 1963; WOLFF et al., 1964), the problem has been further considered in terms of possible relationships between affective states and brain biogenic amines in man (SCHILDKRAUT and KETY, 1967). Some authors, for example, have suggested that, while rage reactions are more closely associated with norepinephrine variations (AX, 1959), fear and anxiety would, instead, be related to both norepinephrine and epinephrine variations (AX, 1959; RAAB, 1966).

Increases in urinary norepinephrine excretion may be observed in many situations, corresponding generally to "emergency" reactions. In this respect, an increase of urinary norepinephrine concentration has been demonstrated in hockey players during competitive games and among psychiatric patients during aggressive attacks (EDLMADJIAN et al., 1957). An increase in urinary norepinephrine level has also been observed in sportsmen who, without actively participating in the game, were observing the competition as spectators (SCHILDKRAUT and KETY, 1967). This finding agrees well with similar observations previously reported for mice. Generally speaking, all those situations in which a subject may become emotionally engaged can result in variations of urinary catecholamine excretion (VON EULER, 1964; FRANKENHAÜSER et al., 1968), even if differences exist between anxious patients and subjects with aggressive components (SILVERMAN et al., 1961). Obviously, any differences that may be found, must not be considered as evidence for a difference in peripheral adjustment mediated by the central nervous system through the hypophyseal-adrenal axis.

On the other hand, a series of experiments (VEARN and STURGIS, 1919; RICHTER, 1940; BASOWITZ et al., 1956; HAWKINS et al., 1960) have shown that epinephrine infusion in man brings about anxiety-like symptoms, while norepinephrine proved to be less efficacious (KING et al., 1952; ROTHBALLER, 1959; HAWKINS et al., 1960). A possible explanation for the effects of epinephrine is that this substance mediates a non-specific excitatory state which is acted upon by the individual's past experiences and the characteristics of the experimental situations; these may serve to determine both the intensity and the type of emotional reaction.

It should not be forgotten that the hemato-encephalic barrier strongly prevents the penetration of epinephrine into the brain, with the possible exception of some hypothalamic areas (WEIL-MALHERBE et al., 1959). Hence, if this catecholamine is released or administered peripherally and brings about variations in affective behavior by means of either a direct action on the hypothalamus or through a series of subjective perceptual variations which resemble excitation conditions, this then constitutes an interpretive problem. This problem is related to the theory of the visceral origin of emotions proposed by JAMES (1890) and initially criticized by CANNON (1927) and, more recently, by BREGGIN (1964).

A great deal of experimental research has been attempted to clarify the possible biochemical correlates of behavior disorders and especially of schizophrenia. The theoretical positions taken in this approach may be summarized on the basis of the following: (a) a hypothesis formulated by OSMOND and SMYTHIES (1952), considered that schizophrenia could be associated with an abnormality of the norepinephrine oxymethylation process with the resulting formation of psychotoxic metabolites, such as dimethoxyphenyl-ethanolamine; (b) a hypothesis suggested by GADDUM (1954) and by WOOLLEY and SHAW (1954), considered that schizophrenia could depend upon abnormalities in serotonin metabolism, with the production of psychotoxic metabolites such as dimethyltryptamine and similar analogs; (c) POLLIN et al. (1961) proposed that behavior disorders could occur if amine metabolism was disrupted at the transmethylation step; this would provide for the formation of abnormal methylated compounds with psychotoxic properties, which would further disrupt neuronal function through the impairment of transmethylation by such methylated derivatives.

Recently HIMWICH et al. (1967) have summarized a series of experimental findings of great interest concerning brain amines and schizophrenia. These considerations provide an up-to-date view of the relationship, indicating, however, that extensive work is necessary for the achievement of greater consistency. However, what now appears to emerge, is that, not only in schizophrenia, but also in several other psychopathological conditions there are biochemical disorders; such alterations have been principally associated with biogenic amine metabolism. In this regard, the analysis of urine from schizophrenic subjects has yielded substances that could not be detected in normal subjects; these have, as yet, not been identified (FRIED-HOFF and VAN WINKLE, 1962; MATTOK et al., 1967a; BOULTON et al., 1967). Parallels between metabolic alterations in tryptophan metabolism and psychosis have been illustrated (BRUNE and HIMWICH, 1963; BRUNE, 1967), and the appearance of a hallucinogenic indoleamine, bufotenine, in the urine of schizophrenic patients has been described (FISCHER et al., 1961; TANIMUKAI et al., 1967). In schizophrenic subjects, a decrease in the urinary excretion of dopamine (MATTOK et al., 1967b) and alterations of catecholamine metabolism have been studied (FRIEDHOFF and VAN WINKLE, 1967). Differences in amine level for the depressive and manic phases of manic-depressive illness have been considered (CATALANO et al., 1966), as well as changes among patients with extrapyramidal disturbances (RINNE et al., 1966). HALEVY et al. (1965) have also attempted to establish correlations between the level of blood serotonin and the behavior of psychiatric patients as evaluated by means of the Minnesota Multiphasic Personality Inventory (MMPI).

Although, for the present, the extensive experimental data available do not yet permit the formulation of clear conclusions concerning the meaning of possible correlations between several metabolic changes and behavioral alterations of psychiatric patients, it is important to emphasize that, despite previously mentioned technical difficulties which retard biochemical assessment in man, progress has been made; this type of experimental-clinical research will, in the hopefully near future be able to provide a more precise definition of those processes responsible for disruption of the normal functional equilibrium of the human brain.

REFERENCES

Aghajanian, G. K. and Bloom F. E., (1967) J. Pharmacol. Exper. Ther. 156, 23.
Akcasu, A., Akcasu, M., and Tumay, S. B., (1960) Nature, London 187, 324.
Andén, N. E., (1964) Acta Pharmacol. Toxicol. 21, 260.
Andén, N. E., Roos, B. E., and Verdinius, B., (1963a) Life Sci. 2, 448.
Andén, N. E., Roos, B. E., and Verdinius, B., (1963b) Experientia 19, 359.

Ansell, G. B. and Beeson, M. F., (1968) Anal. Biochem. **23**, 196.

Anton, A. H. and Sayre, D. F., (1962) J. Pharmacol. Exper. Ther. **138**, 360.

Aprison, M. H. and Hingtgen, J. N., (1965) J. Neurochem. **12**, 959.

Aprison, M. H. and Hingtgen, J. N., (1966) Life Sci. **5**, 1971.

Aprison, M. H., Wolf, M. A., Poulos, G. L., and Folkerth, T. L., (1962) J. Neurochem. **9**, 575.

Ashcroft, G. W. and Sharman, D. F., (1962) Brit. J. Pharmacol. **19**, 153.

Ax, A. F., (1959) Psychosom. Med. **21**, 344.

Basowitz, H., Korchin, S. J., Oken, D., Goldstein, M. S., and Gussaek, H., (1956) A. M. A. Arch, Neurol. Psychiat. **76**, 98.

Bennett, E. L., Diamond, M. C., Krech, D., and Rosenzweig, M. R., (1964) Science **146**, 610.

Bogdanski, D. F., Pletscher, A., Brodie, B. B., and Udenfriend, S., (1956) J. Pharmacol. Exper. Ther. **117**, 82.

Boulton, A. A., Pollit, R. J., and Majer, J. R., (1967) Nature, London **215**, 132.

Bowman, R. L., Caufield, P. A., and Udenfriend, S., (1955) Science **122**, 32.

Breggin, P. R., (1964) J. Nerv. Ment. Dis. **139**, 558.

Brodie, B. B., Costa, E., Dlabac, A., Neff, N. H., and Smookler, H. H., (1966) J. Pharmacol. Exper. Ther. **154**, 493.

Brune, G. G., (1967) in "Amines and Schizophrenia," Himwich, H. E., Kety, S. S., and Smythies, J. R., Eds., Pergamon Press, Oxford p. 87.

Brune, G. G. and Himwich, H. E., (1963) in "Recent Advances in Biological Psychiatry," vol. 5, Wortis, J., Ed., Plenum Press, New York, p. 144.

Callingham, B. A. and Cass, R., (1963) J. Pharm. Pharmacol. **15**, 699.

Cannon, W. B., (1915) "Bodily Changes in Pain, Hunger, Fear and Rage," Appleton-Century, New York.

Cannon, W. B., (1927) Amer. J. Psychol. **39**, 106.

Catalano, A., De Risio, C., Campanini, T., and Ridolo, P., (1966) Sist. Nerv. **18**, 100.

Ciplea, A., Bubyianu, G., and Galasanu, E., (1964) Int. J. Neuropharmacol. **3**, 583.

Consolo, S., Garattini, S., and Valzelli, L., (1965a) J. Pharm. Pharmacol. **17**, 594.

Consolo, S., Garattini, S., and Valzelli, L., (1965b) J. Pharm. Pharmacol. **17**, 53.

Consolo, S. and Valzelli, L., (1970) Europ. J. Pharmacol. **13**, 129.

Costa, E., Gessa, G. L., Hirsch, C., Kuntzman, R., and Brodie, B. B., (1962) Ann. N. Y. Acad. Sci. **96**, 118.

Cranmer, M. F., (1968) Life Sci. **7**, 995.

Crout, J. R., (1961) in "Standard Methods of Clinical Chemistry," vol. 3, Academic Press, New York, p. 62.

Curzon, G. and Green, A. R., (1970) Brit. J. Pharmacol. **39**, 653.

Da Vanzo, J. P., Daugherty, M., Ruchart, R., and Kang, L., (1966) Psychopharmacologia (Berl.) **9**, 210.

Darwin, C., (1874) "The Descent of Man," 2nd ed., Rand McNally, Chicago, p. 53.

Davis, R. B., (1959) J. Lab. Clin. Med. **54**, 344.

Elmadjian, F., Hope, J. M., and Lamson, E., (1957) J. Clin. Endocrinol. Metab. **17**, 608.

Essman, W. B., (1966) Psychol. Rep. **19**, 173.

Essman, W. B., (1968) J. Comp. Physiol. Psychol. **66**, 244.

Essman, W. B., (1969) in "Agressive Behaviour," Garattini, S. and Sigg, E. B., Eds., Excerpta Medica Found., Amsterdam, p. 203.

Essman, W. B., (1970a) in "Maternal-Social Deprivation as Functional Somatosensory Deafferentation in the Abnormal Development of the Brain and Behavior," Riesen, A. H., Ed., Amer. Psychol. Assoc., Washington, D. C., in press.

Essman, W. B., (1970b) in "Maturations of Brain Mechanisms and Sleep Behavior," U.S. Government Printing Office, Washington, in press.

Essman, W. B., (1971) in "Brain Development and Behavior," Sterman, M. B., McGinty, D. J., and Adinolfi, A. M., Eds., Academic Press, New York, p. 265.

Essman, W. B. and Frisone, J. D., (1966) J. Psychosom. Res. 10, 183.

Essman, W. B. and Smith, G. E., (1967) Amer. Zool. 7, 370.

Essman, W. B., Heldman, E., Barker, L. A., and Valzelli, L., (1972) Fed. Proc. Fed. Amer. Soc. Exper. Biol., 31, 232 (Abstr. 121).

Fellman, J. H., (1969) J. Neurochem. 16, 135.

Fischer, E., Fernandez Lagravere, T. A., Vazqez, A. J., and Di Stefano, A. O., (1961) J. Nerv. Ment. Dis. 133, 441.

Fishman, J. R., Hamburg, D. A., Handlon, J. H., Mason, J. W., and Sachar, E., (1962) Arch. Gen. Psychiat. 6, 271.

Fox, H. M., Murawski, B. J., Bartholomay, A. F., and Gifford, S., (1961) Psychosom. Med. 23, 33.

Frankenhäuser, M., Mellis, I., Rissler, A., Björkvall, C., and Pátkai, P., (1968) Psychosom. Med. 30, 109.

Friedhoff, A. J and Van Winkle, E., (1962) Nature, London 194, 897.

Friedhoff, A. J. and Van Winkle, E., (1967) in "Amines and Schizophrenia," Himwich, H. E., Kety, S. S., and Smythies, J. R., Eds., Pergamon Press, Oxford, p. 19.

Fuxe, K., Grobecher, H., Hökfelt, T., and Johnsson, G., (1967) Brain Res. 6, 475.

Fuxe, K., Hökfelt, T., and Ungerstedt, U., (1968) in "Advances in Pharmacology," vol. 6A, Garattini, S. and Shore, P. A., Eds., Academic Press, New York, p. 235.

Gaddum, J. H., (1954) in "Ciba Foundation Symposium on Hypertension," Churchill Ltd., London, p. 75.

Garattini, S., Giacalone, E., and Valzelli, L., (1967) J. Pharm. Pharmacol. 19, 338.

Garattini, S., Giacalone, E., and Valzelli, L., (1969) in "Aggressive Behaviour," Garattini, S. and Sigg, E. B., Eds., Excerpta Medica Found., Amsterdam, p. 179.

Giacalone, E. and Valzelli, L., (1966) J. Neurochem. 13, 1265.

Giacalone, E. and Valzelli, L., (1969) Pharmacology 2, 171.

Giacalone, E. and Valzelli, L., (1972) "Proceedings of the 1st. CIANS International Congress," Pacini-Mariotti, Pisa, 1074

Giacalone, E., Tansella, M., Valzelli, L., and Garattini, S., (1968) Biochem. Pharmacol. 17, 1315.

Glowinski, J., Kopin, I. J., and Axelrod, J., (1965) J. Neurochem. 12, 25.

Goldberg, M. E. and Salama, A. I., (1969) Biochem. Pharmacol. 18, 532.

Gordon, R., Spector, S., Sjoerdsma, A., and Udenfriend, S., (1966) J. Pharmacol. Exper. Ther. 153, 440.

Häggendal, J., (1963) Acta Physiol. Scand. 59, 242.

Halevy, A., Moos, R. H., and Solomon, G. F., (1965) J. Psychiat. Res. 3, 1.

Hanin, I., Jenden, D. J., and Lamb, S. I., (1968) Proc. West. Pharmacol. Soc. 11, 144.

Hawkins, D. R., Monroe, J. T., Sandifer, M. G., and Vernon, C. R., (1960) Psychiat. Res. Rep. 12, 40.

Hercules, D. M., (1966) "Fluorescence and Phosphorescence Analysis," Interscience Publ., New York.

Hess, S. M., Connamacher, R. H., Ozaki, M., and Udenfriend, S., (1961) J. Pharmacol. Exper. Ther. 134, 129.

Himwich, H. E., Kety, S. S., and Smythies, J. R., Eds., (1967) "Amines and Schizophrenia," Pergamon Press, Oxford.

Himwich, W. A. and Costa, E., (1960) Fed. Proc. Fed. Amer. Soc. Exper. Biol. 19, 838.

Jackson, I. J. and Rose, B., (1949) J. Lab. Clin. Med. 34, 250.

James, W., (1890) "Principles of Psychology," Holt Publ., New York.

King, B. D., Sokoloff, L., and Wechsler, R. L., (1952) J. Clin. Invest. **31**, 273.

Koe, B. K. and Weissman, A., (1966) J. Phamacol. Exper. Ther. **154**, 499.

Köhler, W., (1938) "The Place of Value in a World of Facts," Liveright Publ., New York, p. 239.

Kramer, S. Z., Seifter, J., and Bhagat, B., (1968) Nature, London **217**, 184.

Krech, D., Rosenzweig, M. R., and Bennett, E. L., (1960) J. Comp. Physiol. Psychol. **53**, 509.

Krech, D., Rosenzweig, M. R., and Bennett, E. L., (1965) Physiol. Behav. **1**, 99.

Kremzner, L. T. and Pfeiffer, C. C., (1966) Biochem. Pharmacol. **15**, 197.

Kuntzman, R., Shore, P. A., Bogdanski, D., and Brodie, B. B., (1961) J. Neurochem. **6**, 226.

Lindstedt, S., (1964) Clin. Chim. Acta **9**, 309.

Maas, J. W., (1962) Science **137**, 621.

Maas, J. W., (1963) Nature, London **197**, 255.

Mahler, D. J. and Humoller, F. L., (1962) Clin. Chem. **8**, 47.

Maickel, R. P. and Miller, F. P., (1966) Anal. Chem. **38**, 1937.

Marcucci, F. and Giacalone, E., (1969) Biochem. Pharmacol. **18**, 691.

Marcucci, F., Mussini, E., Valzelli, L., and Garattini, S., (1968) J. Neurochem. **15**, 53.

Matray, F. and Moreau, J., (1964) Pathol. Biol. **12**, 1137.

Mattok, G. L., O'Reilly, P. O., and Hughes, R. T., (1967a) Dis. Nerv. Syst. **28**, 396.

Mattok, G. L., Wilson, D. L., and Hoffer, A., (1967b) Nature, London **213**, 1189.

McCaman, R. E., McCaman, M. W., Hunt, J. M., and Smith, M. S., (1965) J. Neurochem. **12**, 15.

McCaman, R. E. and Hunt, J. M., (1965) J. Neurochem. **12**, 253.

Mead, J. A. R. and Finger, K. F., (1961) Biochem. Pharmacol. **6**, 52.

Medina, M. and Shore, P. A., (1966) Biochem. Pharmacol. **15**, 1627.

Osmond, H. and Smythies, J. R., (1952) J. Ment. Sci. **98**, 309.

Palaic, D., Page, I. H., and Khairallah, P. A., (1967) J. Neurochem. **14**, 63.

Pollin, W., Cardon, P. V., Jr., and Kety, S. S., (1961) Science **133**, 104.

Potter, L. T., (1967) J. Pharmacol. Exper. Ther. **156**, 500.

Pujol, J. F., Mouret, J., Jouvet, M., and Glowinski, J., (1968) Science **159**, 112.

Quay, W. B., (1963) Anal. Biochem. **5**, 51.

Raab, W., (1966) Amer. Heart J. **72**, 538.

Rahe, R. H. and Arthur, R. J., (1968) Dis. Nerv. Syst. **29**, 114.

Ramon y Cajal, S., (1895) "Les Nouvelles Idées sur la Structure du Système Nerveux chez l'homme et chez les Vertébrés," Reinwald Ed., Paris, p. 78.

Randrup, A. and Munkvad, I., (1966) Acta Psychiat. Scand. (Suppl. 191) **42**, 139.

Rech, R. H., Borys, H. K., and Moore, K. E., (1968a) J. Pharmacol. Exper. Ther. **153**, 412.

Rech, R. H., Carr, L. A., and Moore, K. E., (1968b) J. Pharmacol. Exper. Ther. **160**, 326.

Richter, D., (1940) Proc. Roy. Soc. Med. **33**, 615.

Rinne, U. K., Sonninen, V., and Palo, J., (1966) Psychiat. Neurol. **151**, 321.

Roos, B. E., Andén, N. E., and Werdinius, B., (1963) Acta Physiol. Scand. (Suppl. 213) **59**, 132.

Rosenzweig, M. R., (1966) Amer. Psychol. **21**, 321.

Rosenzweig, M. R., Krech, D., Bennett, E. L., and Diamond, M. C., (1962) J. Comp. Physiol. Psychol. **55**, 429.

Rothballer, A. B., (1959) Pharmacol. Rev. **11**, 494.

Russell, R. W., (1958) Acta Psychol. 14, 281.

Russell, R. W., (1964) in "Animal Behaviour and Drug Action," Ciba Foundation Symposium, Churchill Ltd., London, p. 144.

Saelens, J. K., Schoen, M. S., and Kovacsics, G. B., (1967) Biochem. Pharmacol. 16, 1043.

Sato, T. L., (1965) J. Lab. Clin. Med. 66, 517.

Scheel-Krüger, J. and Randrup, A., (1967) Acta Pharmacol. Toxicol. 25 (Suppl. 4), 61.

Schildkraut, J. J. and Kety, S. S., (1967) Science 156, 21.

Shore, P. A. and Olin, J. S., (1958) J. Pharmacol. Exper. Ther. 122, 295.

Silverman, A. J., Cohen, S. I., Shmavonian, B. M., and Kirshner, N., (1961) in "Recent Advances in Biological Psychiatry," vol. 3, Wortis J., Ed., Plenum Press, New York, p. 104.

Snyder, S. H. and Hendley, E. D., (1968) J. Pharmacol. Exper. Ther. 163, 386.

Spano, P. F., Devoto, G., and Gessa, G. L., (1967) Boll. Boc. Ital. Biol. Sper. 43, 1265.

Spurzheim, J. G., (1815) "The Physiognomical System of Drs. Gall and Spurzheim," 2nd ed., Baldwin, Cradock and Joy Publ., London, p. 554.

Stevens, D. A., Resnick, O., and Krus, D. M., (1967) Life Sci. 6, 2215.

Sudak, H. S. and Maas, J. W., (1964a) Nature, London 203, 4951.

Sudak, H. S. and Maas, J. W., (1964b) Science 146, 418.

Tanimukai, H., Ginther, R., Spaide, J., Bueno, J. R., and Himwich, H. E., (1967) Life Sci. 6, 1697.

Thierry, A. M., Fekete, M., and Glowinski, J., (1968a) Europ. J. Pharmacol. 4, 384.

Thierry, A. M., Javoy, F., Glowinski, J., and Kety, S. S., (1968b) J. Pharmacol. Exper. Ther. 163, 163.

Thompson, J. H., Spezia, C. A., and Angulo, M., (1970) J. Med. Sci. 3, 197.

Tozer, T. N., Neff, N. H., and Brodie, B. B., (1966) J. Pharmacol. Exper. Ther. 153, 177.

Udenfriend, S., (1962) "Fluorescence Assay in Biology and Medicine," Academic Press, New York.

Udenfriend, S., (1969) "Fluorescence Assay in Biology and Medicine," vol. 2, Academic Press, New York.

Valzelli, L., (1967a) in "Neuropyschopharmacology," Proc. 5th CINP International Congress, Excerpta Medica Foundation, Amsterdam, p. 781.

Valzelli, L., (1967b) in "Advances Pharmacology," vol. 5, Garattini, S. and Shore, P. A., Eds., Academic Press, New York, p. 79.

Valzelli, L., (1969a) in "Aggressive Behaviour," Garattini, S. and Sigg, E. B., Eds. Excerpta Medica Foundation, Amsterdam, p. 70

Valzelli, L., (1969b) Psychopharmacologia (Berl.) 15, 232.

Valzelli, L., (1971a) Actual. Pharmacol. 24, 133.

Valzelli, L., (1971b) Psychopharmacologia (Berl.) 19, 91.

Valzelli, L., (1973) in "The Benzodiazepines," Garattini S. and Randall L. O., Eds, Raven Press, N. Y.

Valzelli, L. and Garattini, S., (1968) in "Advances in Pharmacology," vol. 6B, Garattini, S. and Shore, P. A., Eds., Academic Press, New York, p. 249.

Valzelli, L. and Garattini, S., (1972) Neuropharmacology 11, 17.

Vearn, J. T. and Sturgis, (1919) Arch. Int. Med. 24, 247.

Von Euler, J. S., (1964) Clin. Pharmacol. Ther. 5, 398.

Waalkes, T. P., (1959) J. Lab. Clin. Med. 53, 824.

Wadeson, R. W., Mason, J. W., Hamburg, D. A., and Handlon, J. H., (1963) Arch. Gen. Psychiat. 9, 146.

Weil-Malherbe, H., Axelrod, J., and Tomchick, R., (1959) Science 129, 1226.

Welch, A. S. and Welch, B. L., (1968) Proc. Nat. Acad. Sci. U.S.A. **60**, 478.
Welch, A. S. and Welch, B. L., (1969) Anal. Biochem. **30**, 161.
Wolff, C. T., Hofer, M. A., and Mason, J. W., (1964) Psychosom. Med. **26**, 592.
Woolley, D. W. and Shaw, E., (1954) Proc. Nat. Acad. Sci. U.S.A. **40**, 228.
Woolley, D. W. and Van der Hoeven, T., (1963) Science **139**, 610.
Woolley, D. W. and Van der Hoeven, T., (1965) Int. J. Neuropsychiat. **1**, 529.
Yuwiler, A., Geller, E., and Eiduson, S., (1959) Arch. Biochem. Biophys. **80**, 162.

Chapter VI

THE PSYCHOTROPIC DRUGS

The term psychotropic drug has been used to refer to that series of substances acting upon the higher functions of the central nervous system and inducing changes in either the behavioral and/or cognitive processes of the subject. A further aspect, important for the completion of this definition, is that such modifications should be transitory and reversible, although, current views of the uncontrolled abuse of some of these psychoactive substances indicate that they can provide for prolonged changes in cognition, perception, and personality—even among otherwise normal individuals.

Apart from the question of an "official" acceptance of the term psychopharmacology, which emerged about 1950 as an independent discipline, it should be observed that, the occasional and nonsystematic use of centrally active substances for the mediation of therapeutic effects dates back hundreds of years. From the beginning of this century the clinician has had the first pharmacologically active available therapeutically effective means of dealing with certain types of behavior pathology; this was made possible through the synthesis of barbiturates in 1903. It is also appropriate to indicate that for a span of several years psychiatric therapies utilized several rather unspecific, but sometimes effective, somatic techniques; these essentially consisted of prolonged narcosis, insulin coma, malaria therapy, electroconvulsive therapy, and psychosurgical procedures, such as prefrontal leucotomy and lobotomy. In the light of available chemotherapy for behavior disorders and appearing at a time when serious questions concerning the efficacy and practicality of somatic therapies in psychiatry were being raised, it is perhaps understandable that psychopharmacology gained rapid and wide acceptance, generating active interest and enthusiasm in the clinical environment.

With the wider use, increased frequency of new compounds, and greater public acceptance, the use of psychotropic drugs has created a series of other medical, medico-legal, sociological, and ethical problems, all of which focus around a triad of drug use, misuse, and abuse. This triad, of course, is a consideration of psychotropic drug applications that extends well beyond their clinical or therapeutic use. It certainly takes into account the phenomena of drug-dependence and drug habituation, concepts closely linked with the indicated triad, both in terms of possible cause and of potential effect; dependency usually refers to the need for continued, regular use of a given drug, which when withdrawn, leads to effects—either physiological and/or psychological—that increase the need to reuse this drug. It is, in a sense, similar to those conditions that characterize the physical dependence that develops for narcotic drugs which, when withdrawn, produce profound physical symptoms. A form of dependence of a more behaviorally reinforcing type is quite clearly indicated in the writing of HUXLEY (1960) wherein he has indicated that the pharmacologist can provide something that the majority of people have never had before: such drug-mediated states as happiness, peace, and love are held as drug-state-derived capacities. The world can be transformed by the drug state and doors can be opened to visions of unbelievable and vivid perceptions and insight. Human beings would be able, without any effort, to procure for themselves those things which could previously be obtained only with difficulty, through self-control and spiritual exercises.

At the cost of appearing completely unsympathetic to such hedonistic desires by which man can achieve perfect bliss in his detachment from reality, there is the obvious consideration that the aim of the pharmacologist and particularly the psychopharmacologist is that of providing therapeutic media and to elucidate, perhaps through the use of such media, the mechanisms that underlie and regulate tissue functions—or, more specifically, in the present case—brain functions.

Perhaps from the foregoing general framework within which one aspect of drug abuse was indicated, it may be possible to extract a second concept basic to the triad—drug habituation; by this we refer to the repeated use of a nonnarcotic psychoactive drug in much the same way as the use of a narcotic drug may be considered as addiction. Obviously, in the case of drug habituation there must be some aspect of the drug effect that generates central effects that are pleasant enough to lead thereby, to sustained reuse. Just as the limits of systemic toxicity are indicated for any drug, there are also limits to the behaviorally toxic effects of psychotropic drugs; exceeding such limits can precipitate serious hazards, involving not only the sensory and perceptual effects temporally linked to the drug effect, but the more important transient or longer-lasting cerebral circulatory and metabolic changes and alterations in personality (BURNER and CHISTONI, 1968) that have been connected to drug abuse.

A) CLASSIFICATION OF THE PSYCHOTROPIC DRUGS

A debatable issue in psychopharmacology is the classification of the psychotropic drugs into categories which permit a sufficiently precise characterization of their activities. The problem is further complicated by the consideration that the effects of currently available psychotropic drugs, although principally active upon behavioral components in man, also include a series of complex effects upon the peripheral nervous system as well as upon other organ systems. There are, in fact, a series of relationships among behavioral, neurological, and peripheral vegetative spheres that do not easily lend themselves to a sufficiently descriptive class fication scheme (LATTANZI, 1961). On the other hand, a subdivision of psychotropic agents based upon their chemical structure, although perhaps more scientifically exact, does not prove to be practically suitable. This is, in part, because the pharmacological activity and therapeutic efficacy can differ considerably between compounds of similar structure, and also because such structurally based classifications would involve as yet unexplored structure-activity relationships, thus imposing a difficult burden upon the clinician.

It would seem that for the present it is only possible to accept a classification scheme that can apply in a sufficiently immediate manner to conditions wherein its subdivisions became meaningful; it would require the use of terminology that has both meaning within, and significance for both the clinical situation and the therapeutic process.

Another approach to the classification of psychotropic agents that has proved useful and quite interesting is a consideration of quantitative changes in the electroencephalogram (EEG) of human subjects (FINK, 1961, 1963). EEG analyses by visual description, visual-hand measurement, or electronic frequency analysis were used to describe drug-related changes in frequency pattern, abundance, and the appearance of new waveforms and rhythms. Certain consistent features emerged for specific drugs or classes of compound, so that behavioral characteristics such as tranquilization or somnolence could be defined for some drugs and excitement, illusory sensations, and anxiety could be specified on the basis of EEG measures for others. The use of EEG analysis to evaluate the clinical efficacy of psychotropic drugs, in terms of their presumed category of activity has also been made (ITIL, 1961) and such analyses have been in good agreement with both drug classification and clinical indices of therapeutic gain (AKPINAR et al., 1972).

From a purely practical point of view, the classification scheme that will be used in this book, is that outlined in Figure 28; it must be emphasized that this system is not intended as a strictly definitive one and it certainly possesses both the defects and advantages inherent in any classification.

The most typical representatives of the *sedatives* category are the barbiturates, but certainly there are other substances, not included within this book, which, even with some question about pharmacological potency and clinical significance, are still includable because of their inheritance from classical pharmacology; this would include such substances as valerian, camomile, etc. (AIAZZI-MANCINI and DONATELLI, 1957).

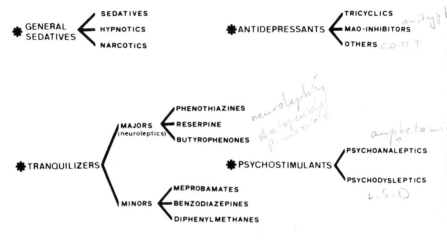

Fig. 28. Psychotropic drug classification.

The *tranquilizers* include those compounds that provided the ground-work for the concept of psychopharmacology, for the first substances introduced in drug therapy for behavior disorders were, as previously mentioned, chlorpromazine and reserpine.

Among the phenothiazine derivatives, of which chlorpromazine is probably the best representative, there are several derivations which has been effectively utilized as antiemetic agents, as media in the treatment of acute alcoholism, and also have been shown to potentiate the action of analgesics. These compounds have been most effectively utilized in the management of disturbed, hyperactive behavior in schizophrenia and in the control of manic excitement.

Reserpine, probably the best representative of the Rauwolfia alkaloids, is best categorized by its effect on the central nervous systems regulating hypertensive disorders, although hypotension produced by this drug can represent an undesirable side effect; sedation and Parkinsonian-like motor involvement also represent possible side effects. Reserpine has been primarily utilized to control hyperactive, disturbed psychotic states. The subdivision into *major* and *minor* tranquilizer is used because the former, within certain dose limits or at certain times within the therapeutic regimen, can produce an apparent, and sometimes intense neurological symptomatology, essentially of the extrapyramidal type; it is from such symptomatology that the term *neuroleptic drug* is derived. The administration of the latter compounds does not lead into such neurological symptoms. Among such agents in current use are the benzodiazepine derivations, which constitute an important group of psychotropic drugs, having potent and often selective axiolytic activity.

Among the *antidepressive agents*, which clearly indicate the intended therapeutic activity, the *monoamine oxidase inhibitors* represent the earliest potential therapeutic alternative, of the pharmacological type, to the use of electro-convulsive therapy for the treatment of depression; currently, these derivatives, because of several untoward side effects, are not frequently used in clinical practice, and have been largely replaced by the more recently developed and effective *tricyclic compounds,* of which one of the most important is imipramine.

Finally, the category of *psychostimulant drugs,* includes a series of compounds, of which the group of *psychoanaleptic drugs* is the oldest, having been described by ALLES in 1927 in a paper concerning the stimulant effects of amphetamine on the central nervous system. Subsequently, amphetamine and many of its derivatives were employed in the treatment of moderate depressive syndromes, with temporary and variable effectiveness.

Amphetamine generally produces an elevation of mood that has been linked with its stimulatory effect upon the sensory cerebral cortex. The administration of this drug and its analogs can produce a number of more specific and individually characteristic effects such as elation, euphoria, irritability, insomnia, etc. The sequelae to amphetamine use usually includes depression and fatigue. One area in which the amphetamines have found unique therapeutic applications is in the treatment of hyperactive disturbed children (GINN and HOHMAN, 1953), and related to this, in the treatment of learning disorders in hyperactive children (CONNERS, 1972).

The category of *psychodysleptic drugs* paradoxically is both the oldest and, at the same time, one of the most recent groups of psychotropic drugs. In fact, among this group there are currently synthesized compounds that have been identified as the active constituents of spices and potions used in some of the mystical and religious rituals in primitive worship. These substances are extremely potent and also quite dangerous; because of their uncontrolled diffusion and increasing abuse, the previously cited problem of drug-dependence again becomes an important aspect of psychopharmacology.

B) ACTIVITY SPECTRUM OF THE PSYCHOTROPIC DRUGS

By this term, the limits of activity for a centrally acting drug in mediating behavioral alterations or exerting a therapeutic effect are defined. In evaluating the specificity of action of a given psychotropic drug, it follows that, from the viewpoint of psychopharmacology, a psychoactive compound is as specific as the limitations and therapeutic selectivity of its activity spectrum. The activity spectrum of a psychotropic agent is, therefore, defined not only in terms of the range of specifiable symptomatology, but also in terms of the range of syndrome manageability.

For example, while the barbiturates possess a wide spectrum of activity, and could be employed to control psychomotor hyperexcitation in neurotic, depressive, and schizophrenic episodes as well as other disorders, imipraminic-like antidepressive agents have been shown to be therapeutically useful only in those patients in whom depressive syndromes represent a selectively characterized diagnostic feature of their symptomatology.

In Figure 29, the distribution of a series of psychotropic drugs as a function of their spectrum of activity is schematically represented.

One of the most important aspects of the psychiatric therapeutic applications, which characterizes the major tranquilizer agents or neuroleptics, is the *antipsychotic* properties through which such agents act upon schizophrenic symptoms such as hallucinations and disordered thought processes. Moreover these drugs, as a particular aspect of their profound and general sedative activity, posesses an obvious hypnogenic activity, by which normal sleep may be restored in the reactive neurotic or psychotic insomnias; the establishment of normal sleep, in the absence of true hypnotic effects as brought about by the barbiturates is a desirable effect in that there are no narcotic effects even at the highest dosages.

From a practical point of view, this suggests that increased frequency of sleep, especially at the beginning of therapy, permits the patient to be easily awakened without dramatic shifts in consciousness, as occurs with the use of barbiturates (DELAY and DENIKER, 1953). Another important aspect of the remarkable clinical value of tranquilizers is represented by the observation that a wide series of these drugs, provide an antipsychotic effect that is inversely proportional to its hypnogenic activity.

As shown in Figure 30, those neuroleptic drugs which induce an intensive

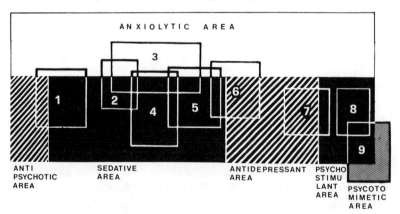

Fig. 29. Activity spectrum of different psychotropic drug categories.

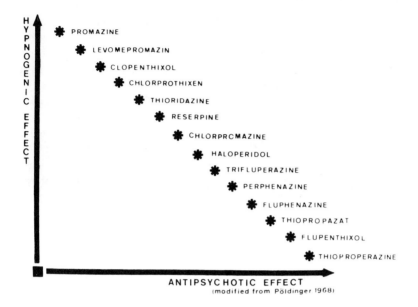

Fig. 30. Hypnogenic versus antipsychotic activity of different major tranquilizers.

initial hypnogenic action possess a relatively poor antipsychotic potency
and seem better suited for the therapy of acute excitatory states of varying
etiology. Those derivatives characterized by a slight hypnogenic effect
possess an intensive antipsychotic activity; these compounds are particularly
useful in maintenance therapy for chronic schizophrenia.

The minor tranquilizer agents can also exert a hypnogenic action that is
especially appropriate for the treatment of psychogenic insomnias. These
drugs often combine a sedative and muscle-relaxant effect, which, for
several members of this class of compounds provides a useful therapeutic
medium for many syndromes characterized by spasticity of the striated
muscles. The efficacy of this series of substances in the control of internal
tension and anxiety is particularly apparent and selective for chlordiazepoxide and its derivatives which constitute the *anxiolytic* drugs.

One classification of the antidepressive agents (PÖLDINGER, 1968) has
been to consider them as either *thymoleptic* drugs, which act mainly on
mood, or *thymeretic* drugs (of the monoamine oxidase inhibitor class),
which act as stimulants. The primary action of these substances is different
for what FREYHAN (1959-1960) has defined as the "guide symptoms" of
depression: depressive dysthymia, blockade of ideation, and psychomotor
inhibition, or anxious excitement. Consequently, the therapeutic success
obtainable with these drugs depends upon other important factors such as
the age of the patient, the duration of the previous illness, the dose of drugs

administered, and the duration of therapy; such success is also related to an exact nosographic characterization of the patient, since the endogenous depressions, manic-depressive states, and involutional conditions are positively influenced by thymoleptics, while the psychoreactive depressions and the depressive dysthymia of the schizophrenic state responds better to neuroleptic drugs or to those antidepressive derivatives that also possess neuroleptic activity.

From a general point of view, if symptomatology is dominated by pathological melancholia and by dulled affect, drugs of the imipramine type are indicated while desipramine appears to be useful when psychomotor inhibition predominates. If anxiety feelings or anxious excitement prevails, such an antidepressive agent as amitryptiline is indicated; this compound possesses a clear sedative component. An interesting observation is that many antidepressive agents have been shown to be useful in the treatment of bronchial asthmas and of vasomotor rhinitis.

The use of several of the psychotropic drugs mentioned in the clinical situation, specifically for therapeutic effects in either schizophrenia, depression, or anxiety neuroses, has been considered in some controlled double-blind studies. These have been reviewed (KLEIN and DAVIS, 1969) and several comparisons have emerged. For example, in Figure 31 the therapeutic efficacy of several psychotropic drugs, in studies in which the clinical improvement for a given behavioral category was indicated, has been expressed in terms of those studies in which the drug proved more effective than a placebo.

Finally, consideration may be given to the psychoanaleptic agents which are employed only sparingly for therapeutic purposes, because of their numerous undesirable side effects and their transitory action, which is merely symptomatic and never curative; the psychodysleptic agents are still the subject of considerable discussion with respect to their therapeutic utility. Currently, some of them, such as lysergic acid diethylamide (LSD) and psylocibine, have been employed under strictly controlled conditions for reducing the duration of psychoanalytic treatment or to induce therapeutically useful psychotic-like states; the advantages of this therapeutic approach according to LEUNER (1962), consists in the induction of states resembling those of spontaneous dreaming, with rapid flash-back to the experiences of an earlier infantile period that provide a rapid release of emotion and affective drives and the induction of "hyperlucidity states." However, the possibility of inducing serious and sometimes persistent psychotic states should provide a real caution in the employment of these substances, at least until certain aspects of their mode of action are studied further and more extensively clarified.

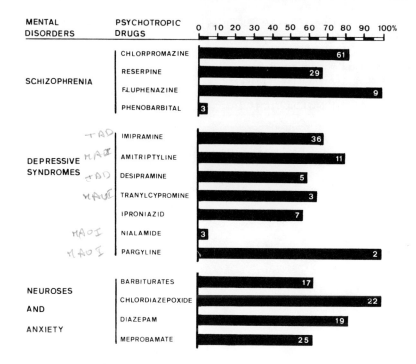

Fig. 31. Percentage of controlled double-blind studies in which psychotropic drug was shown to be more therapeutically effective than placebo. (White figures indicate the number of studies in which the therapeutic effect of the drug was evaluated.)

REFERENCES

Aiazzi-Mancini, M. and Donatelli, L., (1957) "Trattato di Farmacologia," F. Vallardi Publ., Milano.

Akpinar, S., Itil, T., Rudman, S., Hsu, W., and Sletten, I., (1972) Pharmakopsychiatrie, **5,** 25.

Alles, G. A., (1927) J. Pharmacol. Exper. Ther. **32,** 121.

Burner, M. and Chistoni, G. C., (1968) Médecine Hygiène **26,** 506.

Conners, C. K., (1972) in "Drugs, Development and Cerebral Function," Smith, W. L., Ed., Chas. C. Thomas, Springfield, Ill., p. 179.

Delay, J. and Deniker, P., (1953) Thérapie 8, 347.

Fink, M., (1961) Med. Exp. **5,** 364.

Fink, M., (1963) Electroenceph. Clin. Neurophysiol. **15,** 133.

Freyhan, F. A., (1959-60) Amer. J. Psychiat. **116,** 1057.

Ginn, S. A. and Hohman, L. B., (1953) South. Med. J. **46,** 1124.

Huxley, A. F., (1960) "The Doors of Perception," Chatto and Windus Publ., London.
Itil, T. M., (1961) Med. Exp. **5**, 367.
Klein, D. F. and Davis, J. M., (1969) "Diagnosis and Drug Treatment of Psychiatric Disorders," Williams and Wilkins, Baltimore.
Lattanzi, A., (1961) Clinica Ter. **20**, 345.
Leuner, H. C., (1962) "Die Experimentelle Psychose," Springer-Verlag, Berlin.
Pöldinger, W., (1968) Clin. Ter. **44**, 103.

Chapter VII

THE SEDATIVES

The term sedatives refers to a series of substances which induce a modest functional depression of central nervous system activity, resulting in quiescence; this effect is most evident as a function of the level of predrug excitation. One characteristic of sedatives is their ability to induce behavioral effects without bringing about any attenuation of consciousness; the latter event is typical of the action of hypnotics and narcotics, where such effects are dependent upon dose-related increments in pharmacological activity. This is a typical property of most barbiturates, which have dose-dependent sedative, hypnotic, or narcotic effects.

Among the sedatives, extensive consideration has been given to the barbiturates and their derivatives. The psychoactive properties of barbiturates represent a potential source of controversy, particularly since these agents possess a nonselective effect that involves major portions of the central nervous system.

Apart from any other specific consideration, these substances are discussed here only because of their continuing practical therapeutic employment; major details of the barbiturates has been deferred to the more traditional and classical textbooks of pharmacology (AIAZZI-MANCINI and DONATELLI, 1957; GOODMAN and GILMAN, 1970).

A) THE BARBITURATES

The barbiturate derivatives constitute an extensive series of compounds which were originally derived following the synthesis of veronal by CONRAD and GUTHZEID in 1882. Later, in 1903, FISCHER and VON MERING described the hypnotic effect of this compound in man, providing a basis for its introduction into therapeutic use.

1) General Aspects

All of the numerous barbiturate derivations are characterized by their rapid *absorption* by the organism when administered by oral, rectal, intramuscular, and intravenous routes. Based upon their preferential lipid solubility, these compounds show a specific affinity for the nervous system, related to the high lipid content of this structure. The issue of barbiturate *metabolism* presents a number of possible degradative pathways that may provide for the formation of alcohols, ketones, phenols, and carboxylic acids, all of which, unlike the original molecule, are easily eliminated by urinary excretion. The principal basis for metabolic degradation of these compounds lies in the liver, specifically in microsomal sites. It is important to emphasize that the barbiturates are inducers of enzyme activity, so that with repeated administration, they can augment the intensity and the frequency of their own metabolic inactivation by stimulating microsomal enzymes. In this regard, it has been experimentally shown that the repeated administration of phenobarbital, for four days, accelerates the activity of these enzymes by 20 to 50% (CONNEY et al., 1960). The renal *excretion* of barbiturates and the rate at which these substances clear the organism, depend upon their duration of action. The major portion of a single dose of barbiturate, having a brief or moderate duration of action, is eliminated between 36 to 48 hours; with a barbiturate having a long duration of action, the drug's presence in the urinary output of the subject may be observed even twenty days after a single administration. In particular, the half-life of phenobarbital, the time within the initial quantity of the drug measurable from body fluids decreases to half, is approximately three to four days. Other data concerning barbiturate plasma-levels have been reported by MARK (1963).

From the point of view of barbiturate *pharmacology,* these derivatives exert a general depression of all central nervous system activities. Their action is notoriously dose-dependent, so that, generally moderate doses initially affect the highly specialized cerebral cortical areas of the brain, particularly the neocortex, while higher doses lead to effects involving the lower regions of the central nervous system. (Fig. 32).

Electroencephalographically, barbiturates initially produce excitation through a release of cortical activity from the inhibition maintained by subcortical structures and the reticular formation (BRAZIER, 1963); following this, the typical sedation takes place. In other words, the barbiturates induce an imbalance in central inhibitory and activating mechanisms, influencing both the cerebral cortex (BRAZIER, 1954; HIMWICH, 1960) and reticular formation (KING et al., 1957; KING, 1956).

Another well known barbiturate effect is the anticonvulsant properties which some derivatives such as phenobarbital, methylphenobarbital and methylbarbital possess at nonanesthetic doses (MILLICHAP, 1965); this effect may be accounted for by suppression of the excitability of the cortical motor areas (KELLER and FULTON, 1931) as well as by a selective

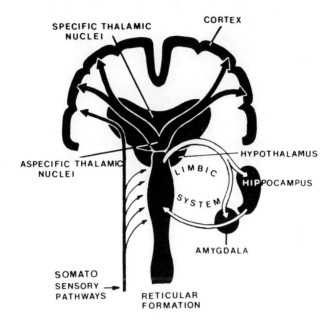

Fig. 32. Brain areas affected by barbiturate activity.

depression exerted upon interneuron activity (DOMINO, 1956). Phenobarbital is the most active barbiturate anticonvulsant, it suppresses convulsions induced by electric shock, pentylenetetrazol, and picrotoxin (SPINKS and WARING, 1963) in experimental animals.

Other aspects of barbiturate pharmacology are concerned with a series of peripheral effects on the cardiovascular, respiratory, and gastrointestinal systems which occur only as a consequence of prolonged treatment or following particularly high doses; such effects, however, are always dependent upon an activity decrement in those brain centers which regulate the activity of the various peripheral organs and systems.

The action of barbiturates upon *neurochemical mediators* still remains unclear since significant data have not been sufficiently available. It seems, however, that barbiturates induce a decreased excitability of both presynaptic and postsynaptic membranes, interfering, in this way, with the release of neurotransmitter molecules following the spread of the neural impulse (CURTIS, 1965). Increases in brain serotonin content following barbiturate administration have been described (BONNYCASTLE et al., 1957; BISIANI et al., 1958; ANDERSON and BONNYCASTLE, 1960; DUBNICK et al., 1962).

Other parameters of *brain biochemistry* affected by barbiturates include the selective depression of respiratory rate and blood flow of the somato-sensory areas (SOKOLOFF and KETY, 1960), inhibition of brain phos-phorylation processes (BAIN, 1957), and a decrease in brain adenosine triphosphate (ATP) level (LEONARD, 1966) after continuing administration.

2) Behavioral Effects

As a logical consequence of their general sedative activity, barbiturates produce a dose-dependent decrement or abolition of *motor activity,* both in animals and man. In mice, these derivations act nonspecifically upon *aggressiveness induced by isolation,* since the intensity of fighting is reduced, as a function of dosage, by the impairment of the animal's muscular tonus (VALZELLI et al., 1967). The *exploratory behavior* of mice is affected by hexobarbital which substantially decreases exploratory drive, both in normal and in aggressive animals (VALZELLI, 1969).

Barbiturates generally produce a detrimental effect upon maze *learning* or in conditioning situations, while they generate a somewhat positive effect in controlling the behavioral alterations produced by *experimental neurosis* (MASSERMAN, 1962).

Barbiturates also consistently impair performance in man in such a way that, as task complexity increases, positive action becomes disrupted by these derivations (MIRSKY et al., 1959); an oral dose of 100 mg of secobarbital can evidently impair the normal car-driving skill of a subject (LOOMIS and WEST, 1958). In general, small doses of barbiturates are reported to increase feelings of elation and activation which are followed, at successively greater doses, by distortions of judgment, clouding of perception, and drowsiness (SMITH and BEECHER, 1959; LEGGE and STEIN-BERG, 1962).

3) Clinical Effects

As previously indicated, barbiturates represented the first pharmacological medium in use for over 60 years, and have been traditionally employed by the psychiatrist for four main purposes; first as a hypnotic for the relief of sleep disorders common to several psychiatric syndromes; secondly, as general sedatives, thirdly, as anticonvulsant agents, and fourthly, as a means of controlling agitated and disturbed behavior in psychoses.

The wide use of barbiturates as hypnotics has the disadvantage of resulting in unpleasant residual effects, which are generally experienced by the patient the morning following use as drowsiness, sluggishness, and a feeling of general prostration. Moreover, several barbiturates consistently reduce REM sleep (OSWALD et al., 1963; BAEKELAND, 1967, HART-MANN, 1968) in such a way as to raise serious question as to their effective utility in the course of a prolonged hypnotic therapy. The effect on REM sleep may perhaps explain why some barbiturates, phenobarbital in particular, depress mood and, can moreover, induce anxious states. Conversely, amobarbital is widely used for its antianxious, sedative, and slightly euphoriant properties: however, the well documented antianxiety activity of this compound (WEATHERALL, 1962; RAYMOND et al., 1957) is only symptomatic and short-lasting.

Phenobarbital has been classically employed as an anticonvulsant (LENNOX et al., 1936; TOMAN and DAVIS, 1949; MILLICHAP, 1965), and this property of the drug is quite consistently utilized in the treatment of major and focal seizures, but less effective in the management of *petit mal* (HENSON, 1964). However, such treatment brings about varying degrees of general sedation and, sometimes, induces adverse or paradoxical behavioral effects, primarily in children and young adults; these include irritability, hostility and aggressive outbursts (SHEPHERD et al., 1968).

Intravenous barbiturate administration has also been used in catatonic schizophrenic patients (BLECKWENN, 1930) where the effect can be dramatic but extremely short-lasting; so that, the antipsychotic or antischizophrenic acitvity of barbiturates may be considered to be quite low.

Several barbiturates have been used therapeutically, or as therapeutic standards against which the efficacy of other psychotropic agents have been evaluated, particularly in studies constituted of patients with neurotic anxiety or anxiety disorders. In such investigations barbiturates have generally produced a greater therapeutic benefit than a placebo. For example, in eleven controlled double-blind studies in which phenobarbital was given, seven studies showed the drug to have a greater therapeutic effect than a placebo, the effect was equal to a placebo in three studies, and in one study the placebo effect exceeded that of the drug. With amobarbital, five controlled double-blind studies indicated that the barbiturate exceeded the therapeutic effect of a placebo.

4) Undesirable Effects

Barbiturates can bring about hypersensitivity reactions, mainly represented by cutaneous sensitization and rashes. Tolerance readily occurs in such a way that a continuous increase in the dosage is required to obtain the same effects: this factor suggests how the development of a drug-dependence situation may be facilitated, particularly in anxious subjects and when prolonged treatment is employed (FRASER et al., 1954). High doses, of from 600 to 800 mg daily, lead to a persistent impairment of mental functions, emotional lability, ataxia, dysarthria, and nystagmus; the withdrawal of barbiturates from addicted subjects can lead to extreme anxiety, tremor, nausea, vomiting, insomnia, weight loss, dizziness, and, sometimes, convulsions and delirium (WULFF, 1959).

Unfortunately, barbiturates are the most frequently employed substances utilized in suicide; in the treatment of barbiturate poisoning, stimulant drugs such as pentylenetetrazol, possessing analeptic properties specific to bulbar respiratory and cardiocirculatory centers, are generally used. Bemegride is also employed in these cases, but none of these stimulant drugs can be considered as a true barbiturate antidote (RICHARDS, 1959; MYSCHETZKY, 1961; GEALL, 1966).

B) NONBARBITURATE SEDATIVES

Among the drugs classically employed as sedatives in the years preceding modern psychopharmacology, the most important of these included the opium derivatives, particularly morphine, as well as other compounds such as paraldehyde, chloral hydrate, alcohol, and bromides. The use of these substances as sedatives is now extremely limited and, mainly found in physicians' prescriptions rather than being prescribed by the psychiatrist.

Among the more recently developed sedatives, there are several derivatives of *crotonylurea* and *isopropyl-crotonylurea,* which are extremely non-toxic and possess a slight sedative activity without any further relaxant or hypnotic effects (ASUNG et al., 1957; FERGUSON and LINN, 1956). Other compounds such as *glutetimide, methyprylon, methaqualone,* and *phenylglutarimide* are sedatives which may be employed, depending upon dosage, as hypnotics (GROSS et al., 1955). Many other hypnotic compounds are now available but they may all be considered as potentially capable of inducing tolerance, dependence, and addiction (ESSIG, 1966).

One of the most recently introduced hypnotic substances utilized in clinical practice is *nitrazepam,* a derivative of the benzodiazepine class. Nitrazepam possess good psychosedative activity which also brings about an anxiolytic effect; this compound has been defined as a "hypnoinducer", because its effect is interpreted as an induction or triggering effect upon the normal sleep process (SHALLEK and KUEHN, 1965; RANDALL et al., 1965).

From a general point of view, every nonspecific sedative effect may be considered as conferring limitations upon the behavioral abilities and activities of the subject; this varies as a function of the magnitude of the sedative effect. At the same time, it is important to emphasize that several psychotropic drugs can behave as selective sedatives as a result of a superimposed action upon different behavioral pathologies, which may be providing a baseline of hyperactive behavior as well as of sleep disturbances.

REFERENCES

Aiazzi-Mancini, M. and Donatelli, L., (1957) "Trattato di Farmacologia," F. Vallardi Publ., Milano.
Anderson, E. G. and Bonnycastle, D. D., (1960) J. Pharmacol. Exper. Ther. 130, 138.
Asung, C. L., Charchowa, A. I., and Villa, A. P., (1957) N. Y. State J. Med. 57, 1911.
Baekeland, F., (1967) Psychopharmacologia (Berl.) 11, 388.
Bain, J. A., (1957) in "Ultrastructure on Cellular Chemistry of Neural Tissue: Progress in Neurobiology," vol. 2, Cassell Publ., London.
Bisiani, M., Garattini, S., Kato, R., and Valzelli, L., (1958) Atti Soc. Lomb. Med. Biol. 13, 345.
Bleckwenn, W. J., (1930) Arch. Neurol. Psychiat., Chicago 24, 365.
Bonnycastle, D. D., Giarman, N. J., and Paasonen, M. K., (1957) Brit. J. Pharmacol. Chemother. 12, 228.
Brazier, M. A. B., (1954) in "Brain Mechanism and Consciousness," Adrian, Bremer, and Jasper, Eds., Blackwell Publ., Oxford, p. 163.
Brazier, M. A. B., (1963) in "Physiological Pharmacology," vol. 1, Root, W. S., and Hofmann, F. G., Eds., Academic Press, New York, p. 219.
Conney, A. H., Davidson, C., Gastel, R., and Burns, J.J., (1960) J. Pharmacol. Exper. Ther. 130, 1.
Curtis, D. R., (1965) Brit. Med. Bull. 21, 5.
Domino, E. F., (1956) Ann. N. Y. Acad. Sci. 64, 705.
Dubnick, B., Leeson, G. A., and Phillips, G. E., (1962) J. Neurochem. 9, 299.
Essig, C. F., (1966) J. Amer. Med. Assoc. 196, 714.
Ferguson, J. T. and Linn, F. V. Z., (1956) Antibiot. Med. Clin. Ther. 3, 329.
Fischer, E. and Von Mering J., (1903) Ther. Gegen. 44, 100.
Fraser, H. F., Isbell, H., Eidenman, A. J., Wilker, A., and Pescor, F. T., (1954) A. M. A. Arch. Internal. Med. 94, 34.
Geall, M., (1966) Hosp. Med. 1, 51.
Goodman, L. S. and Gilman, A., Eds., (1970) "The Pharmacological Basis of Therapeutics," 4th ed., MacMillan, New York.
Gross, F., Tripod, J., and Meier, R., (1955) Schweiz. Med. Wochensh. 85, 305.
Hartmann, E., (1968) Psychopharmacologia (Berl.) 12, 346.
Henson, R. A., (1964) Practitioner 192, 37.
Himwich, H. E., (1960) in "Drugs and Behavior," Uhr, L. and Miller, J. G., Eds., Wiley, New York.
Keller, A. D. and Fulton, J. F., (1931) Amer. J. Physiol. 97, 537.
King, E. E., (1956) J. Pharmacol. Exper. Ther. 116, 404.
King, E. E., Naquet, R., and Magoun, H. W., (1957) J. Pharmacol. Exper. Ther. 119, 48.
Legge, D. and Steinberg, H., (1962) Brit. J. Pharmacol. Chemother. 18, 490.

Lennox, W. G., Gibbs, F. A., and Gibbs, E. L., (1936) A. M. A. Arch. Neurol. Psychiat., Chicago 36, 1236.

Leonard, B. E., (1966) Biochem. Pharmacol. 15, 255.

Loomis, T. A. and West, T. C., (1958) J. Pharmacol. Exper. Ther. 122, 525.

Mark, L. C., (1963) Clin. Pharmacol. Ther. 4, 504.

Masserman, J. H., (1962) J. Neuropsychiat. (Suppl. 1), 3, 104.

Millichap, J. G., (1965) in "Physiological Pharmacology," vol. 2, Root, W. S., and Hofmann, F. G., Eds., Academic Press, New York, p. 97.

Mirsky, A. F., Primac, D. W., and Bates, R., (1959) J. Nerv. Ment. Dis. 128, 12.

Myschetzky, A., (1961) Dan. Med. Bull. 8, 33.

Oswald, I., Berger, R. J., Jaramillo, R. A., Keddie, K. M., Olley, P. C., and Plunkett, G. B., (1963) Brit. J. Psychiat. 109, 66.

Randall, L. O., Shallek, W., Scheckel, C., Bagdon, R. E., and Rieder, J., (1965) Schweiz. Med. Wochensh. 95, 334.

Raymond, M. J., Lucas, C. J., Beesley, M. L., O'Connel, B. A., and Fraser-Roberts, J. A., (1957) Brit. Med. J. 2, 63.

Richards, R. K., (1959) Neurology, Minneapolis 9, 228.

Shallek, W. and Kuehn, A., (1965) Med. Pharmacol. Exper. 12, 204.

Shepherd, M., Lader, M., and Rodnight, R., (1968) "Clinical Psychopharmacology," English Universities Press Ltd., London.

Smith, G. M. and Beecher, H. K., (1959) J. Amer. Med. Assoc. 170, 542.

Sokoloff, L. and Kety, S. S., (1960) Physiol. Rev. (Suppl. 4), 40, 38.

Spinks, A. and Waring, W. S., (1963) in "Progress in Medicinal Chemistry," vol. 3, Ellis, G. P. and West, G. B., Eds., Butterworths, London.

Toman, J. E. P. and Davis, J. P., (1949) Pharmacol. Rev. 1, 425.

Valzelli, L., (1969) Psychopharmacologia (Berl.) 15, 232.

Valzelli, L., Giacalone, E., and Garattini, S., (1967) Europ. J. Pharmacol. 2, 144.

Weatherall, M., (1962) Brit. Med. J. 1, 1219.

Wulff, M. H., (1959) Electroenceph. Clin. Neurophysiol. (Suppl.), 11, 1.

Chapter VIII

MAJOR TRANQUILIZERS OR NEUROLEPTIC DRUGS

The term "tranquilizer" officially initiated modern psychopharmacological therapy, providing a new conceptual dimension for the management of agitated psychiatric patients. Such a term has been widely criticized as being clinically meaningless and essentially irrelevant; however, it still remains as a widely accepted and frequently employed term because of several immediate and implicit differences from the term "sedative"

Tranquilizing activity is characterized by somnolence which, at a sufficient dosage, may eventuate in sleep, from which the patient may be easily aroused. Moreover, with the disappearance of somnolence, the patient appears normal and is quite capable of performing oriented and directed tasks, even if he does not take the initiative or express demands, concern, or preference.

The classical description of chlorpromazine activity in psychotic subjects was made by DELAY (WIKLER, 1957), in which he observed that external stimuli appeared to deflect from the patient, such that it became necessary to repeat questions; these were usually answered after a slight delay, in a neutral tone of voice with lowered eyes and without any active interest. The subject appeared as if plunged into a pleasant indifference that was separated from the environment by an invisible curtain.

From the pharmacological point of view, the major tranquilizers are represented chiefly by the phenothiazines, reserpine and some of its derivatives, and by the butyrophenones. The phenothiazines are basically derivatives of methylene-blue and from some related derivatives that were synthesized in the early years of this century; it was only later that the molecular structure of phenothiazines was evolved and then was employed initially as a veterinary anthelmintic (MASSIE, 1954). Among the phenothiazines, several derivatives, such as promethazine, show obvious antihistaminic and sedative effects, so that, in searching for other compounds that were more intensively endowed with sedative capability (WALKENSTEIN et al., 1958), CHARPENTIER and his co-workers (1951) were able to synthesize chlorpromazine which was initially employed in anesthesiology as an ingredient of the so-called lytique cocktail (LABORIT et al., 1952).

It was observed that under these circumstances chlorpromazine did not impair the patient's consciousness, but that it appeared capable of precipitating a form of pharmacologically induced functional lobotomy, whereby the patient became completely disinterested in his surroundings. These observations led DELAY (DELAY et al., 1952; DELAY and DENIKER, 1953) to utilize chlorpromazine alone in the treatment of psychiatric disorders.

Within the same period, reserpine, an alkaloid isolated by MÜLLER et al. (1952) from the roots of *Rauwolfia Serpentina,* was introduced into pharmacopsychiatric therapy. Preparations of the Rauwolfia Serpentina plant had been traditionally employed in India for many centuries as a means of managing several illnesses including mental disturbances (WOODSON, 1957); quite strangely, however, the clinical activity of Rauwolfia extracts on hypertension and insanity were first described by SEN and BOSE in 1931 in a medical journal, without any subsequent practical consequence of application.

Butyrophenones were more recently synthesized (JANSSEN and NIEMEGEERS, 1959; JANSSEN, 1961). With these compounds the series designated as the major tranquilizers and also defined as neuroleptics has been completed; this latter referent has also been used because these compounds affect the activity of the extrapyramidal system, providing a series of neurological symptoms which closely resemble those characterizing the Parkinsonian syndrome.

A) PHENOTHIAZINES

As a consequence of the therapeutic success of chlorpromazine, its derivatives soon became extremely numerous. These compounds provide for an extensive range of clinical applicability, both from the standpoint of their speed of action, as well as their dose specificity; these derivatives are not, however, essentially different from the general activity of the parent compound. It is not within the scope of this book to examine each of the phenothiazine derivatives, so that chlorpromazine may essentially be considered as a prototype of the entire series.

1) General Aspects

All the phenothiazine derivatives are characterized by their very rapid absorption so that, for example, when administered orally, the maximum serum concentration is reached in man 30 minutes after the drug has been administered (HUANG and RUSKIN, 1964). After oral administration, chlorpromazine (Fig. 33) is rapidly accumulated in the liver from which it is transported, via the bile, to the duodenum, from which reabsorption and re-circulation along the same route occur; in this way a classical enterohepatic circuit is provided. This does not occur after intravenous administration (FYDOROV, 1959).

The *tissue distribution* of chlorpromazine after treatment is characterized by an elevated concentration of the drug in the heart and lungs (GOTHELF and KARCZMAR, 1963); very high concentrations are rapidly obtained in the brain, primarily in the diencephalic structures such as hypothalamus, thalamus, hippocampus, as well as in the basal ganglia, pons, and medulla. Very small amounts are present in the cerebral cortex and in the cerebellum.

A similar tissue distribution is typically obtained after administration of other phenothiazine derivatives such as prochlorperazine and thiethylpera-zine; the latter is only a weak tranquilizer but a potent antiemetic and antivertigo drug and is maximally concentrated in the cerebellum after treatment (DE JARAMILLO and GUTH, 1963). Similar findings have also been reported by others (WASE et al., 1956; CASSANO et al., 1965; GUTH and SPIRTES, 1964).

Studies concerned with the *metabolism* and *excretion* of phenothiazines have been reported by DOMINO (1962), EMMERSON and MIYA (1963), WILLIAMS and PARKE (1964) and the results obtained have substantially indicated that 50 to 60% of a single dose of chlorpromazine is eliminated through urinary excretion, mainly as glycuronated derivatives and to a lesser extent in a hydroxylated form, while only 1% is excreted unchanged (HUANG et al., 1963; POSNER et al., 1963). Much of the remaining 40% is eliminated in the feces, mainly via the bile.

The general *pharmacology* of chlorpromazine is characterized by a wide spectrum of activity including antiadrenergic and anticholinergic effects (COURVOISIER et al., 1953, 1957; COURVOISIER and DUCROT, 1955; VIAUD, 1954). The antiadrenergic activity is such as to reverse the hyper-tensive response to epinephrine administration, while it is also capable of diminishing, but not reversing the hypertensive effect of norepinephrine

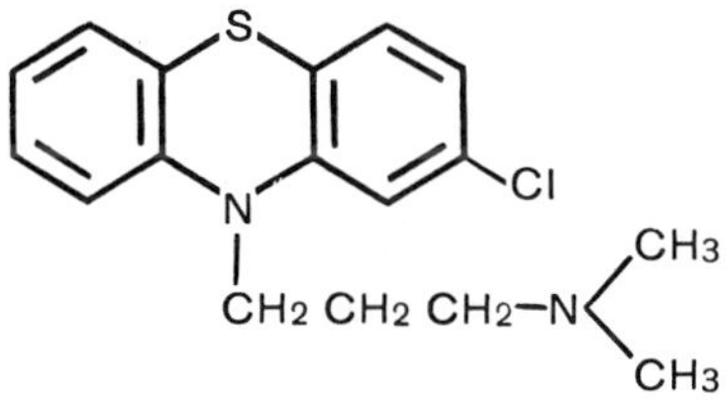

Fig. 33. Chlorpromazine.

administration (BRADLEY, 1963); moreover, chlorpromazine is twenty times more active than promethazine in antagonizing the toxicity caused by the administration of epinephrine or norepinephrine.

The major metabolic effects of epinephrine, such as hyperglycemia, are not altered by chlorpromazine which is a hyperglycemia-inducing agent per se (BONACCORSI et al., 1964). Both the anticholinergic and the antihistaminic properties of this compound are very slight; instead of sufficient intensity, at least on some isolated-tissue preparations such as rat colon, is the antiserotonin activity (GARATTINI and VALZELLI, 1955). Chlorpromazine induces hypotension, often accompanied by a compensatory tachycardia with an increased coronary blood flow (JOURDAN et al., 1958); as previously indicated, this compound exerts a weak spasmolytic effect as well as possessing some local anesthetic activity that is only slightly greater than that of promethazine. A potent antiemetic effect, dependent upon a selective depression of the chemoreceptor emetic trigger areas (BRAND et al., 1954), has been observed with this compound, and a hypothermic effect, the intensity and duration of which are dependent upon ambient temperature (LE BLANC and ROSENBERG, 1957), has been measured.

There have been many experimental observations concerned with the activity of phenothiazine derivatives on hormonal regulation, so that both in animals and man, these compounds can induce pseudopregnancy (BARRACLOUGH, 1957) as a consequence of a reduced availability of hypophyseal gonadotropins, produced by phenothiazine-induced hypothalamic depression (SULMAN and WINNIK, 1956). This observation has been supported by a decreased urinary excretion of estrogens (SCHLITTLER and PLUMMER, 1964) after phenothiazine treatment.

Chlorpromazine and many other phenothiazines possess mammotropic and lactogenic activity (WINNIK and TENNENBAUM, 1955; POLISHUK and KULCSAR, 1956; ROBISON, 1957) which do not correlate with the intensity of tranquilizing activity exerted by different derivatives; in fact, these effects are particularly evident for phenothiazine sulfoxide, which completely lacks any tranquilizing properties (KHAZEN et al., 1968). The antipsychotic activity of chlorpromazine and other phenothiazine derivatives appears to correspond closely with the intensity of the melanocyte-stimulant effect which these compounds show, as a consequence of their ability to release melanocyte-stimulating hormones from the hypophysis (SCOTT and NADING, 1961).

The *neuropharmacology* of phenothiazines is dominated by studies concerned with the activity of these substances on the reticular formation (KILLAM, 1962; BRADLEY, 1963). This structure is known to send projections to all the cortical areas, to the hippocampus, and to several other structures; it receives inputs from the major sensory pathways through collaterals in the mesencephalon and brain stem. The reticular formation maintains cortical arousal through a tonic facilitation exerted on the whole brain. As a consequence, sleep may be attributed to the reduction or a blockage of such a facilitating activity. Unlike barbiturates, chlorpromazine does not depress the reticular formation directly but, as illustrated in the schema shown in Figure 34, it selectively depresses the inputs directed to the reticular formation through collaterals coming from the sensory pathways (BRADLEY, 1963).

As far as the electrical activity of the brain is concerned, phenothiazines are ineffective in modifying the activity of isolated cortical preparations; this further supports the hypothesis that electrocorticographic synchronization induced in living animals by these drugs is essentially dependent upon their action in brain stem structures.

At the synaptic level, phenothiazines directly block the receptor membrane and induce changes in *neurochemical mediators* metabolism. In fact chlorpromazine increases the output of catecholamine basic-oxymethylated (CARLSSON and LINDQVIST, 1963) and of acidic metabolites (ANDÉN et al., 1964); chlorpromazine and other phenothiazines consistently increase the level of homovanillic acid, the major metabolite of dopamine, in the

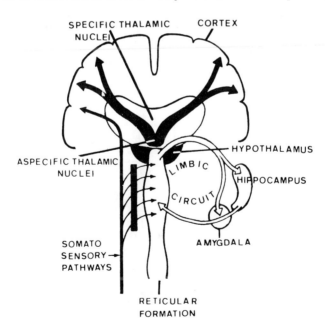

Fig. 34. Brain areas affected by chlorpromazine activity.

corpora striata of experimental animals (SHARMAN, 1963, 1966; JUORIO et al., 1966). These findings depend upon the blocking of the amine reuptake mechanism as well as of the receptor membrane (Fig. 35), leading to increased activity of catecholaminergic terminals (CARLSSON and LINDQVIST, 1963; ANDÉN et al., 1964; ROOS, 1965; CORRODI et al., 1967).

The functional blockage of catecholaminergic neurons results in an increased rate of synthesis of brain catecholamines; this is of minor importance for norepinephrine, but most significant for dopamine (NYBÄCK and SEDVALL, 1967, 1968; NYBÄCK et al., 1967), and not appreciably involved with serotonin metabolism. Such observations are of particular relevance for the neuroleptic activity of phenothiazines since changes in dopamine availability to the receptor occur almost exclusively on the nigro-striatal pathways as well as on the corpora striata (NYBÄCK and SEDVALL, 1969) or, in other words, on the core of the extrapyramidal system.

In *brain biochemistry* chlorpromazine in vitro reduces the rate of the oxidative metabolism (DAWKINS et al., 1959), mitochondrial oxidative phosphorylation (GUTH and SPIRTES, 1964), and glucose utilization (BACHELARD and LINDSAY, 1966), and it impairs aerobic glycolysis (BERNSOHN et al., 1956a; MASURAT et al., 1960) leading, in all likelihood, to the inhibition of cell membrane permeability (McILWAIN, 1962; McILWAIN and GREENGARD, 1957). Chlorpromazine also provides for a slight reduction of adenosine-triphosphate uptake by brain tissue (BERNSOHN et al., 1956b).

All of these phenothiazine effects, as well as several others exerted on

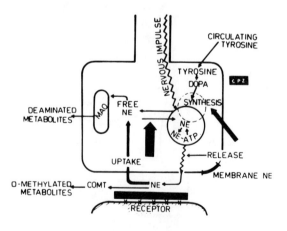

Fig. 35. Chlorpromazine activity upon synaptic mechanism.

neuroenzymatic activity, may be placed into the general framework of altered cell membrane permeability impairing interaction between enzymes and substrates.

2) Behavioral Effects

Chlorpromazine, as many other phenothiazine derivatives, induces a series of characteristic changes in animal behavior, which are essentially dose-dependent. In fact, low doses provide a typical taming effect consisting in an increased animal sociability, while median doses gradually impair *spontaneous motor activity*; high doses markedly reduce motor activity and muscle tonus to such an extent that the animal may fall into a cataleptic state so that it stands motionless and maintains unnatural positions into which it has been placed (BAN, 1969).

Chlorpromazine is very weakly active upon *aggressiveness induced,* in mice, *by isolation*; in fact, a reduction in fighting behavior is provided only at doses which impair peripheral muscle tonus (VALZELLI et al., 1967; VALZELLI, 1971). It seems interesting, however, to observe that aggressive animals are less sensitive to the traditional pharmacological effects of this drug than normal mice (CONSOLO et al., 1965). Chlorpromazine appears to be more effective in blocking the fighting behavior of spontaneously aggressive animals (BOISSIER et al., 1968); this is perhaps due to differences in the type of aggressive behavior characterized by different behavioral models; it has also been observed that chlorpromazine is less active in those animals which have been made hyperemotional by neurosurgical intervention (BAXTER, 1968; KUMADAKI et al., 1967).

Chlorpromazine, as other major tranquilizers, reduces *exploratory behavior* both in rats (MARRIOT and SPENCER, 1965; SHILLITO, 1967; ITOH and TAKAORI, 1968) and mice (BOISSIER et al., 1964; VALZELLI, 1969), and impairs conditioning and *learning* processes, mainly when avoidance techniques are employed (HERZ, 1960), even when the effect of this drug is modified as a function of strain differences (HUFF, 1962; ROYCE and COVINGTON, 1960; FULLER, 1966). However, the effects of chlorpromazine are greater on the acquisition of a conditioned response than upon the extinction of a previously learned task (ADER and CLINK, 1957). The effects upon conditioned response acquisition are probably dependent on a negative effect of chlorpromazine upon attention processes or vigilance (KORNETSKY and BAIN, 1965), which becomes particularly apparent when discriminative learning tests are employed, together with a decrease in reaction time (ITOH and TAKAORI, 1968).

The *interactions* of phenothiazines with other drugs have been observed, such as an intense potentiation of barbiturate activity by chlorpromazine and by many other phenothiazine derivatives; the anticonvulsant and anti-amphetamine activities of the phenothiazines have also been studied, and in this regard, chlorpromazine counteracts both the hyperthermic and activating effects of amphetamine in mice, as a function of its potent antiadrenergic properties. Chlorpromazine, however, also provides for increases in brain amphetamine level, since it impairs hepatic inactivation and degradation of this amine (VALZELLI et al., 1967). This situation may be related to the impairment of cell membrane permeability induced by chlorpromazine such that amphetamine is prevented from contact by liver microsomal metabolizing enzymes; thereby more amphetamine can be provided in the circulation and in the brain of chlorpromazine pretreated animals.

3) Clinical Effects

Chlorpromazine has certainly provided a new therapeutic medium for the clinical management of behavior disorders, mainly because of its pronounced effect upon even the most severe states of excitement and psychomotor syndromes of varied origin; in this way this compound has acquired a designation as a "chemical strait-jacket" (SHEPHERD et al., 1968). In this context, chlorpromazine efficacy is not only supported by an extensive body of experimental clinical results, but also by a series of statistical data based upon such diverse observations as the drastic reduction in the number of broken windows, hours of seclusion, use of restraint, and assault on personnel in psychiatric wards for agitated patients (ANGUS-BOWES, 1956; BRILL, 1959; LABHARDT, 1954).

According to FREYHAN (1959) the indications for the clinical use of phenothiazines pertain principally to the following five main nosographic divisions: (a) schizophrenia, with excitatory states, paranoid components, aggressive outbursts, stereotyped and bizarre activities, noisy and destructive behavior; (b) affective syndromes, manic and hypomanic states, agitated depression, paranoid components in involutional psychoses; (c) acute brain syndromes, delirium and hallucinatory states, intoxication by psychotomimetic drugs; (d) chronic brain syndromes, state of restlessness, confusional situations, violent outbursts, noisy and destructive behavior; and (e) psychoneurotic and personality disturbances, with tension states, tormenting feelings, aggressive tendencies, and poor control of impulsiveness. The efficacy of chlorpromazine is particularly notable in the management of *acute schizophrenic episodes* even though its action, in most cases, may be considered purely symptomatic (AYD, 1957; BRACELAND, 1963; HEILI-ZER, 1960) and only of secondary importance in depressive states (KIN-

ROSS-WRIGHT, 1955). This is also true for other phenothiazine derivatives; however, the piperazine derivatives, such as trifluoperazine, prochlorperazine, perphenazine, and fluphenazine, are more potent tranquilizers and, at the same time, are also more effective as psychomotor stimulants (DELAY and DENIKER, 1964), so that while they can be particularly effective in the management of hypoactive or apathetic psychotic patients, they often produce deleterious effects upon hyperactive states (BUENO and HIMWICH, 1967).

According to the results of a multiple collaborative research program carried out by several different psychiatric institutions (Psychopharmacology Service Center, 1964), phenothiazine derivatives, aside from their properties as tranquilizers, may be considered as true "antischizophrenic drugs" in that they act upon all symptoms and manifestations of schizophrenic psychoses.

The efficacy of chlorpromazine and other phenothiazines is also notable in the management of *chronic schizophrenia* (HEILIZER, 1960) even though, according to some authors (GOLDMAN, 1955; KINROSS-WRIGHT, 1959; LABHARDT, 1954), the clinical activity in such syndromes is less evident. As with other psychotropic drugs, there are a series of clearly observable interactions between phenothiazine therapy, psychosocial therapy, and environmental influences (HORDEN and HAMILTON, 1963; WING and FREUDENBERG, 1961; GRINSPOON and GREENBLATT, 1961). Moreover, many clinical reports deal with the efficacy of phenothiazines in "maintenance therapy" (KATZ and COLE, 1962; GITTELMAN et al., 1964) and as an alternative to restraint of chronic schizophrenic patients (ENGELHARDT et al., 1963, 1964).

Chlorpromazine can be of some help in controlling *hypomanic and manic syndromes* (AYD, 1957; HAMON et al., 1952; LEHMANN, 1954) even though more precise evaluation of the efficacy of this drug for treatment of such conditions remains difficult to achieve, mainly due to spontaneous remission of symptomatology; moreover, hypomanic patients treated with chlorpromazine can become depressed, while in *depressive syndromes* phenothiazine derivatives can aggravate the depression (AYD, 1957). An exception to this general effect is represented by perphenazine (HINTON, 1959, 1965).

Phenothiazines have been described as effective in the management of *epilepsy* with behavioral disturbances (BONAFEDE, 1955), in *posttraumatic psychoses* (BAN, 1969), in the control of *alcohol withdrawal syndrome* (CUMMINS and FRIEND, 1954; VAN GASSE 1958), and in the treatment of *toxic psychoses* produced by mescaline or lysergic acid diethylamide (LSD). These compounds are not indicated for the treatment of *psychoneuroses* which may, as a consequence, be further elaborated (RAYMOND et al.,

1957; PATRIDGE, 1965); the efficacy of phenothiazines in the amelioration of *personality disorders* is still under consideration (JENNER, 1965).

Chlorpromazine has proved useful in the treatment of some nonpsychia-
tric conditions, such as persistent vomiting (FRIEND and CUMMINS, 1953)
and tetanus (WILKINSON, 1961; FAIRLEY, 1963).

4) Undesirable Effects

As with many other drugs, chlorpromazine and other phenothiazines can
induce a series of side effects, which are temporally linked to an exasperation of the pharmacodynamic activity of the molecule or to a possible
hypersensitivity of the subject.

Among those effects in the former category, the most important is the
appearance of Parkinsonian-like *extrapyramidal syndromes* (BORDELEAU,
1961; FRIEDMAN and EVERETT, 1964) which induce akinesia, dyskinesia, slight tremors, festinant gait, mask-like facies, akathisia, dystonic states
with uncoordinated movements, torticollis, grimacing, dysarthria, oculogy-
ric crises, and opisthotonus. FAURBYE et al. (1964) have also described
another syndrome defined as *tardive dyskinesia* which is characterized by
repetitive uncoordinated movements. The occurrence of such disturbances is
dependent upon the dosage employed, the specific phenothiazine derivative
administered, and duration of treatment; some clinicians have suggested that
the induction of extrapyramidal effects represents a necessary condition for
attainment of therapeutic activity for the phenothiazine derivatives (DENI-
KER, 1960; FLÜGEL, 1960, HAASE, 1954; MATTKE, 1968), but the
clinical efficacy of some phenothiazines which possess very mild extrapyramidal activity, such as thioridazine and mesoridazine, does not support such
a theory (COLE and CLYDE, 1961; AST et al., 1967).

Due to an antiadrenergic effect of phenothiazines, *postural hypotension*
with compensatory tachycardia can occur, mainly after parenteral administration (KAPLAN, 1959), as may *nasal congestion* and *inhibition of ejaculation* (BLAIR and SIMPSON, 1966). The anticholinergic effect, particularly
produced by mepazine, can induce dryness of the mouth, urinary retention,
constipation, and paralysis of the ileus (LOMAS et al., 1955; MARGOLIS,
1957).

Among the hypersensitivity reactions resulting from chlorpromazine is
jaundice, which occurs in 0.5-1.5 percent of subjects (KLATSKIN et al.,
1961; BECKER and STAUFFER, 1962; AYD, 1963; SARGANT, 1964);
such jaundice is of the cholostatic type, with minimal cell involvement
(SHERLOCK, 1962). *Blood dyscrasias* have been reported (HIPPIUS and
KANIG, 1958), as well as skin complications, such as *urticaria* and *erythema
multiforme, phototoxic and photoallergic reactions* in which patients under

phenothiazine treatment are encouraged to avoid sunlight whenever possible; contact dermatitis is also a common manifestation (HARTMAN and DICKEY, 1964; KNOX, 1961; SAMS, 1960).

It is beyond the limits of this book to deal with the unique properties of all the numerous phenothiazine derivatives, as well as with their multiple effects and therapeutic indications; several useful sources on this subject may be found in an excellent review by GORDON (1967) and in a recent volume edited by CLARK and DEL GIUDICE (1970).

B) RESERPINE

Reserpine (Fig. 36) is another of those compounds with which the modern era of psychopharmacology was begun. Currently, reserpine is not as widely employed for clinical purposes as previously, but it still retains a degree of importance in experimental laboratory studies, primarily because of its biochemical effects. These extensively involve the central nervous system in such a way that the reserpinized animal has been routinely utilized as a standard test in the investigation of brain chemistry and as a baseline in the evaluation of the activity of psychoactive drugs.

1) General Aspects

Reserpine *absorption* by the animal is a very rapid process; its distribution to different tissues is also rapid, in that the brain takes up this alkaloid at the same rate as other body tissues (PLUMMER et al., 1957). The *metabolism* of reserpine provides for a series of derivatives, the major ones of which include trimethoxybenzoate, methylreserpate, reserpic acid, syryn-

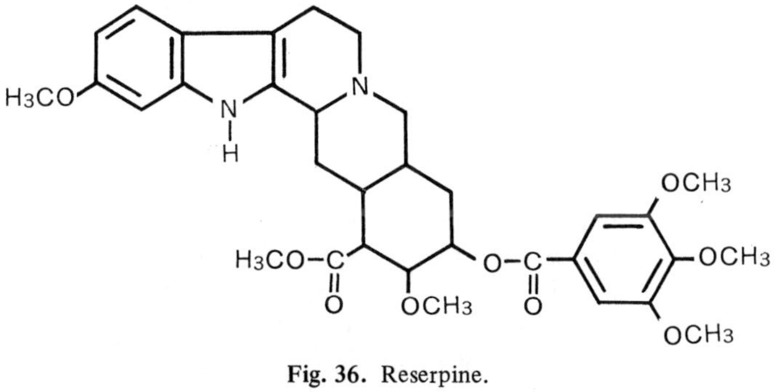

Fig. 36. Reserpine.

goilmethyl-reserpate, syryngic acid and carbonium dioxide; these are all void of any relevant central nervous system activity. Reserpine degradation to methylreserpate and trimethoxybenzoate is reported to be accomplished in the liver and, to a lesser extent, in the intestinal mucosa through an esterase that is mainly concentrated in the microsomal fraction (SHEPPARD and TSIEN, 1955).

The *excretion* of reserpine from the organism is principally accomplished through the intestine, while reserpine metabolites are maximally eliminated through the kidneys. However, several other eliminatory pathways, which are still unclear, seem to be present in man (MARONDE et al., 1963).

The *pharmacology* of reserpine, including its multiple and complex activities, depends upon the ability of this drug to deplete the monoamine stores of the central and peripheral nervous system. In fact, the theory that biochemical mediation of a nerve impulse depends upon specific neurotransmitter substances derives from the elaboration of early experimental data obtained after reserpine administration in animals.

Reserpine symptomatology is essentially represented by sedation, hypothermia, initial muscular hypertonus, and catalepsy; these effects are followed by muscle relaxation, blepharospasm, and diarrhea.

Animals treated with reserpine are initially hyperreactive to stimuli and subsequently become hyporeactive and show bradycardia, hypotension, and a marked reduction of spontaneous motor activity. BEIN (1953) has interpreted the main effects of this substance, such as hypotension, bradycardia, myosis, sedation, relaxation of nictitant membrane, as consequences of reduced activity in those brain structures which regulate sympathetic effects. This theoretical position was further confirmed by other investigators (PLUMMER et al., 1954; SCHNEIDER, 1955; RINALDI and HIMWICH, 1955) while, at the same time, BRODIE and his co-workers placed a primary emphasis upon the marked diminution of serotonin in different organs, the brain included, after reserpine administration, as responsible for the drug activity (SHORE et al., 1955a, b); other scientists have underlined the prominent significance of norepinephrine depletion (CARLSSON and HILLARP, 1956; BERTLER et al., 1956; HOLZBAUER and VOGT, 1956) by reserpine.

A very interesting finding is represented by the observation that, while reserpine seems to disappear in an extremely short time (about half an hour) from nervous tissue, even after the administration of large doses, the multiple pharmacological activities of this alkaloid last for more than 72 hours. Moreover, the pharmacological effects closely parallel the sharp initial decrease and subsequent depletion and gradual restoration of brain serotonin levels, in such a way as to reinforce the hypothesis that reserpine could act through the alterations induced on this putative neurochemical mediator (HESS et al., 1956).

Currently, however, with much more sensitive assay methods and detection techniques, it has been shown that reserpine does not really disappear so rapidly from nervous tissue but instead, after a very rapid initial decay, remains in the brain in very small amounts for a sufficient time to justify its prolonged length of action (MANARA and GARATTINI, 1967; ALPERS and SHORE, 1969). Moreover, the continuous presence of minute amounts of reserpine in some specific and specialized brain areas may serve to sustain both the depletion of brain monoamines as well as the typical drug symptomatology (SCHLITTLER and PLUMMER, 1964).

The mechanism by which reserpine induces the depletion of putative *neurochemical mediators* essentially consists in an impairment of the storage process by which these endogenous substances are sequestered within the synaptic vesicles (see Fig. 37) (PLETSCHER et al., 1955; BERTLER et al., 1956; SHORE, 1962); this effect is so intense that fluorescence microscopy has depicted the complete disappearance of the granular material from neuronal structures (HÖKFELT, 1966; VAN ORDEN et al., 1966).

Contrary to initial assertions, the sedative effects of reserpine are not clearly nor unequivocally related to a modification of the level of a single specific mediator in the brain (HÄGGENDAL and LINDQVIST, 1964), but rather appear to be inversely proportional to the ability of brain tissue to restore, in time, its capacity for again incorporating serotonin, norepinephrine, and other possible mediators into its intraneuronal storage sites (BRODIE et al., 1966; GLOWINSKI et al., 1966).

Some degree of controversy still remains concerning the putative transmitter primarily responsible for the maintenance of reserpine symptomatology; this argument assumes some practical importance in the BRODIE

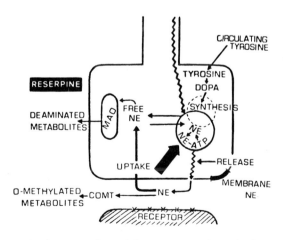

Fig. 37. Reserpine activity upon synaptic mechanism.

hypothesis (1965), wherein the reserpine syndrome has been considered as an analogue of depressive states in man.

As far as other aspects of *brain biochemistry* are concerned, reserpine, unlike other substances such as the phenothiazines or alcohol, does not inhibit glycolysis (McILWAIN and GREENGARD, 1957; WALLGREN, 1963), shows no significant effect on brain phosphatides, and does not modify phosphocreatine levels (KAUL and LEWIS, 1963; LEWIS and VAN PATTEN, 1963), even though it induces a small decrease of the adenosine-triphosphate-adenosinediphosphate ratio (KAUL and LEWIS, 1963).

2) Behavioral Effects

Reserpine, as other psychoactive drugs, has been described as a taming substance in animals (BEIN, 1956; SCHNEIDER and EARL, 1954), which sometimes induces a transitory phase of excitation. The decrease in *spontaneous motor activity* produced by reserpine can result in complete immobility and eventuate in total catalepsy; these effects are even more evident than those induced by phenothiazines.

In *aggressiveness induced by isolation* in mice, reserpine, administered in minimal amounts, apparently without effect upon brain biochemistry, was without behavioral effect; in higher doses, this drug blocked aggressive behavior in the same manner and extent as for other behavioral patterns. Moreover, this alkaloid clearly decreases *exploratory behavior* (BOISSIER et al., 1964), as well as *conditioned avoidance responses* and *learning* (BEIN, 1956; PFEIFFER and JENNEY, 1957; LEVISON and FREEDMAN, 1967). Reserpine acted in the same way in rats that were made hyperemotional by ablation of the olfactory bulbs (KUMADAKI et al., 1967), so that the time required by such animals to again show the presurgical behavior closely paralleled that time period necessary for restoration of brain neurochemical levels.

Generally speaking, the reserpine syndrome includes all of those individual behavioral patterns and biochemical changes which are altered by virtue of the drug effect upon the biochemical substances which pertain to the transmission of the nerve impulse in the brain.

Reserpine also exerts some *endocrine* effects; these essentially consist of a release of lactogenic hormone and ACTH, the inhibition of the menstrual cycle (GAUNT et al., 1954) and the induction of hypothermia (BEIN, 1956). Moreover, this drug acts as proconvulsant at low doses (CHEN and ENSOR, 1954; CHEN et al., 1954) and as an anticonvulsant at high doses (LEWIS, 1963). Clinical dosages of reserpine in man effect the electroencephalogram only minimally and nonspecifically (DENNISON, 1955); it is interesting that reserpine is able to increase the number of REM phases as well as their duration, both in man and in animals (KHAZAN and SAWYER, 1964; HARTMANN, 1966).

The possible *interactions* of reserpine with other drugs, especially those which exert potent effects upon neurotransmitter biochemistry are quite numerous; one example of such interactive molecules are the monoamine-oxidase inhibitors which are able to counteract reserpine activity. Such considerations, however, appear to be much more important in animal studies wherein they may be employed as a tool to offer alternatives to the study of brain functions; they appear to offer little value in the context of clinical use.

Of some clinical interest is the interaction between tricyclic antidepressants, such as imipramine or desipramine, with reserpine which may offer some clinical interest and value; when thus interacted, the hypothermic, sedative and blepharospastic activity of reserpine are temporarily counteracted (GARATTINI et al., 1962; BERNARDI et al., 1965). The potentiation of barbiturate induced sleeping time by reserpine is widely known (BEIN, 1956).

3) Clinical Effects

The therapeutic indications for reserpine resemble in general those of chlorpromazine, so that the clinical use of this alkaloid has been mainly directed toward the manifold aspects of *schizophrenia*. Observations concerned with the course of reserpine action in the clinical situation have indicated a triphasic pattern of activity (BARSA and KLINE, 1955); this course of action includes (a) initial sedation, (b) excitation, which has an onset after approximately one week of treatment, including hyperreactivity and cessation of prominent psychotic symptomatology; the duration of this phase is two to three weeks, (c) a final phase within which the patient demonstrates cooperative behavior and responds favorably to other therapeutic programs.

Reserpine was initially employed in the management of different behavioral and neurological disorders such as involutional psychoses (KLINE, 1954), epilepsy (ZIMMERMAN and BURGMEISTER, 1955), neuroses (LUTTRELL and MORRISON, 1955), depressive psychoses (FLACH, 1955; KINROSS-WRIGHT, 1955) and many others; but, soon after initially enthusiastic evaluations, the negative effects of reserpine upon different syndromes, especially depressive disorders, became evident.

In the management of schizophrenia, several clinical reports (ANGUS-BOWES, 1956; FELDMAN, 1957; KURLAND, 1956; SHEPHERD and WATT, 1956) demonstrated that reserpine was clearly less useful than chlorpromazine or other phenothiazines in general, so that this drug is currently not as widely employed as previously and its use is only limited to the treatment of such cases of *chronic schizophrenia* which have failed to show improvement after treatment with medication. In fact, reserpine is currently employed more frequently in the therapy of hypertension (MOYER, 1954; WILKENS and MALITZ, 1960) than for the management of behavioral disorders. There have been reports in which the therapeutic effects of reserpine, although less positive than those gains achieved with chlorpromazine, have been indicated (PEARL et al., 1956; ABSE et al., 1956; GOLLERO, 1960). There have been several indications from these and other studies that both acute and chronic schizophrenic patients, refractory to chlorpromazine, may show improvement with reserpine treatment. In fact, of those investigations in the literature wherein reserpine and chlorpromazine treatment in schizophrenic patients have been compared, the reduction of psychopathology by reserpine was equal to that of chlorpromazine in at least half of these studies. An evaluation of remission from schizophrenic symptomatology has been made for reserpine and chlorpromazine (BELLAK, 1958); a recovery of 38% was indicated for the former and 25% for the latter. In a comparison of reserpine with several phenothiazines for efficacy in reducing symptomatology in hospitalized schizophrenic patients, agitated depression, excitement, and withdrawal were more poorly managed with reserpine (LASKY et al., 1962).

4) Undesirable Effects

The major undesirable effect of reserpine is represented by a shift of mood to depressive states which can sometimes be quite intense (FREIS, 1954); this may occur in individuals who have previously shown an apparently normal affective state (HOLLISTER, 1961). A depressive state can also persist when drug administration has been terminated for a considerable time, such as to require the subsequent therapeutic use of electroconvulsive therapy (HOLLISTER, 1961). A previous history of depressive illness, even in a very mild form, constitutes a certain and potent contraindication to reserpine administration.

Reserpine can induce seizures in some patients and can aggravate the seizure-susceptible status of epileptic patients (BARSA and KLINE, 1955). Moreover, depending upon various effects exerted by reserpine on the autonomic nervous system, this drug can induce bradycardia, hypotension, salivation, and diarrhea (SCHLITTLER and PLUMMER, 1964) as well as activation and occasional perforation of peptic ulcers (HOLLISTER, 1957). Reserpine, like the phenothiazines, can induce an endocrine disequilibrium which, in man, can develop into feminization with gynecomastia, impotence, and impaired libido (WILKINS, 1954). The extrapyramidal effects of reserpine are also well known; these bring about the appearance of Parkinsonian-like signs which become particularly frequent when a daily dosage of more than 5 mg is employed.

C) BUTYROPHENONES

The butyrophenones constitute a class of tranquilizing and neuroleptic drugs developed more recently than chlorpromazine; they were initially synthesized in Belgium by JANSSEN and co-workers in 1956. These compounds were claimed to be more efficacious than chlorpromazine and other phenothiazines (JANSSEN, 1964); however, they have not been as widely utilized experimentally or clinically employed as the phenothiazines. However, interest in the butyrophenones continues to increase, even though their effects do not appear to differ markedly from the phenothiazines.

1) General Aspects

Haloperidol (Fig. 38) is the main representative of the butyrophenones and constitutes the parent compound of the entire class.

These drugs are readily absorbed and are then distributed uniformly through various organs and tissues. As far as their *pharmacology* is concerned, these derivatives appear similar to the phenothiazines, even though some butyrophenone derivatives, such as haloperidol and *triperidol* in particular, show less intense adrenolytic activity. Butyrophenones induce hypothermia and also exert a taming and sedative effect together with a cataleptic result that is more intense than that effected by phenothiazines.

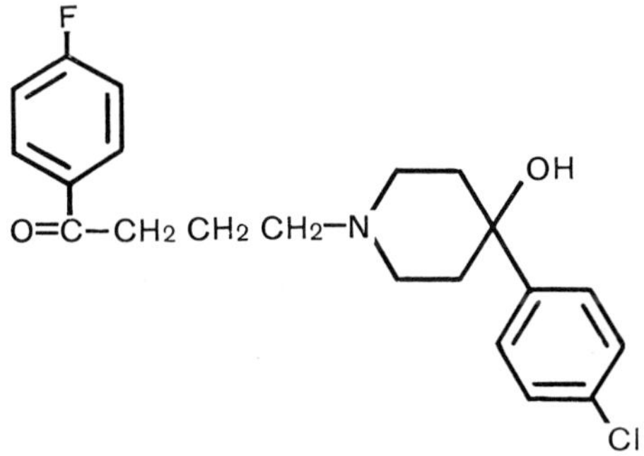

Fig. 38. Haloperidol.

A characteristic feature of butyrophenones given to laboratory animals is that, in small doses, these drugs induce psychomotor excitation that can develop into convulsive episodes; at high doses a true psychomotor inhibition, closely resembling that induced by chlorpromazine, takes place (BEAULNES, 1964).

The *neuropharmacology* of butyrophenones is again similar to the neuropharmacological properties of chlorpromazine. The electroencephalographic effects following active administration, initially consist of the reduction of the arousal reaction to environmental stimuli and in an increased activation after chronic administration (BUENO and HIMWICH, 1967). Triperidol, mainly because of its increased activity on arousal, appears much more similar to imipramine, the parent drug of the tricyclic antidepressant derivatives, than to chlorpromazine (JANSSEN, 1962).

Butyrophenones interfere with the metabolism of several putative *neurochemical mediators* (ROOS, 1964; CARLSSON and LINDQVIST, 1963); these drugs act upon several mechanisms operative at the synaptic level (Fig. 39), markedly affecting dopamine and, to a lesser extent, norepinephrine, while serotonin metabolism remains virtually unaltered.

Haloperidol exerts a potent inhibition on dopaminergic fibers of the corpora striata (VAN ROSSUM, 1966); this effect is quite specific and it is very minimally reflected in the reuptake of norepinephrine into the neuronal terminals (MALMFORS, 1965). This type of interaction between butyrophenones and dopaminergic receptors may account for the intense Parkinsonian-like effects of these compounds which, by means of selective biochemical impairment, abolish the inhibitory control exerted by dopaminergic neurons upon extrapyramidal activity (BUENO and HIMWICH,

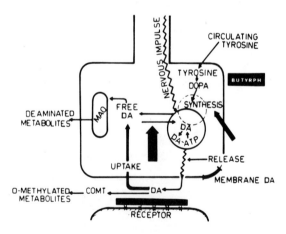

Fig. 39. Haloperidol activity upon synaptic mechanism.

1967). According to other investigators, however, the effect of butyro-phenones on norepinephrine metabolism and noradrenergic neurons may be considered similar to that exerted upon dopamine metabolism (CORRODI et al., 1967); this fact could perhaps account for the increased alerting and arousal effects which follow the chronic administration of butyrophenones.

2) Behavioral Effects

Butyrophenones produce a sharp decrease of *spontaneous motor activity* (CHRISTENSEN et al., 1965; KUMADAKI et al., 1967) and also impair muscular coordination.

These drugs probably act nonspecifically upon *aggressiveness induced by isolation* in both mice and rats (VALZELLI and GARATTINI, 1972; VALZELLI and BERNASCONI, 1971); haloperidol also shows some anti-aggressive activity in spontaneously aggressive mice (BOISSIER et al., 1968) at those doses which have been described as consistently providing for impaired motor activity (CHRISTENSEN et al., 1965; SOFIA, 1969). At the same time, haloperidol decreases the *exploratory behavior* of normal mice (BOISSIER et al., 1964).

This drug blocks a conditioned avoidance response to the same degree as chlorpromazine (CHRISTENSEN et al., 1965; OBERST and CROOK, 1967). As far as *pharmacological interactions* are concerned, haloperidol potentiates barbiturate induced sleeping time, antagonizes strychnine, pen-tamethylentetrazol, and electroshock-induced convulsions, and shows a strong antiamphetamine activity (CHRISTENSEN et al., 1965).

The formation of webs by three varieties of spiders were studied with regard to several parameters by which web production could be assessed. Haloperidol was compared with chlorprothixene and chlorpromazine for effect upon web formation (GROH and LEMIEUX, 1964). Both of the latter drugs inhibited web building activity, whereas haloperidol apparently served to reduce external sources of interference with web building, provid-ing for the construction of a more compact web.

3) Clinical Effects

Butyrophenones show a phenothiazine-like activity that more closely resembles that of the most typical antipsychotic agents rather than being characteristic of sedative compounds of this class. In fact, the clinical activity of butyrophenones, administered in average therapeutic dosages, develops without any gross impairment of consciousness or psychomotor activity in patients (BUENO and HIMWICH, 1967). Moreover, according to

DELAY et al. (1964), haloperidol successfully acts upon the severity of psychotic symptoms in schizophrenic patients; other data emphasize the specificity of action exerted by this drug in the management of psychomotor hyperexcitability and manic syndromes (HUMBEECK, 1960; REES and DAVIES, 1965). In some cases butyrophenones display a typical effect which may be considered as neurodysleptic, characterized by myoclonies, paraesthesia, and states of anxiety (DIVRY et al., 1959, 1960). This syndrome may be induced acutely by intravenous administration of butyrophenone derivatives and it has been proposed as therapeutic support for the treatment of anergic schizophrenic patients (BUENO and HIMWICH, 1967).

The major class of behavior disorders toward which the action of these drugs is directed are the various *schizophrenic syndromes,* but haloperidol and triperidol are also specifically indicated in the management of *hallucinatory* and *delusional syndromes* (DIVRY et al., 1959, 1960; DALAY et al., 1964; ROULEAU and BERNARD, 1964).

Triperidol has been shown to be particularly effective, both in paranoid or nonparanoid schizophrenia, wherein it acts more rapidly and effectively than phenothiazines (BISHOP and GALLANT, 1965); haloperidol, however, is more effective on perceptual, conceptual, and ideational content disorders (BAN and STONEHILL, 1964).

Due to their characteristics, butyrophenones are the most powerful antipsychotic drugs for the management of psychotic symptoms associated with drug abuse.

Another therapeutically useful effect brought about by butyrophenones when given in combination with analgesic drugs is *"neuroleptanalgesia",* this consists of a state in which the patient is sedated and fully anesthetized, although he is completely conscious. Such an effect may provide particular advantages for several neurosurgical procedures (SHEPHARD, 1965).

4) Undesirable Effects

The side effects of the butyrophenones are not very different from those of the phenothiazines. However, extrapyramidal symptoms are more frequently and intensely induced by the butyrophenones and, moreover, as previously indicated, these drugs can induce neurodysleptic syndromes; these can sometimes be caused by some piperazine derivatives of phenothiazines such as thioproperazine (DELAY et al., 1958).

Other side effects are represented by anxiety, akathisia, insomnia (BUENO and HIMWICH, 1967), depressive reactions, loss of appetite (GERLE, 1964), dehydration, increased sweating, and hyperthermia (DELAY et al., 1960).

D) OTHER MAJOR TRANQUILIZERS

It is easy to understand that many factors which include continuously increasing pharmacological research, demands of the clinical situation, and the consolidation of new pharmacotherapy, provide a potent stimulus to the development of new psychoactive drugs; these are not always more active or necessarily better than the older existing compounds. It is also obvious that it becomes impossible to consider all of those compounds released for use as a major tranquilizer since their introduction into current therapeutic use indicates that those surviving clinical trials and warranting continued use are few in number. Several of those clinically employed will be mentioned.

Within these limits, *chlorprothixene* (Fig. 40), which is a thioxanthene derivative similar to the phenothiazines, has been used; it is distributed and metabolized in essentially the same manner as the phenothiazines (MELLIN-GER et al., 1964; PETERSEN and NIELSEN, 1964).

Its pharmacological properties do not differ appreciably from chlorpromazine, except that in addition, there is adrenolytic activity, and a more obvious and powerful peripheral anticholinergic and antiserotonin effect (PELLMONT et al., 1960). Clinical reports have indicated a phenothiazine-like tranquilizing property of chlorprothixene (DENBER et al., 1960; GROSS and KALTENBAECK, 1961; REMVIG and SONNE, 1961); this compound also displays some antidepressant activity (PÖLDINGER, 1960) and minimal extrapyramidal side effects.

Clopentixol is another thioxanthene derivative with a piperazine component; because of its chemical structure it more frequently induces Parkinsonian-like symptoms (HEALEY et al., 1965). It has been compared with perphenazine in the treatment of chronic schizophrenia, wherein it has demonstrated equal efficacy (SUGERMAN et al., 1966; BARTOLUCCI et al., 1966; DEHNEL et al., 1968).

Another tranquilizing drug is *oxypertine* (SKARBEK and JACOBSEN, 1965) which appears to be particularly useful in the management of the acute schizophrenic syndromes (HOLLISTER et al., 1963), as well as for depressed subjects. The antipsychotic properties of this compound are

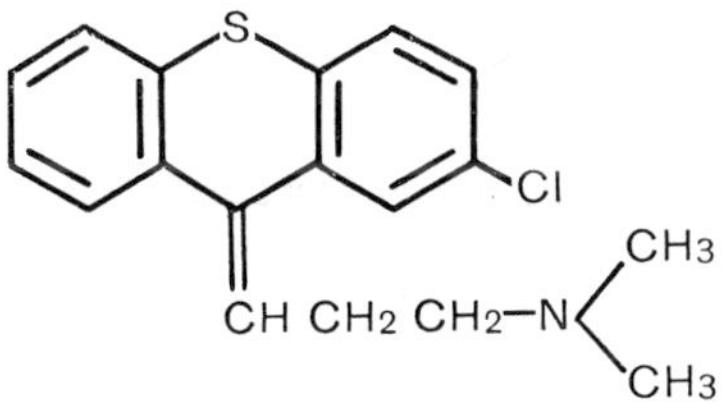

Fig. 40. Chlorprothixene.

similar to chlorpromazine (FLAMENT et al., 1963; FRIEDHOFF and HEKIMIAN, 1963; CALDWELL et al., 1964).

Benzoquinolizines are another chemical class of psychoactive agents showing reserpine-like activities. *Tetrabenazine* (Fig. 41) is the most typical and familiar derivative of this class; it shows all the pharmacological and biochemical characteristics of reserpine, but it is at least 15 times less potent and long-lasting (PLETSCHER et al., 1962).

Tetrabenazine releases biogenic amines from their storage sites, decreases motor activity, inhibits conditioned responses, and induces sedation, hypothermia, and hypotension; the entire symptomatological picture sequentially follows the changes induced in brain neurochemical transmitters. Moreover, it is of interest to note that tetrabenazine counteracts the amine depleting effect of reserpine, perhaps depending upon a competitive interaction between the two drugs for a common receptor site (QUINN et al., 1959).

Tetrabenazine does not pose any particular therapeutic advantage with respect to other tranquilizers, and especially when compared to phenothiazines; the latter have been demonstrated as being more clinically effective (WRIGHT and KYNE, 1960). In possible contrast to this finding, it has been observed that patients, for whom phenothiazines are ineffective, will show a favorable response to tetrabenazine (LINGJAERDE, 1963).

Benzquinamide is another benzoquinolizine derivative that causes release of neurochemical transmitters only when administered at extremely high dose levels (WEISSMAN and FINGER, 1962); its pharmacological activity has been limited to a deconditioning effect on conditioned avoidance responses. From the clinical point of view, benzquinamide does not show any typical tranquilizing effects, even at major doses, but brings about a barbiturate-like effect (SAINZ, 1963). This compound has probably found better therapeutic utility as a minor tranquilizer or sedative.

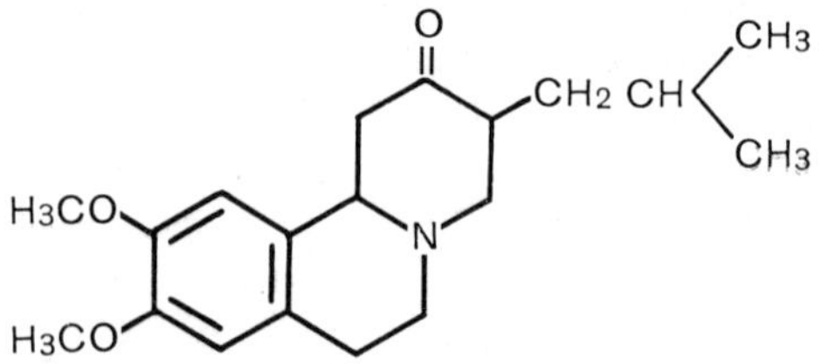

Fig. 41. Tetrabenazine.

REFERENCES

Abse, D. W., Curtis, T. E., Dahlström, W. G., Hawkins, D. R., and Toops, T. C., (1956) J. Nerv. Ment. Dis. 124, 239.

Ader, R. and Clink, D. W., (1957) J. Pharmacol. Exper. Ther. 121, 144.

Alpers, H. S. and Shore, P. A., (1969) Biochem. Pharmacol. 18, 1363.

Andén, N. E., Roos, B. E., and Werdinius, B., (1964) Life Sci. 3, 149.

Angus-Bowes, H., (1956) Amer. J. Psychiat. 113, 530.

Ast, H., Amin, M., Saxena, B. M., Lehmann, H. E., and Ban, T. A., (1967) Curr. Ther. Res. Clin. Exper. 9, 623.

Ayd, F. J., Jr., (1957) in "Psychotropic Drugs," Garattini, S. and Ghetti, V., Eds., Elsevier Publ. Co., Amsterdam, p. 548.

Ayd, F. J., Jr., (1963) J. Amer. Med. Assoc. 184, 51.

Bachelard, H. S. and Lindsay, J. R., (1966) Biochem. Pharmacol. 15, 1053.

Ban, T. A., (1969) "Psychopharmacology," Williams & Wilkins, Baltimore.

Ban, T. A., and Stonehill, E., (1964) in "The Butyrophenones in Psychiatry," Quebec Psychopharmacological Res. Assoc., Montreal, Quebec, p. 113.

Barraclough, C. A., (1957) Anat. Rec. 127, 262.

Barsa, J. A. and Kline, N. S., (1955) J. Amer. Med. Assoc. 158, 110.

Bartolucci, G., Lehmann, H. E., Ban, T. A., and Lee, H., (1966) Curr. Ther. Res. Clin. Exper. 8, 581.

Baxter, B. L., (1968) Int. J. Neuropharmacol. 7, 47.

Beaulnes, A., (1964) in "The Butyrophenones in Psychiatry," Quebec Psychopharmacological Res. Assoc., Montreal, Quebec, p. 1.

Becker, K. L. and Stauffer, M. H., (1962) Amer. J. Med. Sci. 243, 222.

Bein, H. J., (1953) Experientia 9, 107.

Bein, H. J., (1956) Pharmacol. Rev. 8, 435.

Bellak, L., Ed., (1958) "Schizophrenia: A Review of the Syndrome," Lagos Press, New York.

Bernardi, D., Jori, A., Morselli, P., Valzelli, L., and Garattini, S., (1965) J. Pharm. Pharmacol. 18, 278.

Bernsohn, J., Namajuska, I., and Cochrane, M. S. G., (1956a) Arch. Biochem. Biophys. 62, 274.

Bernsohn, J., Namajuska, I., and Boshes, B., (1956b) J. Neurochem. 1, 145.

Bertler, A., Carlsson, A., and Rosengren, E., (1956) Naturwissenschaften 43, 521.

Bishop, M. P. and Gallant, D. M., (1965) Curr. Ther. Res. Clin. Exper. 7, 96.

Blair, J. H. and Simpson, G. M., (1966) Dis. Nerv. Syst. 27, 645.

Boissier, J. R., Grasset, S., and Simon, P., (1968) J. Pharm. Pharmacol. 20, 972.

Boissier, J. R., Simon, P., and Lwoff, J. M., (1964) Thérapie 19, 571.

Bonaccorsi, A., Garattini, S., and Jori, A., (1964) Brit. J. Pharmacol. Chemother. 23, 93.

Bonafede, V. I., (1955) AMA Arch. Neurol. Psychiat. 74, 158.

Bordeleau, J. M., (1961) "Extrapiramidal System and Neuroleptics," Edition Psychiatriques, Montreal.

Braceland, F. J., (1963) Bull. N.Y. Acad. Med. 39, 649.

Bradley, P. B., (1963) in "Physiological Pharmacology," vol. 1, Root, W. S. and Hofmann, F. G., Eds., Academic Press, New York, p. 417.

Brand, E. D., Harris, T. D., Borison, H. L., and Goodman, L. S., (1954) J. Pharmacol. Exper. Ther. 110, 86,

Brill, H., (1959) in "Neuropsychopharmacology" (Proc. 1st CINP Congress, Roma,

1958), vol. 1, Bradley, P. B., Deniker, P., and Radouco-Thomas, C., Eds., Elsevier Publ. Co., Amsterdam, p. 189.

Brodie, B. B., (1965) in "The Scientific Basis of Drug Therapy in Psychiatry," Marks, J. and Pare, C. M. B., Eds., Pergamon Press, Oxford, p. 127.

Brodie, B. B., Comer, M. S., Costa, E., and Dlabac, A., (1966) J. Pharmacol. Exper. Ther. 152, 340.

Bueno, J. R. and Himwich, H. E., (1967) Int. J. Neurol. 6, 77.

Caldwell, W. P. K., Jacobsen, M., and Skabbek, A., (1964) Brit. J. Psychiat. 110, 520.

Carlsson, A. and Hillarp, Å. N., (1956) Kgl. Fysiogr. Saelsk. Lund Foerh. 26, 8.

Carlsson, A. and Lindqvist, M., (1963) Acta Pharmacol. Toxicol. 20, 140.

Cassano, G. B., Sjöstrand, S. E., and Hansson, E., (1965) Arch. Int. Pharmacodyn. Thér. 156, 48.

Charpentier, P., Gaillot, P., and Gaudechon, J., (1951) C. R. Séances Acad. Sci. 232, 2232.

Chen, G. and Ensor, C. R., (1954) Proc. Soc. Exper. Biol. Med. 87, 602.

Chen, G., Ensor, C. R., and Bohner, B., (1954) Proc. Soc. Exper. Biol. Med. 86, 507.

Christensen, J. A., Hernestam, S., Lassen, J. B., and Sterner, N., (1965) Acta Pharmacol. Toxicol. 23, 109.

Clark, W. G. and Del Giudice, J., Eds., (1970) "Principles of Psychopharmacology. A Textbook for Physicians, Medical Students and Behavioral Scientists," Academic Press, New York.

Cole, J. O. and Clyde, D. J., (1961) Rev. Can. Biol. 20, 565.

Consolo, S., Garattini, S., and Valzelli, L., (1965) J. Pharm. Pharmacol. 17, 594.

Corrodi, H., Fuxe, K., and Hökfelt, T., (1967) Life Sci. 6, 767.

Courvoisier, S. and Ducrot, R., (1955) Arch. Int. Pharmacodyn. Thér. 102, 33.

Courvoisier, S., Ducrot, R., and Julou, L., (1957) in "Psychotropic Drugs," Garratini, S. and Ghetti, V., Eds., Elsevier Publ. Co., Amsterdam, p. 373.

Courvoisier, S., Fournel, J., Ducrot, R., Kolsky, M., and Koetschet, P., (1953) Arch. Int. Pharmacodyn. Thér. 92, 305.

Cummins, J. F. and Friend, D. G., (1954) Amer. J. Med. Sci. 227, 561.

Dawkins, M. J. R., Judah, J. D., and Rees, K. R., (1959) Biochem. J. 72, 204.

Dehnel, L. L., Vestre, N. D., and Sehiele, B. C., (1968) Curr. Ther. Res. Clin. Exper. 10, 169.

De Jaramillo, G. A. V. and Guth, P. S., (1963) Biochem. Pharmacol. 12, 525.

Delay, J. and Deniker, P., (1953) Thérapie 8, 347.

Delay, J. and Deniker, P., (1964) in "Neuropsychopharmacology" (Proc. 3rd. CINP Congress, Munich 1962), vol. 3, Bradley, P. B., Flügel, F., and Hoch, P. H., Eds., Elsevier Publ. Co., Amsterdam, p. 529.

Delay, J., Deniker, P., and Harl, J. M., (1952) Ann. Med.-Psychol. 110, 267.

Delay, J., Deniker, P., Ropert, R., Barande, R., and Eurieult, M., (1958) "Comptes Rendus 60th Congress Psychiatry Neurology" (Stransbourg 21-26 juin), Masson Editeur, Paris, p. 675.

Delay, J., Pichot, P., Lempérière, T., Elissalbe, B., and Peigne, F., (1960) Ann. Med.-Psychol. 118, 145.

Delay, J., Pichot, P., Lempérière, T., and Piret, J., (1964) in "Neuropsychopharmacology" (Proc. 3rd CINP Congress, Munich 1962), vol. 3, Bradley, P. B., Flügel, F., and Hoch, P. H., Eds., Elsevier Publ. Co., Amsterdam, p. 89.

Denber, H. C., Rajotte, P., and Roos, E., (1960) Comp. Psychiat. 1, 308.

Deniker, P., (1960) Comp. Psychiat. 1, 92.

Dennison, A. D., (1955) Neurology 5, 56.

Divry, P., Bobon, J., Collard, J., and Demaret, A., (1960) Acta Neurol. Psychiat. Belg. 60, 465.

Divry, P., Bobon, J., Collard, J., Pinchard, A., and Nols, E., (1959) Acta Neurol. Psychiat. Belg. 59, 337.

Domino, E. F., (1962) Clin. Pharmacol. Ther. 3, 599.

Emmerson, J. L. and Miya, T. S., (1963) J. Pharmacol. Sci. 52, 411.

Engelhardt, D. M., Freedman, N., and Mann, D., (1963) Compr. Psychiat. 4, 337.

Engelhardt, D. M., Freedman, N., Rosen, B., Mann, D., and Margolis, R., (1964) Arch. Gen. Psychiat. 11, 162.

Fairley, H. B., (1963) Appl. Ther. 5, 322.

Faurbye, A., Rasch, P. J., Petersen, P. B., Brandborg, G., and Pakkenberg, H., (1964) Acta Psychiat. Scand. 40, 10.

Feldman, P. E., (1957) Amer. J. Psychiat. 113, 589.

Flament, J., Lofft, J. G., and von Mendelssohn, F., (1963) Neuropsychopharmacol. 3, 275.

Flach, F. F., (1955) Ann. N.Y. Acad. Sci. 61, 161.

Flügel, F., (1960) in "Drugs, and Behavior," Uhr, L. and Miller, S. G., Eds., Wiley, New York.

Freis, E. D., (1954) New England J. Med. 251, 1006.

Freyhan, F. A., (1959) Amer. J. Psychiat. 115, 577.

Friedhoff, A. J. and Hekimian, L., (1963) Dis. Nerv. Syst. 24, 241.

Friedman, A. H. and Everett, G. M., (1964) in "Advances in Pharmacology," vol. 3, Garattini, S. and Shore, P. A., Eds., Academic Press, New York, p. 83.

Friend, D. G. and Cummins, J. F., (1953) J. Amer. Med. Assoc. 153, 480.

Fuller, J. L., (1966) Psychopharmacologia (Berlin) 8, 408.

Fydorov, N. A., (1959) in "Proceeding 2nd International Conference Peaceful Uses of Atomic Energy," vol. 24, p. 205.

Garattini, S., Giachetti, A., Jori, A., Pieri, L., and Valzelli, L., (1962) J. Pharm. Pharmacol. 14, 509.

Garattini, S. and Valzelli, L., (1955) Boll. Soc. Ital. Biol. Sper. 31, 1648.

Gaunt, R., Renzi, A. A., Antonchav, N., Miller, G. J., and Gilman, N., (1954) Ann. N.Y. Acad. Sci. 59, 22.

Gerle, B., (1964) Acta Psychiat. Scand. 40, 65.

Gittelman, R. K., Klein, D. F., and Pollack, M., (1964) Psychopharmacologia (Berlin) 5, 317.

Glowinski, J., Iversen, L. L., and Axelrod, J., (1966) J. Pharmacol. Exper. Ther. 151, 385.

Goldman, D., (1955) J. Amer. Med. Assoc. 157, 1274.

Gollero, E. S., (1960) J. Ment. Sci. 106, 1408.

Gordon, M., (1967) in "Psychopharmacological Agents," vol. 2, Gordon, M., Ed., Academic Press, New York, p. 1.

Gothelf, B. and Karczmar, A. G., (1963) Int. J. Neuropharmacol. 2, 39.

Grinspoon, L. and Greenblatt, M., (1961) Proc. 3rd. World Congr. Psychiat. 3, 453.

Groh, G. and Lemieux, M., (1964) in "The Butyrophenones in Psychiatry," Quebec Psychopharmacological Res. Assoc., Montreal, Quebec, p. 53.

Gross, H. and Kaltenbaeck, E., (1961) Wien Klin. Wochenschr. 73, 64.

Guth, P. S. and Spirtes, M. A., (1964) Int. Rev. Neurobiol. 7, 231.

Haase, H. J., (1954) Nervenarzt 25, 486.

Häggendal, J. and Lindqvist, M., (1964) Acta Physiol. Scand. 60, 351.

Hamon, Y., Paraire, R., and Velluz, V., (1952) Annl. Méd.-Psychol. 110, 331.

Hartman, D. L. and Dickey, R. F., (1964) Skin 3, 198.

Hartmann, E., (1966) Psychopharmacologia (Berlin) 9, 242.

Healey, L. A., Harrison, M., and Decker, J. L., (1965) New England J. Med. 272, 526.

Heilizer, F., (1960) J. Chron. Dis. 11, 102.

Herz, A., (1960) Int. Rev. Neurobiol. 2, 229.

Hess, S. M., Shore, P. A., and Brodie, B. B., (1956) J. Pharmacol. Exper. Ther. 118, 84.

Hinton, J. M., (1959) J. Ment. Sci. 105, 872.

Hinton, J. M., (1965) in "Scientific Basis of Drug Therapy in Psychiatry," Marks, J. and Pare, C. M. B., Eds., Pergamon Press, Oxford.

Hippius, H. and Kanig, K., (1958) Arztl. Wochenschr. 13, 501.

Hökfelt, T., (1966) Experientia 22, 56.

Hollister, L. E., (1957) Arch. Intern. Med. 99, 218.

Hollister, L. E., (1961) New England J. Med. 264, 345.

Hollister L. E., Overall, J. E., Kimbell, I. J., Bennett, J. L., Meyer, F., and Caffey, E., Jr., (1963) J. New Drugs 3, 26.

Holzbauer, M. and Vogt, M., (1956) J. Neurochem. 1, 8.

Horden, A. and Hamilton, M., (1963) Brit. J. Psychiat. 109, 500.

Huang, C. L. and Ruskin, B. H., (1964) J. Nerv. Ment. Dis. 139, 381.

Huang, C. L., Sands, F. L., and Kurland, A. A., (1963) Arch. Gen. Psychiat. 8, 301.

Huff, S. D., (1962) Genetics 47, 962.

Humbeeck, L., (1960) Acta Neurol. Psychiat. Belg. 60, 75.

Itoh, H. and Takaori, S., (1968) Jap. J. Pharmacol. 18, 344.

Janssen, P. A. J., (1961) Arzneim.-Forsch. 11, 932.

Janssen, P. A. J., (1962) in "Simposio Internazionale sull'Alloperidol e triperidol," Istituto Luso Farmaco, Milano, p. 9.

Janssen, P. A. J., (1964) in "Neuropsychopharmacology" (Proc. 3rd CINP Congress, Munich 1962), vol. 3, Bradley, P. B., Flügel, F., and Hoch, P. H., Eds., Elsevier Publ. Co., Amsterdam, p. 331.

Janssen, P. A. J. and Niemegeers, C. J. E., (1959) Arzneim.-Forsch. 9, 765.

Jenner, F. A., (1965) "Proceedings of the Leeds Symposium on Behavioral Disorders," May and Baker Publ., Dagenham.

Jourdan, F., Duchène-Marullaz, P., Faucon, G., and Bouverot, P., (1958) Arch. Int. Pharmacodyn. Thér. 117, 341.

Juorio, A. V., Sharman, D. F., and Trajkov, T., (1966) Brit. J. Pharmacol. Chemother. 26, 385.

Kaplan, N. M., (1959) Arch. Intern. Med. 103, 219.

Katz, M. and Cole, J. O., (1962) Arch. Gen. Psychiat. 7, 345.

Kaul, C. L. and Lewis, J. J., (1963) J. Pharmacol. Exp. Ther. 140, 111.

Khazan, N. and Sawyer, C. H., (1964) Psychopharmacologia (Berlin) 5, 457.

Khazen, K., Mishkinsky, J., Ben-David, M., and Sulman, F. G., (1968) Arch. Int. Pharmacodyn. Thér. 171, 251.

Killman, E. K., (1962) Pharmacol. Rev. 14, 175.

Kinross-Wright, V., (1955) Ann. N.Y. Acad. Sci. 61, 174.

Kinross-Wright, V., (1959) in "Psychopharmacology Frontieres," Little, Brown and Co. Publ., Boston.

Klatskin, G., Havems, W. P., Schaffner, H. P. S., and Shay, H., (1961) Bull. N.Y. Acad. Med. 37, 767.

Kline, N. S., (1954) Ann. N.Y. Acad. Sci. 59, 107.

Knox, J. M., (1961) Ann. Allergy 19, 749.

Kornetsky, C. and Bain, G., (1965) Psychopharmacologia (Berlin) 8, 277.

Kumadaki, N., Hitomi, M., and Kumada, S., (1967) Jap. J. Pharmacol. **17**, 659.

Kurland, A. A., (1956) AMA Arch. Neurol. Psychiat. **75**, 510.

Labhardt, F., (1954) Schweiz. Arch. Neurol. Psychiat. **73**, 309.

Laborit, H., Hugenard, P., and Alluaume, R., (1952) Presse Méd. **60**, 206.

Lasky, J. J., Klett, C. J., Caffey, E. M., Bennett, J. L., Rosenblum, M. D., and Hollister, L. E., (1962) Dis. Nerv. Syst. **23**, 698.

Le Blanc, J. and Rosenberg, F., (1957) Proc. Soc. Exper. Biol. Med. **96**, 482.

Lehmann, H. E., (1954) Amer. J. Psychiat. **110**, 856.

Levison, P. K. and Freedman, D. X., (1967) Arch. Int. Pharmacodyn. Thér. **170**, 31.

Lewis, J. J., (1963) in "Physiological Pharmacology," vol. 1, Root, W. S. and Hofmann, F. G., Eds., Academic Press, New York, p. 479.

Lewis, J. J. and Van Patten, G. R., (1963) Brit. J. Pharmacol. Chemother. **20**, 462.

Lingjaerde, O., (1963) Acta Psychiat. Scand. (suppl. 170) **39**, 1.

Lomas, J., Boardman, R. H., and Markowe, M., (1955) Lancet **1**, 1144.

Luttrell, R. R. and Morrison, A. V., (1955) Ann. N.Y. Acad. Sci. **61**, 183.

Malmfors, T., (1965) in "Studies on Adrenergic Nerves," Almqvist and Wiksells, Uppsala, p. 62.

Manara, L. and Garattini, S., (1967) Europ. J. Pharmacol. **2**, 139.

Margolis, L. H., (1957) Ann. N.Y. Acad. Sci. **66**, 698.

Maronde, R. F., Haywood, L. J., Feinstein, D., and Sobel, C., (1963) J. Amer. Med. Assoc. **184**, 7.

Marriott, A. S. and Spencer, P. S. J., (1965) Brit. J. Pharmacol. Chemother. **25**, 432.

Massie, S. P., (1954) Chem. Rev. **54**, 797.

Masurat, T., Greenberg, S. M., Rice, E. G., Herndon, J. F., and Van Loon, E. J., (1960) Biochem. Pharmacol. **5**, 20.

Mattke, D. J., (1968) Dis. Nerv. Syst. **29**, 515.

McIlwain, H., (1962) in "Enzymes and Drug Action," (Ciba Foundation Symposium), Churchill Ltd., London, p. 170.

McIlwain, H. and Greengard, O., (1957) J. Neurochem. **1**, 348.

Mellinger, T. J., Mellinger, E. M., and Smith, W. T., (1964) Amer. J. Psychiat. **120**, 1111.

Moyer, J. H., (1954) Ann. N.Y. Acad. Sci. **59**, 82.

Müller, J. M., Schlittler, E., and Bein, H. J., (1952) Experientia **8**, 338.

Nybäck H. and Sedvall, G., (1967) Acta Pharmacol. Toxicol. (suppl. 4) **25**, 23.

Nybäck, H. and Sedvall, G., (1968) J. Pharmac. Exp. Ther. **162**, 294.

Nybäck, H. and Sedvall, G., (1969) Europ. J. Pharmacol. **5**, 245.

Nybäck, H., Sedvall, G., and Kopin, I. J., (1967) Life Sci. **6**, 2307.

Oberst, F. W. and Crook, J. W., (1967) Arch. Int. Pharmacodyn. Thér. **167**, 450.

Patridge, M., (1965) in "The Scientific Basis of Drug Therapy in Psychiatry," Marks, J. and Pare, C. M. B., Eds., Pergamon Press, Oxford.

Pearl, D., Kamp, H. V., Olsen, A. L., Greenberg, P. D., and Armitage, S. G., (1956) Arch. Neurol. Psychiat. (Chicago) **76**, 198.

Pellmont, B., Steiner, F. A., Besendorf, H., Baechtold, H. P., and Laeuppi, E., (1960) Schweiz. Med. Wochenschr. **90**, 598.

Petersen, P. V. and Nielsen, I. M., (1964) in "Psychopharmacological Agents," vol. 1, Gordon, M., Ed., Academic Press, New York, p. 301.

Pfeiffer, C. C. and Jenney, E. H., (1957) Ann. N.Y. Acad. Sci. **66**, 753.

Pletscher, A., Brossi, A., and Gey, K. F., (1962) Int. Rev. Neurobiol. **4**, 275.

Pletscher, A., Shore, P. A., and Brodie, B. B., (1955) Science **122**, 374.

Plummer, A. J., Earl, A., Schneider, J. A., Trapold, J., and Barrett, W., (1954) Ann. N.Y. Acad. Sci. **59**, 8.

Plummer, A. J., Sheppard, H., and Schulert, A. R., (1957) in "Psychotropic Drugs," Garrattini, S. and Ghetti, V., Eds., Elsevier Publ. Co., Amsterdam, p. 350.

Pöldinger, W., (1960) Praxis 49, 468.

Polishuk, W. Z. and Kulcsar, S., (1956) J. Clin. Endocrinol. Metab. 16, 292.

Posner, H. S., Culpan, R., and Levine, J., (1963) J. Pharmacol. Exper. Ther. 141, 377.

Psychopharmacology Service Center Collaborative Study Group, (1964) National Institute of Mental Health, Arch. Gen. Psychiat. 10, 246.

Quinn, G. P., Shore, P. A., and Brodie, B. B., (1959) J. Pharmacol. Exper. Ther. 127, 103.

Raymond, M. J., Lucas, C. J., Beesley, M. L., and O'Connell, B. A., (1957) Brit. Med. J. 2, 63.

Rees, L. and Davies, B., (1965) Int. J. Neuropsychiat. 1, 263.

Remvig, J. and Sonne, L. M., (1961) Psychopharmacologia (Berlin) 2, 203.

Rinaldi, F. and Himwich, H. E., (1955) Ann. N.Y. Acad. Sci. 61, 27.

Robinson, B., (1957) Med. J. Aust. 2, 239.

Roos, B. E., (1964) Acta Psychiat. Scand. (suppl. 180) 40, 421.

Roos, B. E., (1965) J. Pharm. Pharmacol. 17, 820.

Rouleau, Y. and Bernard, J., (1964) in "The Butyrophenones in Psychiatry," Quebec Psychopharmacological Res. Assoc., Montreal, Quebec, p. 88.

Royce, J. R. and Covington, M., (1960) J. Comp. Physiol. Psychol. 53, 197.

Sainz, A., (1963) Amer. J. Psychiat. 119, 777.

Sams, W. M., (1960) J. Amer. Med. Assoc. 174, 2043.

Sargant, W., (1964) Brit. Med. J. 1, 694.

Schlittler, E. and Plummer, A. J., (1964) in "Psychopharmacological Agents," vol. 1, Gordon, M., Ed., Academic Press, New York, p. 9.

Schneider, J. A., (1955) Amer. J. Physiol. 181, 64.

Schneider, J. A. and Earl, A. E., (1954) Neurology 4, 657.

Scott, G. T. and Nading, L. K., (1961) Proc. Soc. Exper. Biol. Med. 106, 88.

Sen, G. and Bose, K. C., (1931) Indian Med. World 2, 194

Sharman, D. F., (1963) J. Physiol. 169, 95P.

Sharman, D. F., (1966) Brit. J. Pharmacol. Chemother. 28, 153.

Shephard, N. W., Ed., (1965) "The Application of Neuroleptanalgesia in Anaesthetic and Other Practice," Pergamon Press, Oxford.

Shepherd, M., Lader, M., and Rodnight, R., (1968) "Clinical Psychopharmacology," English Universities Press Ltd., London, p. 96.

Shepherd, M. and Watt, D. C., (1956) J. Neurol. Neurosurg. Psychiat. 19, 232.

Sheppard, H. and Tsien, W. H., (1955) Proc. Soc. Exper. Biol. Med. 90, 437.

Sherlock, S., (1962) Brit. Med. J. 2, 1359.

Shillito, E. E., (1967) Brit. J. Pharmacol. Chemother. 30, 258.

Shore, P. A., (1962) Pharmacol. Rev. 14, 531.

Shore, P. A., Silver, S. L., and Brodie, B. B., (1955a) Science 122, 284.

Shore, P. A., Silver, S. L., and Brodie, B. B., (1955b) Experientia 11, 272.

Skarbek, A. and Jacobsen, M., (1965) Brit. J. Psychiat. 111, 1173.

Sofia, R. D. (1969) Life Sci. 8 (1), 705.

Sugerman, A. A., Lichtigfeld, F. J., and Herrmann, J., (1966) Curr. Ther. Res. Clin. Exper. 8, 220.

Sulman, F. G. and Winnik, H. Z., (1956) Nature, London 178, 365.

Valzelli, L., (1969) Psychopharmacologia (Berlin) 15, 232.

Valzelli, L., (1971) Actual. Pharmacol. 24, 133.

Valzelli, L. and Garattini, S., (1972) Neuropharmacol. 11, 17.

Valzelli, L. and Bernasconi, S., (1971) Psychopharmacologia (Berlin) 20, 91.

Valzelli, L., Consolo, S., and Morpurgo, C., (1967) in "Antidepressant Drugs" (Proc.

1st Int. Symp. Milan 1966), Garattini, S. and Dukes, M. N. G., Eds., Excerpta Medica Foundation, Amsterdam, p. 61.
Valzelli, L., Giacalone, E., and Garattini, S., (1967) Europ. J. Pharmacol. 2, 144.
Van Gasse, J. J., (1958) Clin. Med. Surg. 5, 177.
Van Orden, L. C., Bloom, F. E., Barnett, R. J., and Giarman, N. J., (1966) J. Pharmacol. Exper. Ther. 154, 185.
Van Rossum, J. M., (1966) Arch. Int. Pharmacodyn. Thér. 160, 492.
Viaud, P., (1954) J. Pharm. Pharmacol. 6, 361.
Walkenstein, S. S., Knebel, C. M., MacMullen, J. A., and Seifter, J., (1958) J. Pharmacol. Exp. Ther. 123, 254.
Wallgren, H., (1963) J. Neurochem. 10, 349.
Wase, A. W., Christensen, J., and Polley, E., (1956) AMA Arch. Neurol. Psychiat. 75, 54.
Weissman, A. and Finger, K. F., (1962) Biochem. Pharmacol. 11, 871.
Wikler, A., (1957) "The Relation of Psychiatry to Pharmacology," Williams and Wilkins, Baltimore.
Wilkens, B. and Malitz, S., (1960) Amer. J. Psychiat. 117, 23.
Wilkins, R. W., (1954) Ann. N.Y. Acad. Sci. 59, 36.
Wilkinson, J. L., (1961) Brit. Med. J. 1, 1721.
Williams, R. T. and Parke, D. V., (1964) Annu. Rev. Pharmacol. 4, 85.
Wing, J. K. and Freudenberg, R. K., (1961) Amer. J. Psychiat. 118, 311.
Winnik, H. Z. and Tennenbaum, L., (1955) Presse Méd. 63, 1092.
Woodson, R. E. et al., (1957) "Rauwolfia: Botany, Pharmacognosy, Chemistry and Pharmacology," Little, Brown and Co., Publ., Boston.
Wright, R. L. D. and Kyne, W. P., (1960) Psychopharmacologia (Berlin) 1, 437.
Zimmerman, F. T. and Burgmeister, B. B., (1955) Ann. N.Y. Acad. Sci. 61, 215.

Chapter IX

MINOR TRANQUILIZERS

The minor tranquilizers have probably been inaccurately defined in comparison with the major tranquilizing agents; they have been considered, not on the bases of their efficacy, but largely in terms of their comparably milder effects upon the central nervous system. The series of minor tranquilizers originates with the introduction of meprobamate, synthesized by BERGER in 1952. The introduction of this drug into therapeutic use initiated the period during which psychoactive drugs were used, not only by physicians, in the treatment of several syndromes mainly related to its antianxiety properties (BERGER, 1963), but also gave rise to an age when psychoactive drugs were "discovered" by people, who expanded their use and misuse beyond any medical limits.

Meprobamate gave rise to an intense proliferation in the development of several other compounds claimed to possess tranquilizing and antianxiety properties, among which, chlordiazepoxide (RANDALL, 1960; RANDALL et al., 1960), the prototype of the benzodiazepine series, is still the major representative.

These drugs, generally, started a phenomenon of "pill fetishism" which involves a continually growing number of people, who, indiscriminantly use psychotropic drugs as substitutive and corrective measures for the frustrations arising from those obstacles imposed by modern society upon individual self-determination. In this way individuals are exposed to the risk of a psychological drug dependence and to its potentially negative side effects arising from prolonged administration; there are also potential hazards involved with those compounds which are not believed to be dangerous (VISCOTT, 1968; HALBERG and LESSLER, 1964; DAVIS et al., 1968; BURNER and CHISTONI, 1968).

A) MEPROBAMATES

The chemical family of meprobamates derives its name from the parent drug of the series, meprobamate (Fig. 42), which was originally synthesized

161

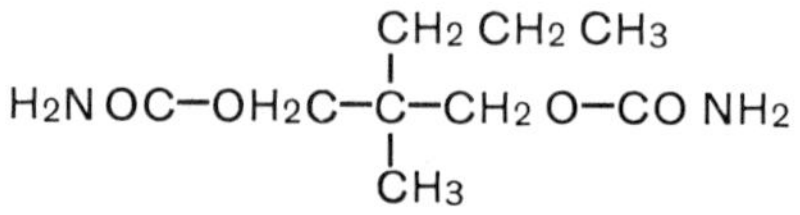

$$H_2N\,OC-OH_2C-\overset{\overset{\displaystyle CH_2\,CH_2\,CH_3}{|}}{\underset{\underset{\displaystyle CH_3}{|}}{C}}-CH_2\,O-CO\,NH_2$$

Fig. 42. Meprobamate.

by BERGER (1952) in a series of studies concerned with a search for new muscle relaxant drugs that were more effective and longer lasting than those available.

Meprobamate is a derivative of mephenesin, which belongs to a group of muscle relaxing drugs, from which, meprobamate probably derives its effects on muscle. Meprobamate, which is currently less frequently utilized than in past years, rapidly became very successful not only because of the emphasis given to its antianxiety effects (BERGER, 1963), but also probably in part, to its effective promotion (LASAGNA, 1962).

More recently several derivatives have been evolved from meprobamate, these include *carisoprodol*, which mainly possesses a muscle relaxant activity (BERGER et al., 1959), *mebutamate*, which has hypotensive activity (BERGER et al., 1961), and *tybamate*, which has the same general activity spectrum as *meprobamate* with a more pronounced antianxiety effect (BERGER et al., 1964).

1) General Aspects

Meprobamate *absorption* occurs very rapidly in the gastrointestinal tract and the drug concentrates both in the brain and in visceral organs (WALKENSTEIN et al., 1958). A major portion of the drug is eliminated through the urinary route within 24 hours, leaving about 10% in its original form but to a major extent as hydroxymeprobamate and as a conjunction product formed with glycuronic acid (BERGER, 1954; DOUGLAS and LUDWIG, 1959; LUDWIG et al., 1961). The *metabolism* of this drug is accelerated by itself and by the presence of other drugs such as aminopyrine, phenylbutazone, chlorpormazine, orphenadrine, and phenobarbital (CONNEY and BURNS, 1960; KATO, 1960; KATO and VASSANELLI, 1962; DOUGLAS et al., 1963).

The observation that meprobamate can accelerate its own metabolic inactivation represents one biochemical basis for explaining the development of tolerance towards this compound after its prolonged administration (PHILLIPS et al., 1962).

The metabolism of the other meprobamate derivatives does not appreciably differ from that of the parent compound and the derivatives maximally undergo hydrolysis (DOUGLAS et al., 1964; BAN, 1969).

The general *pharmacology* of meprobamate is largely represented by its depressant effects upon interneurons (BERGER, 1952), which are those neuronal elements which connect the sensory and motor pathways to the peripheral organs. Some authors (LEAR, 1966) have formulated the hypothesis that the drug may affect thalamic structures and consequently alter emotional responses which, mediated by the limbic system, reach the reticular system through the thalamus and the hypothalamus (SILVESTRINI and KOHN, 1958). Thus, meprobamate can effect a sedative action upon the central nervous system, without any appreciable anticholinergic, antiadrenergic or antihistaminic activity (DOMINO, 1962); this action has been defined by BERGER (1957) as a "central relaxing effect".

Insofar as *neuropharmacology* is concerned (Fig. 43) meprobamate does not affect ascending reticular system function (BERGER et al., 1957; KLETZKIN and BERGER, 1959), but it does cause a decrease in the spontaneous electrical activity of the thalamus and caudate nucleus (BAIRD et al., 1957; HENDLEY et al., 1954, 1955); moreover, it shortens the duration of seizures produced by hippocampal stimulation (BAN, 1969) but it does not exert any direct effect upon the cerebral cortex, even at very high doses (BERGER et al., 1964). SILVESTRINI and KOHN (1958) were able to show that meprobamate produced a synchronizing effect upon brain electrical activity and caused an increase in the threshold for alarm escape responses produced by hypothalamic stimulation.

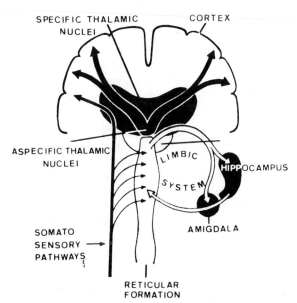

Fig. 43. Brain areas involved by meprobamate activity.

Moreover, meprobamate, selectively depresses polysynaptic reflexes while it is only slightly effective upon monosynaptic pathways (DE SALVA and ERCOLI, 1959), unless they are in a state of hyperactivity (BERGER and LUDWIG, 1964).

Insofar as *brain neurochemical mediators* and the general *biochemistry* of the central nervous system are concerned, there does not appear to be experimental evidence for any activity upon the usual parameters. Only for those subjects who underwent mental stress, a decrease of norepinephrine in urine, after meprobamate administration was reported (FRANKENHÄUSER and KAREBY, 1962).

2) Behavioral Effects

The muscle relaxant effect of meprobamate appears to serve as a basis for its reduction of *motor activity* (CHRISTENSEN et al., 1965) particularly in laboratory animals; moreover, depending upon dose, this compound can cause the disappearance of the righting reflex, as a consequence of flaccid paralysis. However, even if administered in very large doses, it never induces either narcosis or the appearance of extrapyramidal-like effects, as caused by major tranquilizers (BAN, 1969). One of the most characteristic effects of this drug is its taming properties in spontaneously aggressive animals (BERGER, 1954; HENDLEY et al., 1955); this, however, varies in accordance with the dose and the animals studied, and is not always constant (GROSS and WEISKRANTZ, 1961). On the contrary, meprobamate is completely ineffective on *aggressiveness* induced *by isolation,* except for doses which reduce the animal's muscle tone (VALZELLI et al., 1967); the drug has been described as active in altering the aggressive responses of hyperirritable septal rats (HUNT, 1957). The integration of these observations seems to suggest that this drug may decrease the reactive responses to stimuli, without modifying aggressive drives.

The *exploratory behavior* of mice is impaired by meprobamate (BOISSIER et al., 1964), while *conditioning* and *learning* processes may or may not be affected depending upon the dose administered; very small doses are inactive, while performance is gradually impaired by an increased dosage. Meprobamate is also only slightly effective in altering experimentally induced hyperactive behavior in laboratory animals (KUMADAKI et al., 1967; BAXTER, 1968) even though it seems to have some effect in controlling fear reactions and escape behavior (HESS, 1957). It has been demonstrated that meprobamate can alter an *experimental neurosis* induced in rats with a conflict situation (GELLER and SEIFER, 1960). Moreover, this drug reduces REM sleep phases in man (FREEMON et al., 1965) while its withdrawal after repeated administration induces a rebound increase in the percent of REM sleep (OSWALD et al., 1969).

Insofar as *pharmacological interactions* are concerned, meprobamate potentiates barbiturate-induced sleeping time and it antagonizes the convulsions produced by either electroshock, pentylentetrazol, amphetamine, or strychnine (BAN, 1969).

3) Clinical Effects

The major therapeutic indications for meprobamate are those instances in which it is desirable to effect (1) a generally mild sedation, and especially in those *psychoneuroses* in which (2) psychic tension and anxiety are associated with hyperirritability and hyperemotive responses (BORRUS, 1955; GARDNER, 1957; McCLENDON, 1958; RICKELS et al., 1959), (3) in *psychosomatic headache* (BLUMENTHAL and FUCHS, 1957; DIXON, 1957; FRIEDMAN, 1957), and (4) for *insomnia* (DIXON, 1957; PRIGOT et al., 1957; LASAGNA, 1956).

Tybamate appears to be even more affective for the treatment of anxious psychoneurotic patients and in chronic anxiety (SEEHERMAN, 1964; RICKELS et al., 1967; CHIEFFI, 1965), especially for those patients who show a high degree of somatizations (RAAB et al., 1964). Meprobamate derivatives appear to be useless in the treatment of schizophrenic and manic-depressive illness, except as therapeutic adjuncts in those cases characterized by restlessness and agitation (GRAFFAGNINO et al., 1957; McLAUGHLIN, 1957; TUCKER and WILENSKY, 1957); these derivatives can be utilized in the treatment of *chronic brain syndromes* of the elderly, where tybamate, especially, acts to reduce agitation, anorexia, anxiety, behavior disorders, tension, and insomnia (CHESROW et al., 1965; STERN, 1964). Aside from a strict psychiatric point of view, meprobamate is useful in the treatment of premenstrual tension, functional gastrointestinal and cardiovascular disorders, and muscle distrubances. In this latter case, carisoprodol is particularly suitable for the symptomatic treatment of muscle pain, spasms and functional muscle disorders involving inflammation, trauma, or degeneration (COOPER and EPSTEIN, 1959; PROCTOR, 1959; SPEARS, 1959; TRIMPI, 1959; WEIN, 1959). Mebutamate has an antihypertensive action (DUARTE et al., 1960; CAMPBELL and KAYE, 1962), which, however, is still in controversy; the antihypertensive effect is believed to be due to a reduction of activity in the pressor areas of the medulla oblongata (BERGER and MARGOLIN, 1961; MARGOLIN et al., 1963). Furthermore, meprobamate is effective in the treatment of central paralysis and petit-mal seizures (PERLSTEIN, 1956; AYD, 1957; LIVINGSTONE and PAULI, 1957; MILLEN, 1957; SPARUP, 1957). However, in routine medical practice, it is important to remember that meprobamate, even when administered at average doses, can cause a decrement in normal automobile-driving ability (LOOMIS and WEST, 1958) and, at higher doses, it induces a prolonged visual- and auditory-motor reaction time, an interference with motor coordination, and a decrease in learning ability (KORNETSKY, 1958).

4) Undesirable Effects

The most common side effects induced by meprobamate are somnolence and, at very high dosages, ataxia and states of confusion; it is important to consider that the use of these drugs with phenothiazines can induce epileptic-like seizures (BARSA and SAUNDERS, 1963).

More unusual but more serious side effects of meprobamate include an intolerance phenomena consisting in anaphylactoid reactions; these include angioneurotic oedema, urticarioid or maculapapular eruptions, dermatitis bullosa (CHARKES, 1958; DIXON, 1957), purpura, peripheral oedema (CARMEL and DANNENBERG, 1956), fever, bronchial spasms, hypotensive crisis, anuria, and stomatitis (ADLIN et al., 1958; BERNSTEIN and KLOTZ, 1957; CHARKES, 1958; BRACHFELD and BELL, 1959).

Meprobamate can induce tolerance as well as physical and psychological dependence (ESSIG, 1964, 1966) and the withdrawal of the drug can induce a syndrome characterized by insomnia, restlessness, tremors, anxiety, ataxia, and occasionally a reaction resembling delirium tremens (HAIZLIP and EWING, 1958).

B) BENZODIAZEPINES

Metaminodiazepoxide or *chlordiazepoxide* was introduced into pharmacotherapy about ten years ago and since then this compound has probably been prescribed, administered, and spontaneously taken more frequently than any other psychotropic drug. Chlordiazepoxide (Fig. 44) can be considered as the parent compound of the benzodiazepine series of which there are now at least another ten derivatives available.

The interpretations of the mode of action of these derivatives range from psychodynamic views, according to which chlordiazepoxide induces a weakening of ego to allow psychotic projections, similar to some extent to the psychotomimetic drugs (OSTOW, 1962), to the more strictly neurophysiological interpretations.

In most cases, however, this drug has a major anxiolytic effect, without compromising arousal. This fact depends on its relatively high specificity for the limbic system structures and its minimal effect upon the brain stem

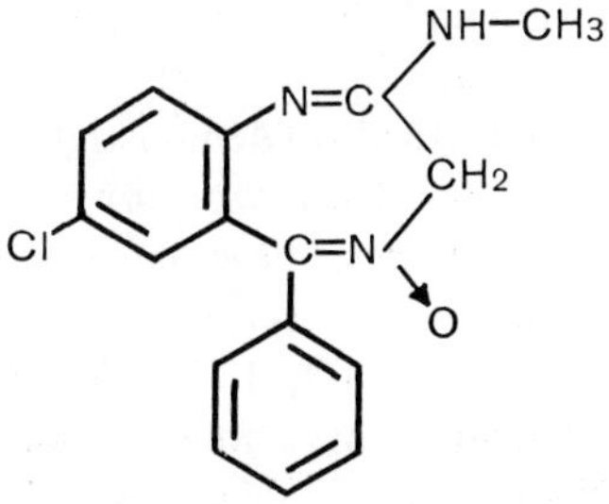

Fig. 44. Chlordiazepoxide.

reticular activating system (SCHALLEK, 1960; SCHALLEK and KUEHN, 1963, 1965a, b; SCHALLEK et al., 1962, 1964).

1) General Aspects

Benzodiazepine *absorption* is very rapid and occurs as easily either through the gastrointestinal or the parenteral route, even though maximal concentration peaks in blood are reached about eight hours following oral administration. Blood concentrations remain rather high over a fairly long period of time, declining to 50% of the initial concentration only after 24 hours (SMYTH and PENNINGTON, 1963; STERNBACH et al., 1964).

The *metabolism* of this drug occurs by demethylation, hydroxylation, or conjugation. Particularly in man, chlordiazepoxide is hydrolyzed, leading to the formation of a lactam derivative (SMYTH and PENNINGTON, 1963; KOECHLIN et al., 1965). Benzodiazepines are maximally cleared through the intestinal route in the rat, while in man urinary *excretion* accounts for maximal disposition (BAN, 1969). A series of studies have shown that it is possible to identify several degraded benzodiazepine products present in urine for about two weeks after the administration (BAUMLER and RIPPSTEIN, 1961; RANDALL, 1961; KOECHLIN and D'ARCONTE, 1963).

The *pharmacology* of benzodiazepines, and of chlordiazepoxide in particular, is dominated by the taming and antiaggressive properties of these compounds, which are more potent and specific than for other substances such as pentobarbital, chlorpromazine, or meprobamate (NORTON, 1957). This behavioral effect is characterized by a decrease of aggressive or defensive expression which parallels an increase in sociability. Very high drug doses can induce ataxia, but taming and antiaggressive effects appear at doses very much below toxic levels, unlike the conditions under which such effects are obtained with pentobarbital, chlorpromazine, and meprobamate (VALZELLI, 1967, 1973; VALZELLI et al., 1967, 1971; BAN, 1969).

The range of effects initiated by these compounds generally is much more dependent upon their action at the central nervous system level than for other drugs, so that, it is difficult to demonstrate a direct peripheral site of action for the benzodiazepines. Only *diazepam* and *oxazepam*, and, more recently, *medazepam* and *prazepam* have been shown to have a weak sympatholytic activity, which is, however, of central origin (ROBICHAUD et al., 1970; AHTEE and SHILLITO, 1970; SCHALLEK et al., 1970). Chlordiazepoxide is also known to have an antiinflammatory and appetite-stimulating effect (RANDALL et al., 1960; RANDALL, 1961; SUPER-STINE and SULMAN, 1966), as well as effective protective properties against experimental gastric ulcerations induced by stress (HAOT et al., 1964).

The *neuropharmacology* of these compounds is typically focused upon the limbic system (RANDALL and SCHALLEK, 1968; RANDALL et al., 1969, 1970; MALICK, 1970), which has been extensively studied and analyzed for chlordiazepoxide effects by SCHALLEK et al., (SCHAL-LEK, 1960; SCHALLEK and KUEHN, 1963, 1965a, b; SCHALLEK et al., 1962, 1964).

This drug was shown to exert a depressing effect upon septal structures and on the amygdala and hippocampus, without any impairment of arousal. In particular, diazepam and notably *nitrazepam,* reduce and attenuate the electrical activity of amygdala much more than chlordiazepoxide does and it is believed that this more potent effect may serve as a basis for the hypnogenic effect exerted by these two derivatives in general and by nitrazepam in particular (BAN, 1969). Moreover, benzodiazepines have an inhibitory effect upon hypothalamic nuclei and upon thalamic structures (Fig. 45), the latter effect resembles that exerted by other typical anticonvulsant drugs such as trimethadione and diphenylhydantoin (SCHALLEK and KUEHN, 1963). It has been possible to observe an inhibitory effect of benzodiazepines upon spinal reflexes and also at the extrapyramidal level, such to justify a postive effect produced by these compounds upon decerebrate rigidity; in addition, their muscle-relaxant effect in accord with the derivative considered, is more or less apparent depending upon the administered dosage.

Electroencephalographic studies have shown that these derivatives induce some characteristic changes of the record, accelerating activity and increasing synchronization; these modifications, which occur caudal to the frontal areas, arise earlier for diazepam than for chlordiazepoxide and persist for a certain period of time after the treatment (BAN, 1969).

From this point of view, benzodiazepine action differs from that of barbiturates, chlorpromazines, meprobamate or imipramine (REQUIN et al., 1963).

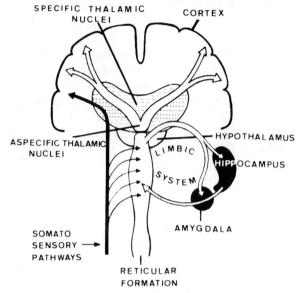

Fig. 45. Brain areas involved by benzodiazepine activity.

Apparently benzodiazepines derivatives do not alter the levels of brain *neurochemical mediators* (VALZELLI, 1973), even though chlordiazepoxide has been both reported to interfere to a certain extent with the conversion of DOPA into dopamine, and to counteract the effects of this neurotransmitter (SHARMAN, 1966; BAN, 1969).

Moreover, recently TAYLOR and LAVERTY (1969) reported that chlordiazepoxide, diazepam, and nitrazepam decrease norepinephrine turnover in the thalamus-midbrain, cortical, and cerebellar regions and dopamine turnover in the striate region.

With regard to other aspects of *brain biochemistry*, benzodiazepines exert an inhibitory effect upon oxygen utilization in brain tissue and liver mitochondria, and they also induce a transitory increase in glucose level.

2) Behavioral Effects

Low doses of benzodiazepines do not impair *spontaneous activity* to any great extent; in particular, chlordiazepoxide does not affect either muscle coordination or spontaneous activity except at very high doses (CHRISTEN-SEN et al., 1965; GOLDBERG et al., 1967). This observation probably relates to the specificity and efficacy of chlordiazepoxide and other benzodiazepine derivatives such as medazepam upon either spontaneous (BOIS-

SIER et al., 1968; HOROVITZ et al., 1965) or induced *aggressiveness* (RANDALL, 1960; HOROVITZ, 1965; VALZELLI et al., 1967, 1971; VALZELLI, 1973).

Chlordiazepoxide, medazepam, and oxazepam, at very low doses, are effective in modifying *aggressiveness* induced *by isolation* in mice, while for other derivatives such as diazepam, *N-methyloxazepam, demethyldiazepam,* and nitrazepam, the antiaggressive activity coincides with the impairment of muscle tonus (VALZELLI, 1973; VALZELLI et al., 1971).

Chlordiazepoxide as well as other benzodiazepines acts differently upon *exploratory behavior* depending upon the emotional baseline of the experimental animal (VALZELLI, 1971); for instance, very low doses of chlordiazepoxide (1 mg/kg) do not interfere, or only minimally alter, the exploratory behavior of normal mice, while at these same doses the performance of aggressive animals is significantly improved (VALZELLI, 1969). The drug probably acts upon emotional elements which inhibit the exploratory pattern in these animals. Diazepam decreases exploratory behavior in normal mice more than chlordiazepoxide does (BOISSIER et al., 1964), and in rats, it reduces (BOISSIER et al., 1964) this parameter more for those animals that had previous exploratory experience than in those tested for the first time (ITOH and TAKAORI, 1968). In this case the emotional level of the animal as well as previous experience contribute to the effect.

On the other hand, the emotional modulation of a benzodiazepine effect is easily demonstrated and rather specific, such that in rats made hyperemotive with olfactory bulb ablation, chlordiazepoxide markedly modifies the animal behavioral symptomatology at doses ineffective in altering spontaneous activity (KUMADAKY et al., 1967).

In experimental conflict situations in rats, oxazepam seems to be more effective in altering the disrupted behavior than either diazepam or chlordiazepoxide, despite the profound effects of these latter compounds under such conditions (GELLER, 1964). Furthermore, chlordiazepoxide seems to accelerate and to support the preservation of *learning* of conditioned avoidance responses (SACHS et al., 1966) and decreases the decision time latency in discriminative learning situations (LIBERSON et al., 1963). This observation is still controversial (HUGHES et al., 1963; KAMANO and ARP, 1964; CICALA and HARTLEY, 1965), probably because of different doses and experimental conditions utilized in such experiments.

Benzodiazepines have obvious anticonvulsant properties, which exceed those of meprobamate; the anticonvulsive efficacy of these derivatives for convulsions induced by electroshock is, in decreasing order of potency, diazepam, *flurazepam,* and chlordiazepoxide; diazepam is the most effective of the benzodiazepines for antagonizing convulsions induced with pentylentetrazol or strychnine (RANDALL et al., 1965; BANZINGER, 1965). The effect of benzodiazepines upon amphetamine-induced excitation is very weak; recently, however, a new derivative, 0-chloroxazepam or *lorazepam*, has been synthesized, which exerts an extremely potent anticonvulsant effect, both in experimental animals and in man (BELL et al., 1968; SCHILLINGS et al., 1971; SCHRAPPE, 1971; MARCUCCI et al., 1972). The potentiation of barbiturate-induced sleeping time is irrelevant except at very high doses of benzodiazepine.

In man chlordiazepoxide modifies sleep patterns, producing a subjective feeling of particularly vivid dreams which may be experienced in colors; it can also lead to the production of nightmares (TOLL, 1960; STANFIELD, 1961; MAGGS and NEVILLE, 1964). Even though all of the benzodiazepines have a sleep facilitating effect, the most effective hypnotic of the series is nitrazepam (CAMPAN and ESPAGNO, 1964; DAVIES and LEVINE, 1967; LANOIR and KILLAM, 1968; HAIDER, 1968), which decreases REM cycles and shows a rebound effect with a prolongation of these cycles when the drug is withdrawn (OSWALD, 1968). In contrast to nitrazepam, flurazepam withdrawal does not produce any rebound effect on REM cycles (KALES et al., 1970).

3) Clinical Effects

The major clinical indications for benzodiazepines in general, and for chlordiazepoxide and medazepam in particular, are *anxiety syndromes* (AZIMA et al., 1962; JENNER et al., 1961a; McNAIR et al., 1965; BOLZANI and SLIVAR, 1969; RANDALL et al., 1969; FOKSTUEN, 1970; RICKELS et al., 1971). For these conditions, chlordiazepoxide has been shown to be more effective than amobarbital (JENNER et al., 1961b; GORE and McCOMISKY, 1961) and meprobamate (BOBON et al., 1962). In spite of some generally negative opinions (SHEPHERD et al., 1968) the efficacy of benzodiazepines in *anxiety psychoneurosis, dissociative* and *conversion syndromes,* and in *peripheral psychosomatic disturbances,* such as gastrointestinal, cardiovascular, muscular, respiratory, gynecological, and neurological syndromes, has been widely demonstrated in a large number of clinical experimental studies, which have been extensively reviewed by STERNBACK et al. (1964) and by COHEN et al. (1967).

Aside from clinical data concerned with the therapeutic efficacy of chlordiazepoxide (WILLIAMS, 1961; LANGSTON, 1962; ROSENSTEIN and SILVERBLATT, 1961; REINHARDT, 1962; ELIA, 1962; PERNI-KOFF, 1960; SCHERBEL, 1961), many other data have recently become available on the efficacy of diazepam, oxazepam, flurazepam, medazepam, nitrazepam, *promazepam, temazepam,* and prazepam (BURDINE, 1964;

CLECKLEY, 1965; DEAN, 1965; KRAKOWSKI, 1965; ISHAM, 1966; THOMAS, 1966; KINGSTONE et al., 1966; RANDALL et al., 1970; SCHALLEK et al., 1970; FOKSTUEN, 1970; KALES et al., 1970).

Chlordiazepoxide has also been widely utilized in the management of alcohol withdrawal and it is effective in the management of both *delirium tremens* and *acute alcoholic hallucinations* (TICKTIN and SCHULTZ, 1960; FISHBEIN, 1961; CHAMBERS et al., 1962; KOUTSKI and SLETTEN, 1963; BAN et al., 1965), as well as in controlling *chronic alcoholism* (MOONEY et al.; 1961; SMITH, 1961); it has been shown to be a useful adjunct to psychotherapeutic practice (DEAN, 1962; LORR et al., 1962).

Benzodiazepines are also widely employed for their muscle-relaxant properties in the treatment of *epilepsy* (BRODIE and DOW, 1962; LE VANN, 1962; LEHMANN and BAN, 1968; NICOL et al., 1969), where diazepam and lorazepam are best indicated. Beneficial effects have also been obtained in controlling petit-mal, grand-mal, myoclonia, psychomotor epilepsies, as well as in the treatment of infantile syndromes wherein convulsive symptomatology is not evident but in which character disorders are coincident with modifications of the electroencephalographic record (KRAFT et al., 1965; BAN, 1969). Benzodiazepines are also capable of exerting effects upon the "epileptic personality" where they improve the characteristic slowness, perseveration, "stickness", the emotional inadequacy, the motor restlessness, and decreased attention span (BAN, 1969).

Other minor indications for chlordiazepoxide, diazepam, and all the benzodiazepine derivatives in general, are as adjuncts in the treatment of depressions presenting hypomanic excitation, such as in the involutive melancholies and psychotic syndromes with anxious-paranoid components (FELDMAN, 1962; McCRAY, 1965; STONEHILL et al., 1966).

Aside from their psychiatric indications, benzodiazepines are remarkably helpful and widely used in general medical practice since, because of their mood stabilizing properties and their strong antianxiety effects, they can successfully be employed directly or as adjuncts to the treatment of a wide range of general medical syndromes. From a practical point of view, it is useful to remember that the most effective antianxiety effects as shown in decreasing order, are provided by medazepam, temazepam, chlordiazepoxide, oxazepam and prazepam; the muscle relaxant effects are brought about by lorazepam, diazepam and oxazepam, while the hypnotic effect is maximally produced by nitrazepam and flurazepam.

It may also be observed that a widely extended range of application represents the major utility of these derivatives, but paradoxically also increases their potential risk probability as it more easily induces the physician to prescribe them with the increased permissivity which can lead to uncontrolled, irrational and long-lasting self-administration, with the dangers of personality changes (BURNER and CHISTONI, 1968) as well as abnormal and toxic reactions.

4) Undesirable Effects

Unwanted effects from benzodiazepines only occur at high doses administered over a long period of time, or in cases of some individual and specific sensitivities. Such effects mainly consist of asthenia, somnolence, ataxia, disorientation, and paradoxical states of confusion, in decreasing order of occurrence. These effects are generally quite infrequent (SVENSON and HAMILTON, 1966), while those arising from a true dependence, that can partially be of a pharmacological nature but are mostly of psychological type, are more dangerous. Such dependence results from heavy, continuous, and uncontrolled benzodiazepine administration over several years and it can degenerate into paradoxical reactions such as hallucination, restlessness, and hostile-aggressive tendencies (VISCOTT, 1968; DI MASCIO et al., 1969; DI MASCIO, 1973; GARDOS et al., 1968; SALZMAN et al., 1969). Similar paradoxical aggression-inducing effects are also manifested in laboratory animals chronically fed with different benzodiazepine derivatives (FOX and SNYDER, 1969; FOX et al., 1970, 1972; GUAITANI et al., 1971; VAL-ZELLI et al., 1971). Other effects may consist of excessive weight increase, constipation, decreased sexual activity, dryness of the mouth, dizziness, hypotension and variations in heart rate (BAN, 1969).

C) DIPHENYLMETHANE DERIVATIVES

The diphenylmethane drugs consist of a series of tranquilizing derivatives which are clinically effective for their anxiety effects. They are employed with comparatively less frequency in therapeutic practice because of the heavy competition from the two previously cited series of drugs. Among the most effective representatives of this chemical family is *azacyclonol* which shows a good general tranquilizing activity (KRÜEGER and McGRATH, 1964) allowing its successful employment in the treatment of agitated and aggressive patients and in toxic psychosis (FABING, 1955; LASCELLES and LEVENE, 1959; RINALDI et al., 1955, 1956; SARWER-FONER and KORANYI, 1956); it has also been employed to antagonize both the clinical and electroencephalographic symptoms induced by lysergic acid diethylamide (LSD) and mescaline (FABING and HAWKINS, 1956).

Another derivative in this category is *benactyzine,* which is characterized by a central anticholinergic property which can inhibit some central nervous system functions. In this context, it was hypothesized that this drug acts on hypothalamic structures, elevating the emotional threshold to the environmental stimulation, but this hypothesis was not confirmed by its clinical activity, which appears to be quite minimal. It is to be emphasized that, at high doses, benactyzine is capable of inducing psychotomimetic effects, which range from a simple difficulty in concentration with associated indecision to clear depersonalization symptoms (AYD, 1957; JACOBSEN, 1958; KINROSS-WRIGHT and MOYER, 1957; FINK, 1960).

Hydroxyzine is the most widely used diphenylmethane compound. It has adrenolytic, anticholinergic, antihistaminic, antiematic, antispastic, hypothermic and hypotensive properties. It induces an elevation of the arousal threshold in the structures of the reticular formation (KALINOWSKY and HOCH, 1961). Hydroxyzine possesses anxiolytic activity, with a tranquilizing component which is particularly valuable in the management of agitated subjects; this activity does not effect either the patient's lucidity or wakefulness (DARMSTADTER and MOCK, 1965; SETTEL, 1957). In particular, this drug has been shown to be useful in the treatment of psychoneuroses with or without anxiety components, psychosomatic diseases (DOLAN, 1958; SCHRAM, 1959; MIDDLEFELL, 1960; GIBBON, 1961), alcoholism, behavior disorders, and dermatological diseases (BAYART, 1956; FREEDMAN, 1958; GOLDMAN, 1961).

Orphenadrine is an antihistaminic drug with central stimulant properties which is useful in the treatment of psychasthenia and drug-induced extrapyramidal-like syndromes (ZAKRZEWSKA et al., 1965); *benztropine* has been similarly employed in the treatment of extrapyramidal-like syndromes induced by drugs and *captodiamine* has some effects in attenuating hyperexcitability in children.

Other compounds, which do not belong to the drug categories outlined, have been and are described in the medical literature as having useful therapeutic properties. Among these are methyprylon, glutethimide, and methaqualone, which all have typical sedative and hypnotic effects; therefore, they do not have such specific characteristics as to justify a further detailed description.

REFERENCES

Adlin, E. V., Sher, P. B., and Berk, N. G., (1958) Arch. Intern. Med. 102, 484.
Ahtee, L. and Shillito, E., (1970) Brit. J. Pharmacol. 40, 361.
Ayd, F. J., (1957) New England J. Med. 257, 669.
Azima, H., Arthurs, D., and Silver, A., (1962) Can. Psychiat. Assoc. J. 7, 44.
Baird, H. W., Szekely, E. G., Wycis, H. T., and Spiegel, E. A., (1957) Ann. N.Y. Acad. Sci. 67, 873.

Ban, T. A., (1969) "Psychopharmacology," Williams & Wilkins, Baltimore.

Ban, T. A., Lehmann, H. E., Matthews, V., and Donald, M., (1965) Clin. Med. 72, 59.

Banziger, R. F., (1965) Arch. Int. Pharmacodyn. Thér. 154, 131.

Barsa, J. A. and Saunders, J. C., (1963) Amer. J. Psychiat. 120, 492.

Baumler, J. and Rippstein, S., (1961) Helv. Chim. Acta 44, 2208.

Baxter, B. L., (1968) Int. J. Neuropharmacol. 7, 47.

Bayart, J., (1956) Acta Pediat. Belg. 4, 164.

Bell, S. C., McCaully, R. I., Gochman, C., Childress, S. J., and Gluckman, M. I., (1968) J. Med. Chem. 11, 475.

Berger, F. M., (1952) J. Pharmacol. Exper. Ther. 104, 468.

Berger, F. M., (1954) J. Pharmacol. Exper. Ther. 112, 413.

Berger, F. M., (1957) Ann. N.Y. Acad. Sci. 67, 685.

Berger, F. M., (1963) Clin. Pharmacol. Ther. 4, 209.

Berger, F. M., Campbell, G. L., Hendley, C. D., Ludwig, B. J., and Lynes, T. E., (1957) Ann. N.Y. Acad. Sci. 66, 686.

Berger, F. M., Douglas, J. F., Kletzkin, M., Ludwig, B. J., and Margolin, S., (1961) J. Pharmacol. Exper. Ther. 134, 356.

Berger, F. M., Kletzkin, M., and Margolin, S., (1964) Med. Exper. 10, 327.

Berger, F. M., Kletzkin, M., Ludwig, B. J., Margolin, S., and Powell, L. S., (1959) J. Pharmacol. Exper. Ther. 127, 66.

Berger, F. M. and Ludwig, B. J., (1964) in "Psychopharmacological Agents," vol. 1, Gordon, M., Ed., Academic Press, New York, p. 103.

Berger, F. M. and Margolin, S., (1961) Fed. Proc. Fed. Amer. Soc. Exper. Biol. 20, 113.

Bernstein, C. and Klotz, S. D., (1957) J. Amer. Med. Assoc. 163, 930.

Blumenthal, L. S. and Fuchs, M., (1957) South Med. J. 50, 1491.

Bobon, J., Collard, J., and Kerf, J., (1962) Rev. Méd. Liège 17, 9.

Boissier, J. R., Grasset, S., and Simon, P., (1968) J. Pharm. Pharmacol. 20, 973.

Boissier, J. R., Simon, P., and Lwoff, J. M., (1964) Thérapie 19, 571.

Bolzani, L. and Slivar, G., (1969) Int. Pharmacopsychiat. 2, 197.

Borrus, J. C., (1955) J. Amer. Med. Assoc. 157, 1596.

Brachfeld, J. and Bell, E. C., (1959) J. Amer. Med. Assoc. 169, 1321.

Brodie, R. E. and Dow, R. S., (1962) Nord West Med. 61, 513.

Burdine, W. E., (1964) Amer. J. Psychiat. 121, 589.

Burner, M. and Chistoni, G. C., (1968) Méd. Hyg. 26, 506.

Campan, L. and Espagno, M. T., (1964) Ann. Anesth. Franç. 5, 711.

Campbell, D. K. and Kaye, M., (1962) Appl. Ther. 4, 143.

Carmel, W. J. and Dannenberg, T., (1956) New England J. Med. 255, 770.

Chambers, J. F., D'Agostino, A., Sheriff, W. H., Jr., and Schultz, J. D., (1962) Can. Med. Assoc. J. 86, 1112.

Charkes, N. D., (1958) Arch. Intern. Med. 102, 584.

Chesrow. E. J., Kaplitz, S. E., Vetra, H., Breme, J. T., and Marquardt, G. H., (1965) Clin. Med. 72, 1001.

Chieffi, M., (1965) Dis. Nerv. Syst. 26, 369.

Christensen, J. A., Hernestam, S., Lassen, J. B., and Sterner, N., (1965) Acta Pharmacol. Toxicol. 23, 109.

Cicala, G. A. and Hartley, D., (1965) Psychol. Rec. 15, 435.

Cleckley, H. M., (1965) J. S. Carolina Med. Assoc. 61, 1.

Cohen, S., Ditman, K. S., and Gustafson, S. R., (1967) "Psychochemotherapy," Western Medical Publications, Los Angeles.

Conney, A. H. and Burns, J. J., (1960) Ann. N.Y. Acad. Sci. 86, 167.

Cooper, C. D. and Epstein, J. H., (1959) in "The Pharmacology and Clinical Usefulness of Carisoprodol," Wayne State University Press, Detroit.
Darmstadter, H. J. and Mock, J. E., (1965) Dis. Nerv. Syst. **26**, 236.
Davies, C. and Levine, S., (1967) Brit. J. Psychiat. **113**, 1005.
Davis, J. M., Bartlett, E., and Termini, B., (1968) Dis. Nerv. Syst. **29**, 157.
Dean, S. R., (1962) Dis. Nerv. Syst. **23**, 1.
Dean, S. R., (1965) Dis. Nerv. Syst. **26**, 181.
De Salva, S. J. and Ercoli, N., (1959) Proc. Soc. Exper. Biol. Med. **101**, 250.
Di Mascio, A., (1973) in "The Benzodiazepines," Garattini, S. and Randall, L. O. Eds., Raven Press, New York.
Di Mascio, A., Schader, R. I., and Harmatz, J., (1969) Psychosomatics (Suppl. 3) **10**, 46.
Dixon, N. M., (1957) Ann. N.Y. Acad. Sci. **67**, 772.
Dolan, C. M., (1958) Calif. Med. **88**, 443.
Domino, E. F., (1962) Annu. Rev. Pharmacol. **2**, 215.
Douglas, J. F., Edelson, J., Schlosser, A., Ludwig, B. J., and Berger, F. M., (1964) Fed. Proc. Fed. Amer. Soc. Exper. Biol. **23**, 489.
Douglas, J. F. and Ludwig, B. J., (1959) Fed. Proc. Fed. Amer. Soc. Exper. Biol. **18**, 385.
Douglas, J. F., Ludwig, B. J., and Smith, N., (1963) Proc. Soc. Exper. Biol. Med. **112**, 436.
Duarte, C., Brest, A. N., Kodama, R., Naso, F., and Moyer, J. H., (1960) Curr. Ther. Res. **2**, 148.
Elia, J. C., (1962) Clin. Med. **69**, 49.
Essig, C. F., (1964) Clin. Pharmacol. Ther. **5**, 334.
Essig, C. F., (1966) J. Amer. Med. Assoc. **196**, 714.
Fabing, H. D., (1955) Dis. Nerv. Syst. **16**, 10.
Fabing H. D. and Hawkins, J. R., (1956) Science **123**, 886.
Feldman, R. S., (1962) J. Neuropsychiat. **3**, 254.
Fink, M., (1960) Electroenceph. Clin. Neurophysiol. **12**, 359.
Fishbein, R. E., (1961) Curr. Ther. Res. **3**, 345.
Fokstuen, T., (1970) Int. Pharmacopsychiat. **3**, 130.
Fox, K. A. and Snyder, R. L., (1969) J. Comp. Physiol. Psychol. **69**, 663.
Fox, K. A., Tuckosh, J. R., and Wilcox, A. H., (1970) Europ. J. Pharmacol. **11**, 119.
Fox, K. A., Webster, J. C., and Guerriero, F. J., (1972) Europ. J. Pharmacol., in press.
Frankenhäuser, M. and Kareby, S., (1962) Percept. Motor Skills **15**, 571.
Freedman, A. M., (1958) Pediat. Clin. N. Amer. **12**, 573.
Freemon, F. R., Agnew, H. W., and Williams, R. L., (1965) Clin. Pharmacol. Ther. **6**, 172.
Friedman, A. P., (1957) Ann. N.Y. Acad. Sci. **67**, 822.
Gardner, A., (1957) Amer. J. Psychiat. **114**, 524.
Gardos, G., Di Mascio, A., Salzman, C., and Shader, R. I., (1968) Arch. Gen. Psychiat. **18**, 757.
Geller, I., (1964) Arch. Int. Pharmacodyn. Thér. **149**, 243.
Geller, I. and Seifer, J., (1960) Psychopharmacologia (Berlin) **1**, 482.
Gibbon, J., (1961) Dis. Nerv. Syst. (Suppl.) **22**, 81.
Goldberg, M. E., Manian, A. A., and Efron, D. H., (1967) Life Sci. **6**, 481.
Goldman, H. I., (1961) Southwest. Med. **42**, 276.
Gore, C. P. and McComisky, J. G., (1961) Proc. 3rd. World Conf. Psychiat. **2**, 979.
Graffagnino, P. N. et al., (1957) Conn. Med. **21**, 1047.

Gross, C. G. and Weiskrantz, L. A., (1961) Quart. J. Exper. Psychol. **13**, 34.

Guaitani, A., Marcucci, F., and Garattini, S., (1971) Psychopharmacologia (Berlin) **19**, 241.

Haider, I., (1968) Brit. J. Psychiat. **114**, 337.

Haizlip, T. M. and Ewing, J. A., (1958) New England J. Med. **258**, 1181.

Halberg, R. and Lessler, K., (1964) Amer. J. Psychiat. **121**, 188.

Haot, J., Djahanguiri, B., and Richelle, M., (1964) Arch. Int. Pharmacodyn Thér. **148**, 557.

Hendley, C. D., Lynes, T. E., and Berger, F. M., (1954) Proc. Soc. Exper. Biol. Med. **87**, 608.

Hendley, C. D., Lynes, T. E., and Berger, F. M., (1955) Fed. Proc. Fed. Amer. Soc. Exper. Biol. **14**, 351.

Hess, E. H., (1957) Ann. N.Y. Acad. Sci. **67**, 724.

Horovitz, Z. P., (1965) Psychosomatics **6**, 281.

Horovitz, Z. P., Ragozzino, P. W., and Leaf, R. C. (1965) Life Sci. **4**, 1909.

Hughes, F. W., Rountree, C. B., and Forney, R. B., (1963) J. Genet. Psychol. **103**, 139.

Hunt, H. F., (1957) Ann. N.Y. Acad. Sci. **67**, 712.

Isham, A. C., (1966) Int. J. Neuropsychiat. **2**, 111.

Itoh, H. and Takaori, S., (1968) Jap. J. Pharmacol. **18**, 344.

Jacobsen, E., (1958) J. Pharm. Pharmacol. **10**, 273.

Jenner, F. A., Kerry, R. J., and Parkin, D., (1961a) J. Ment. Sci. **107**, 575.

Jenner, F. A., Kerry, R. J., and Parkin, D., (1961b) J. Ment. Sci. **107**, 583.

Kales, A., Kales, J. D., Scharf, M. B., and Ling-Tan, T., (1970) Arch. Gen. Psychiat. **23**, 219.

Kalinowsky, L. B. and Hoch, P. H., (1961) "Somatic Treatments in Psychiatry," Grune & Stratton, New York.

Kamano, D. K. and Arp, D. J., (1964) Psychopharmacologia (Berlin) **6**, 112.

Kato, R., (1960) Med. Exper. **3**, 95.

Kato, R. and Vassanelli, P., (1962) Biochem. Pharmacol. **11**, 779.

Kingstone, E., Villeneuve, A., and Kossatz, I., (1966) Curr. Ther. Res. **8**, 159.

Kinross-Wright, V. and Moyer, J. H., (1957) Amer. J. Psychiat. **114**, 703.

Kletzkin, M. and Berger, F. M., (1959) Proc. Soc. Exper. Biol. Med. **100**, 681.

Koechlin, B. A. and D'Arconte, L., (1963) Analyt. Biochem. **5**, 195.

Koechlin, B. A., Schwartz, M. A., Krol, G., and Oberhansli, W., (1965) J. Pharmacol. Exper. Ther. **148**, 399.

Kornetsky, C., (1958) J. Pharmacol. Exper. Ther. **123**, 216.

Koutsky, C. D. and Sletten, I. W., (1963) Minn. Med. **46**, 354.

Kraft, I. A., Ardali, C., Duffy, J. H., Hart, J. T., and Pearce, P., (1965) Int. J. Neuropsychiat. **1**, 433.

Krakowski, A. J., (1965) Amer. J. Psychiat. **121**, 807.

Krüeger, G. L. and McGrath, W. R., (1964) in "Psychopharmacological Agents," vol. 1, Gordon, M., Ed., Academic Press, New York, p. 225.

Kumadaki, N., Hitomi, M., and Kumada, S., (1967) Jap. J. Pharmacol. **17**, 659.

Langston, W. B., Jr., (1962) Southwest. Med. **43**, 295.

Lanoir, J. and Killam, K. E., (1968) Electroenceph. Clin. Neurophysiol. **25**, 530.

Lasagna, L., (1956) J. Chron. Dis. **3**, 122.

Lasagna, L., (1962) "The Doctor's Dilemmas," Victor Gollancz, London.

Lascelles, C. F. and Levene, L. J., (1959) J. Ment. Sci. **105**, 247.

Lear, E., (1966) "Chemistry and Applied Pharmacology of Tranquilizers," C. C. Thomas Publ., Springfield, Ill.

Lehmann, H. E. and Ban, T. A., (1968) Int. J. Clin. Pharmacol. 1, 231.

Le Vann, L. J., (1962) Can. Med. Assoc. J. 86, 123.

Liberson, W. T., Kafka, A., Schwarz, E., and Gagnon, V., (1963) Int. J. Neuropharmacol. 2, 67.

Livingstone, S. and Pauli, L., (1957) Amer. J. Dis. Child. 94, 277.

Loomis, T. A. and West, T. C., (1958) J. Pharmacol. Exper. Ther. 122, 525.

Lorr, M., McNair, D. M., and Weinstein, G. J., (1962) J. Psychiat. Res. 1, 257.

Ludwig, B. J., Douglas, J. F., Powell, L. S., Meyer, M., and Berger, F. M., (1961) J. Med. Pharmacol. Chem. 3, 53.

Maggs, R. and Neville, R., (1964) Brit. J. Psychiat. 110, 540.

Malick, J. B., (1970) Arch. Int. Pharmacodyn. Thér. 186, 137.

Marcucci, F., Mussini, E., Airoldi, L., Guaitani, A., and Garattini, S., (1972) J. Pharm. Pharmacol. 24, 63.

Margolin, S., Plekss, O. J., and Fedor, E. J., (1963) J. Pharmacol. Exper. Ther. 140, 170.

McClendon, S., Jr., (1958) Arch. Pediat. 75, 101.

McCray, W. E., (1965) J. La. State Med. Soc. 117, 232.

McLaughlin, B. E., (1957) Pa. Med. J. 60, 989.

McNair, D. M., Goldstein, A. P., Lorr, M., Cibelli, L. A., and Roth, I., (1965) Psychopharmacologia (Berlin) 7, 256.

Middlefell, R., (1960) Abstr. World Med. 27, 6.

Millen, F. J., (1957) Wis. Med. J. 56, 198.

Mooney, H. B., Ditman, K. S., and Cohen, S., (1961) Dis. Nerv. Syst. (suppl.) 22, 44.

Nicol, C. F., Tutton, J. C., and Smith, B. H., (1969) Neurology, Minneapolis 19, 332.

Norton, S., (1957) in "Psychotropic Drugs," Garattini, S. and Ghetti, V., Eds., Elsevier Publ., Amsterdam, p. 73.

Ostow, M., (1962) "Drugs in Psychoanalysis and Psychotherapy," Basic Books, New York.

Oswald, I., (1968) Pharmacol. Rev. 20, 273.

Oswald, L., Evans, J. I., and Lewis, S. A., (1969) in "Scientific Basis of Drug Dependence," Steinberg, H., Ed., Churchill Ltd., London.

Perlstein, M. A., (1956) J. Amer. Med. Assoc. 161, 1040.

Pernikoff, M., (1960) Clin. Med. 7, 2313.

Phillips, B. M., Miya, T. S., and Yim, G. K. W., (1962) J. Pharmacol. Exper. Ther. 135, 223.

Prigot, A., Garnes, A. L., and Barnard, R. D., (1957) Harlem Hosp. Bull. 10, 63.

Proctor, R. C., (1959) in "The Pharmacology and Clinical Usefulness of Carisoprodol," Wayne State University Press, Detroit.

Raab, E., Richels, K., and Moore, E., (1964) Amer. J. Psychiat. 120, 1005.

Randall, L. O., (1960) Dis. Nerv. Syst. (suppl. 1) 21, 7.

Randall, L. O., (1961) Dis. Nerv. Syst. (suppl. 7) 22, 1.

Randall, L. O. and Schallek, W., (1968) in "Psychopharmacology: A Review of Progress 1957-1967," Efron, D. H., Ed., Public Health Ser. Publ. no. 1836, Washington, D.C., p. 153.

Randall, L. O., Schallek, W. B., Heise, G. A., Keith, E. F., and Bagdon, R. E., (1960) J. Pharmacol. Exper. Ther. 129, 163.

Randall, L. O., Schallek, W., Scheckel, C. L., Stefko, P. L., Banziger, R. F., Pool, W., and Moe, R. A., (1969) Arch. Int. Pharmacodyn. Thér., 178, 216.

Randall, L. O., Scheckel, C. L., and Banziger, R. F., (1965) Curr. Ther. Res. 7, 590.

Randall, L. O., Scheckel, C. L., and Pool, W., (1970) Arch. Int. Pharmacodyn. Thér. 185, 135.

Reinhardt, D. J., (1962) Del. Med. J. 34, 171.

Réquin, S., Lanoir, J., Plas, R., and Naquet, R., (1963) C. R. Soc. Biol. 157, 2015.

Rickels, K., Clark, T. W., Ewing, J. H., Klingensmith, W. C., Morris, H. M., and Smock, C. D., (1959) J. Amer. Med. Assoc. 171, 1649.

Rickels, K., Downing, R. W., and Howard, K., (1971) Clin. Pharmacol. Ther. (part 1) 12, 263.

Rickels, K., Raab, E., De Silverio, R., and Etemad, B., (1967) J. Amer. Med. Assoc. 201, 675.

Rinaldi, F., Rudy, L. H., and Himwich, H. E., (1955) Amer. J. Psychiat. 112, 343.

Rinaldi, F., Rudy, L. H., and Himwich, H. E., (1956) Amer. J. Psychiat. 113, 678.

Robichaud, R. C., Gylys, J. A., Sledge, K. L., and Hillyard, I. W., (1970) Arch. Int. Pharmacodyn. Thér. 185, 213.

Rosenstein, I. N. and Silverblatt, C. W., (1961) J. Amer. Geriat. Soc. 9, 1003.

Sachs, E., Weingarten, M., and Klein, N. W., Jr., (1966) Psychopharmacologia (Berlin) 9, 17.

Salzman, C., Di Mascio, A., Shader, R. I., and Harmatz, J. S., (1969) Psychopharmacologia (Berlin) 14, 38.

Sarwer-Foner, G. J. and Koranyi, E. K., (1956) Can. Psychiat. Assoc. J. 1, 92.

Schallek, W., (1960) Dis. Nerv. Syst. (suppl.) 21, 64.

Schallek, W., Kovacs, J., Kuehn, A., and Thomas, J., (1970) Arch. Int. Pharmacodyn. Thér. 185, 149.

Schallek, W. and Kuehn, A., (1963) Proc. Soc. Exper. Biol. Med. 112, 813.

Schallek, W. and Kuehn, A., (1965a) in "Progress in Brain Research," vol. 18 "Sleep Mechanisms," Akert, K., Bally, C., and Schadé, J. P., Eds., Elsevier Publ., Amsterdam, p. 231.

Schallek, W. and Kuehn, A., (1965b) Med. Pharmacol. Exper. 12, 204.

Schallek, W., Kuehn, A., and Jew, N., (1962) Ann. N.Y. Acad. Sci. 96, 303.

Schallek, W., Zabransky, F., and Kuehn, A., (1964) Arch. Int. Pharmacodyn. Thér. 149, 467.

Scherbel, A. L., (1961) Amer. Pract. Dig. Treat. 12, 275.

Schillings, R. T., Shrader, S. R., and Ruelius, H. W., (1971) Arzneim.-Forsch. 21, 1059.

Schram, W. S., (1959) Dis. Nerv. Syst. 20, 3.

Schrappe, O., (1971) Arzneim.-Forsch. 21, 1079.

Seeherman, R., (1964) Del. Med. J. 36, 213.

Settel, E., (1957) Amer. Pract. Dig. Treat. 8, 1584.

Sharman, D. F., (1966) Brit. J. Pharmacol. 28, 153.

Shepherd, M., Lader, M., and Rodnight, R., (1968) "Clinical Psychopharmacology," The English University Press, London.

Silvestrini, B. and Kohn, R., (1958) Rec. Ist. Sup. Sanità 21, 328.

Smith, R. G., (1961) J. New Drugs 1, 59.

Smyth, D. and Pennington, G. W., (1963) Arch. Int. Pharmacodyn. Thér. 145, 154.

Sparup, K. H., (1957) Lancet 2, 807.

Spears, C. E., (1959) in "The Pharmacology and Clinical Usefulness of Carisoprodol," Wayne State University Press, Detroit.

Stanfield, C. E., (1961) Psychosomatics 2, 179.

Stern, F. H., (1964) J. Amer. Geriat. Soc. 12, 1006.

Sternbach, L. H., Randall, L. O., and Gustafson, S. R., (1964) in "Psychopharmacological Agents," vol. 1, Gordon, M., Ed., Academic Press, New York, p. 138.

Stonehill, E., Lee, H., and Ban, T. A., (1966) Dis. Nerv. Syst. 27, 411.

Superstine, E. and Sulman, F. G., (1966) Arch. Int. Pharmacodyn. Thér. 160, 133.

Svenson, S. E. and Hamilton, R. G., (1966) Curr. Ther. Res. 8, 455.

Taylor, K. M. and Laverty, R., (1969) Europ. J. Pharmacol. 8, 296.

Thomas, J. C., (1966) cited by Cohen, S., Ditman, K. S., and Gustafson, S. R., in "Psychochemotherapy," Western Medical Publ., Los Angeles.

Ticktin, H. E. and Schultz, J. D., (1960) Dis. Nerv. Syst. 21, suppl., 49.

Toll, N., (1960) Dis. Nerv. Syst. 21, 264.

Trimpi, H. D., (1959) in "The Pharmacology and Clinical Usefulness of Carisoprodol," Wayne State University Press, Detroit.

Tucker, K. and Wilensky, H., (1957) Amer. J. Psychiat. 113, 698.

Valzelli, L., (1967) in "Advances in Pharmacology," vol. 5, Garattini, S. and Shore, P. A., Eds., Academic Press, New York, p. 79.

Valzelli, L., (1969) Psychopharmacologia (Berlin) 15, 232.

Valzelli, L., (1971) in "Atti della Tavola Rotonda Sulle Associazioni Psicofarmacologiche" (Simp. "Il Ciocco", November 1970) Di Carlo, F. and Germano, G., Eds., Pacini Editore, Pisa, p. 62.

Valzelli, L., (1973) in "The Benzodiazepines", Garattini, S. and Randall, L. O., Eds., Raven Press, New York.

Valzelli, L., Giacalone, E., and Garattini, S., (1967) Europ. J. Pharmacol. 2, 144.

Valzelli, L., Ghezzi, D., and Bernasconi, S., (1971) Totus Homo 3, 73.

Viscott, D. S., (1968) Arch. Gen. Psychiat. 19, 370.

Walkenstein, S. S., Knebel, C. M., MacMullen, J. A., and Seifter, J., (1958) J. Pharmacol. Exper. Ther. 123, 254.

Wein, A. B., (1959) in "The Pharmacology and Clinical Usefulness of Carisoprodol," Wayne State University Press, Detroit.

Williams, M. W., (1961) South Med. J. 54, 922.

Zakrzewska, F., Sujecka-Szymkiewicz, H., and Grabowski, K., (1965) Neurol. Neurochir. Psychiat. Pol. 15, 107.

Chapter X

THE ANTIDEPRESSANT DRUGS

One of the most important considerations in current pharmaco-psychiatric therapy is the availability of compounds for the treatment of depressive disorders and the stabilization of mood. Every physician who, even to a limited degree, has encountered these types of disorders, is aware of the profound difficulty with which the treatment of the symptoms of such disorders may be managed.

One of those factors which contributes to the complexity of the therapeutic problem is that in depressive illness it is common to observe a spontaneous remission of symptomatology as a typical characteristic of its cyclic course. However, an accurate analysis of this issue by LEHMANN (1966a) indicated that over a one month period, approximately 20 to 25% spontaneous remission occurred; a placebo increased the incidence of remission from 25 to 50%, while an effective antidepressant drug brought about remissions in 50 to 75% of the cases.

From a semantic point of view, it is useful to remember that the term "depression" has two meanings which do not necessarily overlap one another in the clinical and pharmacological areas. In fact, in a pharmacological context, depressing, depressant, and sometimes, less properly, "depressive agents" are defined as all those drugs or drug-induced mechanisms capable of decreasing the functional activity of an organ or of a system; while in a psychiatric context depression indicates a pathological sequence characterized by a particular orientation of individual mood modulation, accompanied by either a psychological or physiological symptomatological sequence; in general, this term in this context does not necessarily imply the existence of a depression in the pharmaco-physiological sense involving some particular organ or system. From this general approach and use of the term it becomes apparent that the necessity of stimulant properties for an antidepressant drug is obviated, even though the term itself might suggest the need for stimulation.

With the complexities of mood disorders characterized by manic-depressive syndromes, it should also be recalled that the classic alternation between manic and depressive episodes, from which this behavior disorder acquired its name, may not always be quite clearly separable, since it is possible to have a series of episodes in which one phase predominates; this is more often the depressive one (Fig. 46). All these considerations are further complicated by the distribution of patients under consideration into homogenous categories for the purpose of pharmaco-therapeutic experiments; this, to an equal extent, complicates the evaluation of the clinical efficacy of a given drug being used as antidepressant.

Another source of uncertainty in the systematization of the data obtained derives from the lack of uniform agreement concerning the eti-

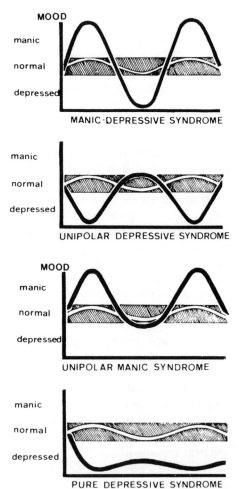

Fig. 46. Different types of manic-depressive syndromes.

ology of the outburst of the depressive manifestations; these are mainly considered as the reactive or the exogenous form and the endogenous form, depending upon the possible identification of some causative external events. This distinction has been historically preserved (LEWIS, 1934), and accepted as a contemporary distinction (KILOH and GARSIDE, 1963) not irrelevant to pharmaco-therapeutic consideration, when it is remembered that some antidepressant agents seem to be more suitable for the treatment of one type of syndrome rather than another one.

Finally, it may also be considered that there are no experimental models at the animal level which reproduce or represent a laboratory analogue of all aspects of human depression.

From this very rapid and superficial evaluation of the problem of depressive syndromes, it should become evident that this issue, when presented earlier to the experimenter or to the clinician, is beset with complexities which point to the importance of pharmacological management of the manifold aspects of the varieties of depressive disorders.

A) MONOAMINE OXIDASE INHIBITORS (MAOI)

The use of monoamine oxidase inhibitors in the treatment of depressive disorders derives from observation that the treatment of tubercular pneumonia with isoniazid induced an elevation of the patient's mood (ROBITZEK et al., 1952). This finding prompted clinicians to test the antidepressive properties of this compound (DELAY et al., 1952), which was not conventionally employed in psychiatric treatment because of its dangerous side effects. Clinical and experimental experiments were initiated and carried out subsequent to the synthesis of the isoniazid isopropilic derivative, iproniazid, which immediately showed its efficacy as an antidepressant and euphoriant (SELIKOFF et al., 1952), while ZELLER et al. (1952) demonstrated its potent inhibitory effect upon the activity of the monoamine oxidases; it is from these two observations that the interpretation of depressive disorders was considered in biochemical terms.

This attractive but over-simplified a posteriori hypothesis was initially proposed by KLINE et al. (1957) on the basis of observations that the antidepressive effect of iproniazid was associated with a large increase in brain serotonin and norepinephrine levels, whereas the depressant activity of reserpine was coincident with a very pronounced decrease in the brain levels of these neurochemical mediators. Moreover, a biochemical interpretation of the affective disorders provided a fertile ground upon which several psychodynamic interpretations were suggested; according to OSTOW (1962) the action of MAOI induces an overabundance of Id energies which provide feelings of joy and optimism experienced by patients. With increasing doses, a further increase of such energies occurs which compromises Ego integrity with the appearance of anxiety. More massive doses induce such intense Id energies as to induce a collapse of Ego defenses, and the appearance of neurotic or psychotic manifestations which seldom occur during the course of treatment with these derivatives.

Iproniazid, mainly because of its toxicity, provided impetus to the synthesis of a series of active derivatives whether of the hydrazine type, such as isocarboxazid, nialamide, and phenelzine, or of the nonhydrazine type, such as phenylcyclopropylamine. However, the side effects of these substances, also defined as thymeretics because of their mood stimulating activity, are so numerous that their therapeutic utilization gradually diminished in favor of a second category of antidepressant drugs, the so-called imipraminic or tricyclic compounds (or also "thymoleptics" for their mood-stabilizing activity) which are safer to use and more specific in action.

From a practical point of view, iproniazid will be taken as a representative of the hydrazine MAOI category and *tranylcypromine* will be selected as a representative of the nonhydrazines.

1) General Aspects

The *absorption* of either hydrazine or nonhydrazine MAOI derivatives is very rapid, so that after just twenty minutes following a single dose of iproniazid it is possible to find the highest concentrations in the brain (HESS et al., 1958; NAIR, 1959) from where it disappears after twenty minutes, whereas 48 hours are required for complete *excretion* of this substance from the body to occur; the elimination of tranylcypromine is more rapid and may be considered complete within 24 hours following administration (ALLEVA, 1963). The enzymatic blockade induced by these substances obviously takes place in all those tissue sites which have mono-aminergic activity. However, aside from the generality of this concept, there is a certain degree of selectivity of the inhibitor for a final target depending upon the route of administration; intraperitoneal administration has an equal affinity for both the hepatic and cerebral enzymes, the oral route provides the greatest blockade of hepatic enzymes as compared with cerebral ones, while subcutaneous administration exerts a more potent inhibition upon brain than upon hepatic enzymatic activity (BAN, 1969). In any case, the inhibitory effects of MAOI persist for a period of time beyond that required for the elimination of the drug from the body, so that after a single administration of iproniazid cerebral monoamine oxidase activity is inhibited for more than six days (KOECHLIN and ILIEV, 1959). Inhibition persisting for as long as 30 days has been demonstrated for other compounds of this class of drugs and there is also the reported possibility of an irreversibly induced inhibition of enzyme activity (BIEL et al., 1964).

Generally, the degradative products of these drugs consist of (a) isonicotinic acid, (b) hippuric acid, and (c) monobenzoate glycuronic acid for the hydrazine derivatives, while for tranylcypromine the main metabolites consist of (a) hydroxycinnamic acid and (b) benzoic acid; the *excretion* of all these metabolic products occurs through the kidneys.

As in the case of reserpine, the *pharmacology* of these substances may be generally interpreted as the consequence of metabolic impairment in the metabolism of specific neurochemical mediators. The changes in these amine's biochemistry are in the opposite direction to those resulting from reserpine treatment; i.e., norepinephrine and serotonin levels are elevated in the brain. MAO inhibitors may be subdivided into (1) reversible, short-lasting derivatives (direct stimulants), (2) irreversible, long-lasting derivatives (indirect stimulants), and (3) derivatives with intermediate activity (bimodal stimulants). Typical of this last category are the hydrazine derivatives in general, such as iproniazid, *isocarboxazid, phenyprazine, phenelzine, nialamide* and, among the nonhydrazine derivatives, tranylcypromine, the harmane derivatives, such as *harmine* and *harmaline* which belong to the first cateogry, but are rarely employed in clinical practice (PLETSCHER, 1963) (Fig. 47).

The inhibition of monoamine oxidase activity in mitochondria induced by these substances obviously cause effects upon all the metabolic events associated with *neurochemical mediators*. As previously considered in Chapter III, the more obvious and significant effects in the brain upon putative transmitters involve serotonin, since monoamine oxidase action thereon

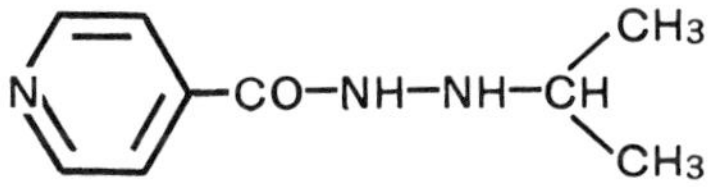

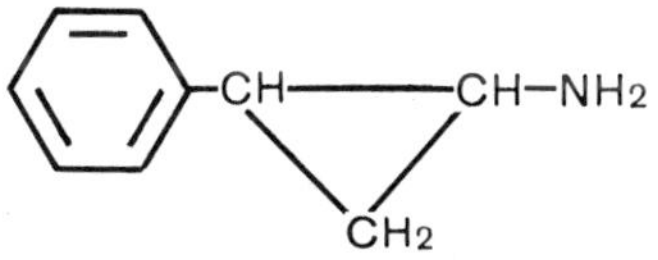

Fig. 47. (A) Iproniazid; (B) tranylcypromine.

represents the main degradative pathway; brain catecholamines, on the other hand, can be metabolized extraneuronally by COMT (Fig. 48). The consequence of MAO inhibition is an increase in brain serotonin level and in norepinephrine and dopamine content in all tissue sites where these amines are stored, yet the magnitude of the increase is greater for serotonin than for the other two neurochemical molecules.

This finding suggests that the metabolic fate of many other endogenous substances or administered drugs may be modified considerably when their inactivation is partially or totally dependent upon the functional integrity of monoamine oxidase enzymes. Many of the pharmacological interactions of MAOI with other drugs are based upon this contingency; such effects observed in clinical practice may be dependent upon the potentiation of a biologically active constituent, such as tyramine, which is present in some foods and capable of inducing very serious interactive side effects.

The effects induced by these drugs is largely of the sympathomimetic type which are, however, difficult to clearly observe after only a single administration; they instead become evident after some days of treatment. Generally the only signs that are quite easily observable in experimental animals consist of hyperthermia and hyperexcitation; both of these parameters become much more evident when the precursors of brain monoamines are administered together with the MAO inhibitors (GARATTINI and VALZELLI, 1960).

With respect to other more general aspects of *brain biochemistry,* some compounds initiate the inactivation of other oxidative enzymes such as diamine oxidases methylamino oxidases, and choline oxidases, or may cause an increase in glycolysis processes; phenyprazine also induces an inhibition of hypothalamic succinic-dehydrogenases (BAN, 1969).

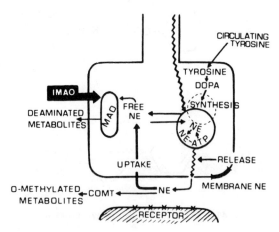

Fig. 48. MAOI activity upon synaptic mechanism.

The *neuropharmacology* of MAO inhibitors is mainly represented by a blockade of nerve transmission at the levels of the autonomic ganglia and by a depression of neural transmission at the spinal level. Moreover, some derivatives such as phenyprazine, have local anaesthetic properties, and others, particularly the hydrazines, possess some clear analgesic effects (BAN, 1969). HIMWICH (1965) was able to demonstrate an alerting effect of these substances on the components of the reticular formation, arguing against central activation related to serotonin increase at the bulbar level; some experimental studies have suggested, as well, that MAO inhibitors induce an increase in the excitability of the nuclei of the amygdala (SCHALLEK and KUEHN, 1963; KUEHN and SCHALLEK, 1965). Electro-encephalographic activity is affected differently by these substances, so that either desynchronization or synchronization of the record may both occur, as well as a succession of both effects. In any case, the effects are considered to be dependent upon the relative variations in brain monoamine levels, particularly as far as the relationship between norepinephrine and serotonin levels as well as their rate of synthesis and degradation or their turnover (COHEN et al., 1967) are concerned.

2) Behavioral Effects

The behavioral effects of the monoamine oxidase inhibitors are neither very intense nor clearly observable, and they only become generally evident after repeated drug treatment in animals, mainly as sympathomimetic effects, such as a slight hyperthermia, hyperactivity and mydriasis; these effects may be considered as dependent upon an increase in brain norepi-nephrine (BRODIE et al., 1959). There are no obvious effects of MAO inhibitors on learning, aggressiveness, exploratory behavior, or other related parameters, while the *pharmacological interactions* of these inhibitors with other substances are certainly more apparent. For instance, the administra-tion of reserpine to animals previously treated with iproniazid, produces a complete reversal of the typical effects induced by this alkaloid, so that sedation is transformed to excitation, miosis to mydriasis, hypothermia to hyperthermia, while blepharospasm, hypotension and bradycardia disappear and piloerection and hyperactivity emerge (CHESSIN et al., 1957; SHORE and BRODIE, 1957; GARATTINI et al., 1960). All these effects have been interpreted as being dependent upon the biochemistry of neurotransmitters massively released from their storage by reserpine, and not being inactivated by the blocked monamine oxidase enzymes they continuously flow onto the receptors, acting there for a prolonged time and causing a sustained stimulation.

The intensity of the antireserpine effect of MAO inhibitors varies depending upon the specific compound considered and, generally, only becomes evident when the monoamine oxidase inhibitor is administered preceding the reserpine. Moreover, the antireserpine effect is not exclusive to MAO inhibitors but may also be induced by the tricyclic antidepressant drugs of the imipramine type; these are completely void of any monoamine oxidase blocking activity.

Interactions also occur between the MAOI and other substances, such as barbiturates, the narcotic properties of which are potentiated due to a block of their intrahepatic oxidation (FOUTS and BRODIE, 1956).

It is well known that MAO inhibitors interact metabolically with many other substances such as aminopyrine, acetanilide, cocaine, and meperidine (BIEL, 1964; JARVIK, 1965; PLETSCHER, 1965; SOURKES, 1962). Two specific metabolic interactions, which are very important because of their extremely hazardous effects during the course of clinical treatment, are the association of the monoamine oxidase inhibitors with tricyclic antidepressants or with the intake of some exogenous substances such as tyramine.

In the case of the former, some very serious behavioral alterations have been observed, both in the experimental animal (HIMWICH and PETERSEN, 1961) and in man (AYD, 1961), with the appearance of vertigo, perspiration, hyperthermia, restlessness, and excitement, probably due to the action of the imipramine derivatives which alter the function of the membrane pump (see Fig. 50) and, consequently, modify the reuptake of neurochemical mediators into the synaptic terminal. This effect augments the action of the monoamine oxidase inhibitors which, as previously described, lead to increases in the absolute level of brain monoamines at the synaptic endings.

In the second instance, tyramine, which is present in several foods such as cheeses, beer, Chianti wine, bird liver, snails, yeast extracts, milk, cream, and others, can induce some dangerous side effects in patients under treatment with MAOI, notably hypertension (BLACKWELL and MARLEY, 1964, 1966) which may even result in strokes and death. This effect is due to the fact that tyramine, which does not normally cause any troublesome effects because it is rapidly inactivated by monoamine oxidase, accumulates rapidly when these enzymes are blocked. It is also important to emphasize that such negative reactions may occur even after the cessation of therapy with MAOI while the enzymatic blockade of several such inhibitors may persist.

Moreover, these substances cause a potentiation of the convulsive activity of tryptamine, another exogenous molecule that is normally inactivated by monoamine oxidases (TEDESCHI et al., 1959), while they antagonize the convulsions induced by electroshock and pentylentetrazole (PROCKOP et al., 1959).

The monoamine oxidase inhibitors exert a direct effect upon the cycles of paradoxical or REM sleep, which are reduced in duration (TOYODA, 1964) or completely abolished by some of these compounds (JOUVET et al., 1965). Such effects, in accord with the prolonged duration of action of these substances, persists for a long time without causing any rebound effects as have been observed with other drugs (JOUVET, 1967).

3) Clinical Effects

The introduction of monoamine oxidase inhibitors into psychiatric practice, provoked a surprising interest in the clinical as well as the basic properties of these compounds. It has, in fact, been estimated that in the first ten months between 1957 and 1958, 380,000 patients were treated with iproniazid (HORDERN, 1965). Subsequently, with more stringently designed clinical studies and application of clear clinical criteria the clinical efficacy of these derivatives was redefined.

In psychiatric use, the most important indications for the MAOI are the *depressive syndromes,* ranging from the neurotic type to the reactive and catatonic-like varieties; the greatest efficacy of MAOI has been achieved in the management of atypical depressions (WEST and DALLY, 1959). Such drugs are, however, minimally active in the agitated-depressed patient. According to GALLINEK (1959), the most ideal subjects for iproniazide therapy are the inhibited depressed patients with somatizations and a neurotic profile. Favorable therapeutic results have also been obtained in manic-depressed subjects, while isocarboxazide has been best indicated in the treatment of the *involutional* and *neurotic depressions* (KLINE and STANLEY, 1959); phenelzine, on the other hand, is effective in the treatment of *reactive* and *atypic depressions* with hysteric foundations or components (SARGANT and SLATER, 1963); tranylcypromine has been mainly indicated in the treatment of psychoneurotic and reactive depressions, and for therapy in *involutional melancholia* and manic-depressive syndromes.

The monoamine oxidase inhibitors have been shown to even have positive effects for treatment of *psychoneuroses,* especially in cases with phobic-anxious components and hysterical conversion symptoms and in "psychasthenic-anhedonic" syndromes (ALEXANDER and BERKELEY, 1959), characterized by a chronic depressive state, hyperactivity, and absense of self-confidence (BAN, 1969).

These drugs have had little utility in the treatment of *functional schizophrenic psychoses* (SCHIELE et al., 1963).

The MAOI, as with many other psychotropic drugs, have found a series

of therapeutic indications outside of the psychiatric field, especially in the
treatment of *cardiovascular pathology*, Reynaud's disease, angina pectoris,
and essential hypertension (MODELL, 1962; HOROWITZ and
SJOERDSMA, 1963; GESSA et al., 1963). These vascular effects should not
be interpreted as dependent upon modification of monoamine levels, but
rather a consequence of the previously mentioned ganglionic blocking
action, and the bretylium-like properties shown by these drugs (GESSA et
al., 1963). Favorable therapeutic effects with MAOI have also been reported
in many inflammatory disorders such as rheumatoid arthritis, sclerodermia,
lupus erythematosus, ulcerative colitis, dermatomyositis, as well as several
other dermatological syndromes (BAN, 1969).

4) Undesirable Effects

Unfortunately, the monoamine oxidase inhibitors, aside from their useful
effects in many areas of human pathology, possess a number of dangerous
side effects which have contributed to the withdrawal from the pharmaceutical market of most of these compounds for use as antidepressant drugs.
Some of such negative effects constitute an absolute contraindication in all
cases of hepatic or renal damage, as well as in pheochromocitomas and in
overt manic syndromes.

Less hazardous contraindications are represented by cardiac failures,
cerebrovascular disturbances, schizophrenic syndromes and epilepsy; however, in these cases as well, the potential danger considerably outweighs the
expectation of therapeutic efficacy. Among the most seriously negative
effects there are those previously mentioned combinations with other drugs,
such as the tricyclic antidepressants, narcotics, alcohol, analgesics and anti-
pyretic drugs, epinephrine, amphetamine, or any pharmaceutical preparations containing amphetamine and barbiturates; besides this there is also the
need to carefully regulate diet, which must be maintained for some pre-
cautionary period of time after the interruption of any therapeutic treatment with MAOI.

Other more typically recognized side effects consist of orthostatic hypotension, blurring of vision, delay in micturition and ejaculation, impotence,
vascular headaches, and migraine exacerbation.

The side effects upon the central nervous system may differ as a function
of the inhibitor administered, so that, for instance, phenelzine can produce
somnolence while tranylcypromine has stimulant effects, due to its amphetamine-like structure, and can induce insomnia, pharmacological dependence
and abuse (LE GASSICKE et al., 1964), toxic pyschoses, and reactivation of
schizophrenic symptoms.

B) TRICYCLIC ANTIDEPRESSANTS

The tricyclic antidepressants, so called for their molecular configuration in which two benzene rings are bound with an heterocyclic ring, may be considered the present successors of the monoamine oxidase inhibitors for the treatment of the depressive disorders. These drugs have also been designated as thymoleptics or mood equilibrators, or iminodibenzyl derivatives from their basic chemical structure. It is quite interesting to note that for several years the theoretical bases for such derivatives were available and it has been only recently that the most chemically effective compounds have come into routine psychopharmacological use; the first chemical synthesis and description of tricyclic compounds was in 1899 (THIELE and HOLZINGER, 1899). It was only later on, however, that some derivatives of this original nucleus were studied for their antihistaminic, anti-Parkinsonian, hypnotic, and sedative properties (SCHINDLER and HÄFLIGER, 1954). These studies came from an analogue of chlorpromazine structure, an iminodibenzyl derivative of promazine, *impramine* (Fig. 49), that was introduced for clinical experimentation and evaluation for its possible tranquilizer and antipsychotic properties.

It is well known that imipramine is relatively ineffective in the treatment of schizophrenic disorders, but is very chemically active in the treatment of depressions, particularly in the endogenous ones (KUHN, 1957, 1958). These observations have been confirmed by several investigators (LEHMANN et al., 1958) and initiated research to evolve other agents capable of potentiating imipramine activity; this led to the synthesis of several other compounds which have been described pharmacologically as imipramine-like.

Generally the action of these compounds has been interpreted from a psychodynamic point of view as leading to the induction of a different projective orientation for aggressive drives of the patient from inside to outside, with a secondary reorganization of the libido, a decrease of guilt

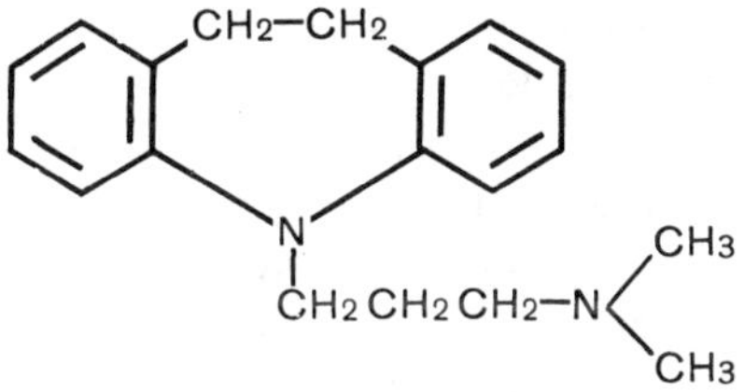

Fig. 49. Imipramine.

feelings, and a shift of attention from the inner to the outer environment, allowing for the dissolution of the depressive syndrome (AZIMA, 1961).

As previously mentioned, the many forms which the depressive syndromes display, together with the availability of antidepressive agents having both stimulant as well as sedative properties, emphasize the need for an accurate evaluation and diagnostic conclusion for each clinical case before therapeutic treatment is initiated; in such a way, only the most appropriate compounds are utilized to obtain a maximum clinical effect with a minimum of undesirable side effects.

1) General Aspects

From a general point of view there are some similarities between tricyclic antidepressants and phenothiazines insofar as absorption, tissue distribution, and metabolism.

The *absorption* of the tricyclic antidepressants occurs easily and rapidly, within about five to ten minutes following intraperitoneal administration and not more than 30 to 60 minutes following oral intake (BERNHARD and BEER, 1962; HAYDU et al., 1962; HERRMANN and PULVER, 1960). These drugs concentrate mainly in the brain and kidneys, while the liver appears to take up only small quantities. The *metabolism* of these drugs is very active, so that only small quantities are eliminated as unaltered compounds (KLERMAN and COLE, 1965) while the maximum portion is demethylated, oxidized to the nitrogen, hydroxylated, and conjugated (GILLETTE et al., 1960; PSCHEIDT, 1962; DINGELL et al., 1964).

The demethylation is particularly important, not only from a quantitative point of view, but also because for some derivatives, such as imipramine and *amitryptiline,* this metabolic process provides for pharmacologically active derivatives, which are among the tricyclic derivatives available for psychiatric use. Such derivatives are, respectively, *desmethylimipramine* or DMI and *noramitryptiline* (GILLETTE et al., 1961; BURT et al., 1962). However, several differences in the metabolism of these drugs occur depending upon the species treated, so that while rabbits and mice metabolize either imipramine or desmethylimipramine at the same intensity, rat and man metabolize desmethylimipramine more slowly than imipramine. This finding explains why DMI accumulates in rat and human tissues but not in those of rabbit and mouse (SULSER and DINGELL, 1966). Moreover, while human hepatic microsomes metabolize imipramine maximally to DMI, those of the rabbit transform it essentially to 2-hydroxyimipramine (DINGELL et al., 1962, 1964).

Metabolite *excretion* occurs maximally through the urinary route while elimination through the intestinal route accounts for only one-third of the total amount. From a clinical point of view it has been observed that low levels of plasma concentration and elimination of these drugs are present for those patients who respond favorably to the treatment, while both the plasma and excretory levels remain relatively elevated for those subjects who do not respond to the therapy (BAN, 1966, 1967).

The general *pharmacology* of imipramine is characterized by a series of anticholinergic effects including hypotension, compensatory tachycardia and mild mydriasis (SIGG, 1959); associated with an antiserotonin effect are hypothermia and antiemesis which are less marked than those produced by chlorpromazine, as well as antihistaminic activity which is more intense than that produced by the phenothiazines (DOMENJOZ and THEOBALD, 1959). Moreover, the tricyclic drugs induce a slight sedative effect in experimental animals (VERNIER, 1961; MAXWELL and PALMER, 1961; THEOBALD et al., 1964), as well as obvious analgesic activity (CHARPEN-TIER and SOULAIRAC, 1963; OPITZ and BORCHERT, 1968); some of them produce an anorexigenic effect in animals (SANTI and FASSINA, 1965). The *neuropharmacology* of these substances is characterized by their depressing effect upon the alarm reaction of reticular origin, while in animals they effect a convulsant rhinencephalic activity originating in the hippocampus, and increase the excitability of the amygdala (SCHMITT, 1967). These observations are of importance in that they may provide an interpretive basis for depressive syndromes by emphasis upon an increase of the inhibitor activity of the amygdala over the hypothalamus (HOROVITZ, 1967; BARRATT and PRAY, 1965; STEIN, 1967). Tricyclic derivations were also shown to exert a desynchronizing effect on electronencephalographic activity with the appearance of specific signs of cortical excitation which resemble those induced by anticholinergic psychotomimetic substances (FINK, 1959).

Of great interest are the effects of the tricyclic drugs on brain *neurochemical mediators*, since they are believed to be important bases for both the experimental and therapeutic effects of these derivatives. Of those different mechanisms which regulate the biochemical mediation of the nerve impulse, the tricyclic antidepressants act by effecting a blockade of the membrane pump and thereby altering the reuptake of neurochemical mediators into the synaptic endings. The effect depends upon a type of "impermeability" exerted by these substances upon the external membrane of different animal cells (CARLSSON, 1966a), where they are believed to accumulate and impair the retrieval of the mediators by the cell (BOULLIN and O'BRIEN, 1968) (Fig. 50).

This situation generally brings about an augmentation and a prolongation of the effects of serotonin, norepinephrine, and, probably, of other biologically active molecules; the potentiation of some of the peripheral proper-

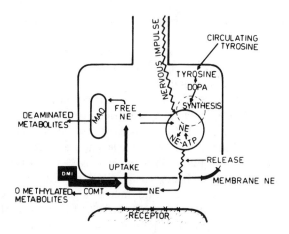

Fig. 50. Desipramine (DMI) activity upon synaptic mechanism.

ties of serotonin induced by imipramine derivatives (GYERMEK and POSSEMATO, 1960; BESENDORF et al., 1962; SABELLI and SINAY, 1960) may therefore be referred to as a block in uptake of the circulating serotonin by the platelets (STACEY, 1961; AXELROD and INSCOE, 1963; COCKRILL et al., 1968). A similar situation also seems to be present in the central nervous system (SABELLI and SINAY, 1960; LAPIN et al., 1968), primarily for some specific agents such as *chlorimipramine* (MEEK et al., 1970).

It is through the same mechanism that these drugs potentiate the effects of the catecholamines, both peripherally and centrally (SCHAEPPI, 1960; SIGG, 1959; FEKETE and MACSEK, 1968; JORI and GARATTINI, 1965; GLOWINSKI, 1967), and, in accord with the concept of "feedback" by which monoamine metabolism is automatically regulated, an increase of their synthesis rate would occur in the brain (NEFF and COSTA, 1967). Studies of ROSS and CARLSSON seem to exclude the dopaminergic endings from effects by the tricyclic antidepressants (ROSS and RENYI, 1967; CARLSSON, 1966b); moreover, these drugs do not show any inhibitory activity on monoamine oxidase (PLETSCHER and GEY, 1959; KIVALO et al., 1961).

The biochemical effect of tricyclic antidepressants in the brain implies that a greater quantity of catecholamines are present at adrenergic receptors; this would agree with and support biochemical theories of the affective disorders and depression in man (SCHILDKRAUT et al., 1964; SCHILD-KRAUT, 1965; DEWHURST, 1965) which have essentially interpreted depression as dependent on the impairment of brain noradrenergic functions. Such an interpretation is not completely arbitrary, since in patients undergoing spontaneous remission of their depressive illness, it may be observed that there is an increased urinary elimination of normetanephrine (SCHILDKRAUT, 1965) similar to what occurs during the course of therapy with imipramine, which also induces a reduction of urinary vanillylmandelic acid (SCHILDKRAUT et al., 1964). These observations assume some importance when they are linked to the fact that vanillylmandelic acid derives from the metabolism of intraneuronal norepinephrine (and is therefore not utilized in the synaptic transmission), while normetanephrine, produced by the extraneuronal inactivation of norepinephrine through COMT, reflects that fraction of the mediator which comes in contact with the receptor (SCHANBERG et al., 1967; KOPIN, 1966); so that, the changes observed in depressed patients may be interpreted as a better utilization, either spontaneous or induced by the antidepressant drugs, of norepinephrine which coincides with an improvement of symptomatology. With respect to other parameters of brain *biochemistry,* imipramine and amitryptiline increase the levels of cerebral adenosinetriphosphate which has been related to the antidepressive activity exerted by these drugs (LEWIS and VAN PETTEN, 1963).

2) Behavioral Effects

The behavioral effects of the tricyclic antidepressants in laboratory animals are generally not obvious or particularly significant, especially at low and medium dosages, whereas high doses of these drugs can induce changes not unlike those typical of the phenothiazines.

The *motor activity* in animals is minimally affected by imipramine (ITOH and TAKAORI, 1968), while at higher doses of this compound or of desipramine a moderate reduction of locomotor behavior is induced (KUMADAKI et al., 1967). These drugs have little effect on the *hyperemotional behavior* of rats induced by surgical ablation of the olfactory bulbs (KUMADAKI et al., 1967) or with electrical stimulation of the hypothalamus (BAXTER, 1968). *Exploratory behavior* in the mouse (BOISSIER et al., 1964) tends to be affected more in the normal mouse than in the aggressive one (VALZELLI, 1969). Imipramine and desipramine are also mildly effective in attenuating the intensity of *aggressiveness induced by isolation* in mice (VALZELLI, 1967; VALZELLI et al., 1967) as well as reducing the behavior of spontaneously aggressive mice (BOISSIER et al., 1968); these compounds block muricide behavior, both in genetically selected muricidal rats (HOROVITZ, 1965) and in those obtained after prolonged isolation (VALZELLI, 1971; VALZELLI and BERNASCONI, 1971). The difference in action exerted by the drugs in these two experimental models of altered behavior, suggest that the etiology and expression of aggressive behavior in the rat and mouse are not based upon single factors, so that a common behavioral response may be expected from tricyclic antidepressants.

Neither imipramine nor desipramine have been shown to have any important effect upon *learning* processes; with avoidance techniques, it has been possible to observe, at the highest doses, a performance decrement in experimental animals, which is more intense with amitriptyline than for the two previous substances (SIGG, 1959; DEWS, 1962; HANSON, 1961; KORNETSKY, 1963). However, the minimal effects induced by tricyclic antidepressants in "normal" animals generally corresponds to a comparable lack of effects of such compounds in the normal man (DI MASCIO et al., 1964), emphasizing in both cases, the necessity for the presence of evident psychopathology to completely reflect their action.

The *interactions* of imipramine and other tricyclic derivatives with other drugs have been more obvious experimentally; the first indication of this has come from the observation that imipramine prevents and antagonizes some aspects of reserpine symptomatology in the rat (GARATTINI, 1958; COSTA et al., 1960).

Such effects are common to other thymoleptics and are also generally developed toward other reserpine-like derivatives such as tetrabenazine and benzquinolizine. From a practical point of view, there are several characteristic symptoms induced by reserpine including inhibition of ptosis (MAXWELL and PALMER, 1961; WILSON and TISLOW, 1962) and hypothermia (ASKEW, 1963; VERNIER et al., 1962; BERNARDI et al., 1966; GARATTINI and JORI, 1967) which are much more specific effects in the experimental evaluation of the efficacy of thymoleptics than their action upon other parameters, such as, for example, the reduction of motor activity (SCHANBERG et al., 1967). Another experimental procedure for the evaluation of the activity of the imipramine-derivatives consists of the potentiation of the behavioral effects of amphetamine, which is considered as indicative of thymoleptic activity in contrast to the tranquilizing effect exerted by phenothiazines (WEISSMAN, 1961; SCHECKEL and BOFF, 1964; MORPURGO and THEOBALD, 1965); this is especially apparent when techniques such as conditioning (JOHNSON and GOLDBERG, 1965) or hypothalamic self-stimulation (STEIN and SEIFTER, 1961) are employed. Recent data indicate that such potentiation suggests the importance of cell membrane impermeability to imipramine derivatives, so that contact with liver microsomal enzymes by circulating amphetamine is prevented; otherwise the drug cannot be metabolized, and persists in the body for an extended time with consequently prolonged activity (CONSOLO et al., 1967).

Tricyclic antidepressants also exert an anticholinergic effect (BENESOVA and TRINEROVA, 1964; CARLSSON et al., 1957) which is however not indicative of their antidepressive properties (RATHBUN and SLATER, 1963; BENNET, 1962; ZETLER, 1968; BRIMBLECOMBE and GREEN, 1967).

A very good critical review of these problems has recently been summarized by JORI (1972).

Tricyclic antidepressants have been reported to reduce REM cycles in man (OSWALD, 1968).

3) Clinical Effects

The tricyclic antidepressant drugs have been successfully employed in the treatment of a series of behavior disorders, which range from the functional psychoses to the neuroses and the personality disorders. All of the imipramine derivatives, including imipramine and desipramine as well as amitriptyline, *nortriptyline, trimipramine,* and *protriptyline* have been shown to exert their greatest efficacy in the treatment of *endogenous depressions;* recent work has also indicated the possibility of positive results in the treatment of *reactive depressions.* A series of clinical observations indicates that the best therapeutic results are obtained in those forms of depression that are objectified by the patient with accompanying physical discomfort, insomnia, and loss of appetite.

From comprehensive critical reviews by KLERMAN and COLE (1965) and LEHMANN (1966b) dealing with clinical research with antidepressant drugs, it has been concluded that imipramine, desipramine, and nortriptyline are all superior in efficacy to a placebo and are at least equal to the effects of electroconvulsive shock treatment in the management of depressive illness (OLTMAN and FRIEDMAN, 1961; WILSON et al., 1963). Moreover, studies have indicated that amitriptyline possesses a therapeutic efficacy greater than that of imipramine (BURT et al., 1962; HOENIG and VISRAM, 1964; HOLLISTER et al., 1964; HORDERN et al., 1964; SNOW and RICKELS, 1964) while there do not seem to be any significant differences between imipramine and desipramine (ROSE and WESTHEAD, 1964; WILSON et al., 1963). The manifold aspects of *schizophrenia* have also been considered with regard to tricyclic compounds; amitriptyline and desipramine can be useful in the treatment of the schizo-affective and cyclophrenic psychoses and in the depressive hypochondrial syndromes that are present in some schizophrenic subjects, while imipramine and trimipramine appear to be less effective in this area.

It is however, important to note that chronic anergic schizophrenic patients may become hostile, aggressive and agitated when treated with imipramine, which can reactivate delusions and hallucinations (FELDMAN, 1959).

With respect to the *psychoneuroses*, WITTENBORN (1962, 1967) maintains that the therapeutic efficacy of imipramine is comparable to that of electroconvulsive shock therapy in the treatment of neurotic depressions. Amitriptyline and trimipramine are particularly suitable in the treatment of those depressive syndromes in which an axiety component is dominant; particularly, patients with somatizations, respond favorably to nortriptyline while desipramine is more appropriate in psychoasthenic subjects.

Although tricyclic antidepressants have been most typically utilized for behavior disorders characterized in some respects by depressive pathology, conditions of less clinical importance have also been favorably managed with these drugs. Some of these are child behavior disorders, such as nocturnal enuresis, nail biting, hostility outbursts, exaggerated disobedience, and school-phobias (BAN, 1969).

The therapeutic indications for the major representatives of the tricyclic antidepressants, can be generally listed as follows (BAN, 1966): *imipramine,* in endogenous depressions, without an anxiety component or thought disturbances (especially in young men); *trimipramine,* in depressive syndromes in which an anxiolitic and sedative effect is required, and particularly in involutional melancholia; *desipramine,* in the depressions with psychomotor blockade and an absence of internal drives; *opipramol* in psychoneuroses in which a sedative and tranquilizing effect is required; *carbamazepine* in epileptic disorders with affective psychopathological components; *amitriptyline,* in endogenous depressions with psychopathological variations of perceptive and cognitive functions, particularly in older patients; *protriptyline,* in neurotic depressions and *nortriptyline* in reactive depressions, and in psychosomatic disturbances.

4) Undesirable Effects

Therapy with the tricyclic antidepressants, particularly when utilized at high doses, can produce a series of side effects, involving different organs and systems, which range from a slight functional impairment to a series of more serious manifestations.

Insomnia, restlessness and excitement or feeling of weakness, fatigue, and somnolence can become equally evident; this occurs normally in a transitory manner during the earliest phases of therapy. Hypomanic excitation or toxic confusional psychosis can also occur, as well as possible reactivation of a latent schizophrenia (LEYBERG and DENMARK, 1959; FULLERTON and BOARDMAN, 1959). The tricyclic antidepressants do not induce any extra-pyramidal-like effects but in some patients they can induce a slight, rapid and persistent tremor (DELAY et al., 1959); moreover, the possible appearance of muscular hypotonia, tics, uncoordination, ataxia and, in particularly sensitive individuals, epileptiform seizure episodes have been reported (SHEPHERD et al., 1968).

Other side effects include dryness of the mouth, mydriasis, disturbances of visual accommodation, appearance of a latent glaucoma or further pathology of an already existing glaucoma; in the cardiovascular system, especially that of elderly patients with circulatory disturbances or functional decrements, tricyclic antidepressants can induce tachycardia, arhythmia, a quinidine-like effect with prolongation of the QT interval, flattening of the T wave, and signs of vagal blockade, resulting in ventricular tachycardia and fibrillation (BAN, 1969). Also, episodes of postural hypotension are not infrequently seen as side effects.

The digestive system can reflect the side effects of tricyclic compounds with nausea, dyspepsia, epigastric palsy, diarrhea, and constipation; in this regard, it should be recalled that the interaction of tricyclics with phenothiazines or anti-Parkinsonian drugs augments constipation and can even result in a paralytic ileum (WARNES et al., 1967).

Difficulty in micturition and impotence with a loss of erection can be induced in man by these drugs, while women can have side effects which manifest as either an increase or a decrease of libido.

Among those tricyclic-induced side effects which may be considered as essentially allergic, are either mild cholestatic jaundice, which generally starts after two to three weeks of treatment, as well as a series of cutaneous reactions, and, more rarely, agranulocytosis.

The most serious hazard to the patient arises from the possible association of tricyclics with other drugs, and the resulting consequences of the numerous pharmacological interactions already mentioned. The use of tricyclic antidepressants with monoamine oxidase inhibitors can produce serious consequences such as anxiety, periodic cephalgia, nausea, abdominal pains, vomiting, psychomotor excitation, tremor, clonic convulsions, dyspnea, hallucinations, delirium, pressor lability, circulatory collapse, coma and death. Moreover, as a precaution tricyclic antidepressants should never be administered for at least three weeks after cessation of any previous MAO inhibitor therapy.

Finally, it should be pointed out that the tricyclic drugs also potentiate the effects of atropine, amphetamine, thyroid hormone, and alcohol.

C) OTHER ANTIDEPRESSANTS

The pharmaco-therapy of depressive illness has more recently included compounds which are completely unrelated to the structural classification within which the MAO inhibitors or tricyclic compounds have previously been considered; among these are the lithium salts.

In clinical use lithium had been employed since 1850 for the treatment of gout and in cardiocirculatory failure as a substitute for sodium chloride; these salts, however, fell into disuse because of their toxicity. However, in 1897 LANGE first described the utility of lithium salts for the treatment of depressive syndromes; it was not until 1949, that CADE, in Australia, again demonstrated their efficacy in the control of the agitated psychotic patients (CADE, 1949). However, it was SCHOU et al. (1954) who described the first systematic and clinical controlled drug-placebo, double-blind study of the therapeutic effects of lithium in the treatment of several positive clinical experimental evaluations (SCHOU, 1956, 1959, 1963, 1967; GERSHON and YUWILER, 1960; MAGGS, 1963; STRÖMGREN and SCHOU, 1964; JACOBSON, 1965) which emphasized the preventive efficacy of the drug for clinically recurrent depressive episodes (HARTIGAN, 1963; BAAS-TRUP, 1964, 1966; STOLT, 1965; HERLOFSEN, 1965; BAASTRUP and SCHOU, 1967).

The importance of such prophylactic treatment is that, when clinically confirmed, it would establish exceptional value for lithium among those psychotropic drugs utilized in psychoaffective therapy (FIEVE, 1970-1971).

The *general aspects* of lithium effects depend upon the ability of this element to substitute for sodium and potassium ions, altering the organic balance of these ions, and acting as their antagonist under some experimental conditions (VON KORFF, 1953; ALDRIGE, 1962; SKOU, 1964; WHITTAM and AGER, 1964). Consequently, lithium can interfere with many enzymatic reactions which normally take place in the presence of sodium or potassium.

Obviously the ability of lithium to interfere with electrolyte balance raises questions regarding membrane excitability, ion transport, and basically, the issue of nerve impulse generation and transmission (COPPEN, 1965; SCHOU, 1967).

All these processes cannot be considered independently of other neurochemical parameters, specifically with respect to the *neurochemical mediators,* even though their absolute levels in the whole brain do not seem to be appreciably changed as a consequence of lithium treatment in experimental animals (KURIYAMA and SPEKEN, 1970). In this context it has recently been stated that lithium either increases the activity of cerebral noradrenergic neurons and norepinephrine synthesis (CORRODI et al., 1967; STERN et al., 1969; SCHILDKRAUT et al., 1966, 1969), or that lithium decreases both norepinephrine and serotonin content in synaptosomes (KURIYAMA and SPEKEN, 1970).

Serotonin level in the hypothalamus and in the brain stem were found to be decreased by lithium, with a reduction of serotonin synthesis in hypotalamic structures (HO et al., 1970); moreover, this element inhibits the liberation of norepinephrine and serotonin which normally occurs in the brain after slight electrical stimulation (KATZ et al., 1968). The *absorption* of lithium occurs through the gastro-intestinal route, and this ion does not show any particular affinity for specific organs or systems or particularly for the brain; transport of lithium across the blood-brain barrier is more difficult than for sodium or potassium (SCHOU, 1958b). Lithium *excretion* occurs principally through the renal system (SCHOU, 1958a; STEFFEN et al., 1962) and it is regulated by sodium and fluid intake (PLATMAN and FIEVE, 1969); the *pharmacology* of this substance is not particularly remarkable, being practically void of any obvious neuroleptic, tranquilizing or antidepressant effects in those tests commonly used to evaluate these properties in experimental animals.

The *clinical effects* of lithium may be referred to the previously mentioned biochemical effects and emphasize the indications used in the treatment of effective disorders to the degree that significance may be attributed to electrolytes in such disturbances (BAER et al., 1970). However, careful attention should be given to the therapeutic use of lithium salts, for all possess some degree of toxicity apparent in a series of unwanted side effects. Of these, mention may be made of the appearance of a slight tremor of the hands, diarrhea, vomiting, tinnitus, somnolence, ataxia, blurred vision, thirst, and polyuria. These early toxic symptoms become apparent at plasma concentrations of lithium around 2 to 3 meq/liter, while at higher plasma concentrations, of the order of 3 to 4 meq/liter, there are muscle spasms, nystagmus, confusional states and convulsive episodes, which with slightly higher concentrations can cause the death of the patient (GLESINGER, 1954; SCHOU, 1959) as a consequence of an irreversible renal damage. Such dangers make frequent evaluation of plasma lithium concentrations indispensable during the course of treatment, so that safe levels of around 3 meq/liter are not exceeded.

The observer who superficially views the general area of affective disorder therapy, cannot fully appreciate the profound changes that have taken place over the past few years. From a practical point of view, there is a range of available therapeutic means that is sufficiently broad as to be adaptable to multiple clinical manifestations of the pathological states, and thereby allow several types of corrective intervention, sufficiently flexible to meet the requirements of any single patient.

Many available drugs possess potential for a certain number of unwanted effects, which can be dangerous to the patient, but which can be reduced to a negligible degree when they are appropriately utilized; this employment

includes the clinical and pharmaco-therapeutic aspects, but also consideration of the evaluation of the intensity of modifications of emotional-
affective factors induced by the administration of such drugs.

In this connection it is sufficient to recall the danger represented by the
possibility of suicide attempts, manifest during the first week of therapy
with imipramine or desipramine in those subjects suffering from blocked
depressive syndromes; this may occur as a consequence of occasionally rapid
withdrawal of the affective blockade, or from depression expressed as mania
or even delirium following an inadequately controlled drug administration.
Similar considerations should discourage the use of these compounds, as
well as other pyschotropic drugs, without a previous accurate diagnostic
evaluation, supported by an adequate case history. These are obtainable
only through a vigilant consideration of data resulting from the experimental evaluation of the manifold aspects of psychopharmacology.

REFERENCES

Aldrige, W. N., (1962) Biochem. J. 83, 527.

Alexander, L. and Berkeley, A. W., (1959) Ann. N. Y. Acad. Sci. 80, 669.

Alleva, J. J., (1963) J. Med. Pharm. Chem. 6, 621.

Askew, B. M., (1963) Life Sci. 2, 725.

Axelrod, J. and Inscoe, J. K., (1963) J. Pharmacol. Exper. Ther. 141, 161.

Ayd, F. J., Jr., (1961) J. Neuropsychiat. (suppl. 1) 2, 119.

Azima, H., (1961) J. Ment. Sci. 107, 74.

Baastrup, P. C., (1964) Comp. Psychiat. 5, 396.

Baastrup, P. C., (1966) 7th Scandinavian Congress of Psychopharmacology Copen-
hagen, March 1966.

Baastrup, P. C. and Schou, M., (1967) Arch. Gen. Psychiat. 16, 162.

Baer, L., Platman, S. R., and Fieve, R. R., (1970) Arch. Gen. Psychiat. 22, 108.

Ban, T. A., (1966) Appl. Ther. 8, 779.

Ban, T. A., (1967) Appl. Ther. 9, 66.

Ban, T. A., (1969) "Psychopharmacology," Williams and Wilkins Co., Baltimore.

Barratt, E. S. and Pray, S. L., (1965) Exper. Neurol. 12, 173.

Baxter, B. L., (1968) Int. J. Neuropharmacol. 7, 47.

Benesova, O. and Trinerova, I., (1964) Int. J. Neuropharmacol. 3, 473.

Bennet, I. F., (1962) J. Nerv. Ment. Dis. 135, 59.

Bernardi, D., Jori, A., Morselli, P., Valzelli, L., and Garattini, S., (1966) J. Pharm.
Pharmacol. 18, 278.

Bernhard, K. and Beer, H., (1962) Helv. Physiol. Pharmacol. Acta 20, 114.

Besendorf, H., Steiner, F. A., and Hürlimann, A., (1962) Schweiz. Med. Wochenschr.
92, 244.

Biel, J. H., (1964) in "Molecular Modification in Drug Design," Gould, R. F., Ed.,
Amer. Chem. Soc., Washington.

Biel, J. H., Horita, A., and Drukker, A. E., (1964) in "Psychopharmacological Agents,"
vol. 1, Gordon, M., Ed., Academic Press, New York, p. 359.

Blackwell, B. and Marley, E., (1964) Lancet 1, 530.

Blackwell, B. and Marley, E., (1966) Brit. J. Pharmacol. 26, 120.

Boissier, J. R., Simon, P., and Lwoff, J. M., (1964) Thérapie 19, 571.

Boissier, J. R., Grasset, S., and Simon, P., (1968) J. Pharm. Pharmachol. 20, 972.

Boullin, D. J. and O'Brien, R. A., (1968) J. Pharm. Pharmacol. 20, 583.

Brimblecombe, R. W. and Green, D. M., (1967) Int. J. Neuropharmacol. 6, 133.

Brodie, B. B., Spector, S., and Shore, P. A., (1959) Ann. N. Y. Acad. Sci. 80, 609.

Burt, C. G., Gordon, W. F., Holt, N. F., and Horden, A. (1962) J. Ment. Sci. 108, 711.

Cade, J. F. J., (1949) Med. J. Aust. 2, 349.

Carlsson, A., (1966a) Pharmacol. Rev. 18, 541.

Carlsson, A., (1966b) Acta Physiol. Scand. 67, 481.

Carlsson, A., Rosengren, E., Bertler, A., and Nilsson, J., (1957) in "Psychotropic Drugs," Garattini, S. and Ghetti, V., Eds., Elsevier Publ., Amsterdam, p. 363.

Charpentier, J. and Soulairac, A., (1963) C. R. Soc. Biol. 157, 1002.

Chessin, M., Kramer, E. R., and Scott, C. C., (1957) J. Pharmacol. Exper. Ther. 119, 453.

Cockrill, S., Sommerville, A. R., and Whittle, B. A., (1968) Arch. Pharmakol. Exper. Pathol. 259, 159.

Cohen, S., Ditman, K. S., and Gustafson, S. R., (1967) in "Psychochemotherapy," Remmen, E., Ed., Western Med. Publ., Los Angeles.

Consolo, S., Dolfini, E., Garattini, S., and Valzelli, L., (1967) J. Pharm. Pharmacol. 19, 253.

Coppen, A., (1965) Brit. J. Psychiat. 111, 1133.

Corrodi, H., Fuxe, K., Hökfelt, T., and Schou, M., (1967) Psychopharmacologia (Berlin) 11, 345.

Costa, E., Garattini, S., and Valzelli, L., (1960) Experientia 16, 461.

Delay, J., Laine, B., and Buisson, J. F., (1952) Ann. Méd.-Psychol. 110, 689.

Delay, J., Deniker, P., Lemperiere, T., Ropert, M., Colin, W., and Ogrizek, B., (1959) Ann. Méd.-Psychol. 117, 521.

Dewhurst, W. G., (1965) J. Psychosom. Res. 9, 115.

Dews, P. B., (1962) Int. J. Neuropharmacol. 1, 265.

Di Mascio, A., Heninger, G., and Klerman, G. L., (1964) Psychopharmacologia (Berlin) 5, 361.

Dingell, J. V., Sulser, F., and Gillette, J. R., (1962) Fed. Proc. Fed. Amer. Soc. Exper. Biol. 21, 184.

Dingell, J. V., Sulser, F., and Gillette, J. R., (1964) J. Pharmacol. Exper. Ther. 143, 14.

Domenjoz, R. and Theobald, W., (1959) Arch. Int. Pharmacodyn. Thér. 120, 450.

Fekete, M. and Macsek, I., (1968) J. Pharm. Pharmacol. 20, 327.

Feldman, P. E., (1959) J. Clin. Exper. Psychopathol. 20, 235.

Fieve, R. R., (1970-1971) Int. J. Psychiat. 9, 375.

Fink, M., (1959) Can. Psychiat. Assoc. J. (suppl. 1) 4, 166.

Fouts, J. R. and Brodie, B. B., (1956) J. Pharmacol. Exper. Ther. 116, 480.

Fullerton, A. G. and Boardman, R. H., (1959) Lancet 1, 1209.

Gallinek, A., (1959) Amer. J. Psychiat. 115, 1011.

Garattini, S., (1958) Schweiz. Arch. Neurol. Psychiat. 84, 8.

Garattini, S., Fresia, P., Mortari, A., and Palma, V., (1960) Med. Exper. 2, 252.

Garattini, S. and Jori, A., (1967) in "Antidepressant Drugs" (Proc. 1st. Int. Symp., Milan 1966) Garattini, S. and Dukes, M. N. G., Eds., Excerpta Medica Foundation, Amsterdam, p. 179.

Garattini, S. and Valzelli, L., (1960) in "Le Sindromi Depressive" (Symp. Rapallo 1960), Minerva Medica, Torino, p. 7.

Gershon, S. and Yuwiler, A., (1960) J. Neuropsychiat. 1, 229.

Gessa, G. L., Cuenca, E., and Costa, E., (1963) Ann. N. Y. Acad. Sci. 107, 935.

Gillette, J. R., Dingell, J. V., and Quinn, G. P., (1960) Fed. Proc. Fed. Amer. Soc. Exper. Biol. 19, 137.

Gillette, J. R., Dingell, J. V., Sulser, F., Kuntzman, R., and Brodie, B. B., (1961) Experientia 17, 417.

Glesinger, B., (1954) Med. J. Aust. 1, 277.

Glowinski, J., (1967) in "Antidepressant Drugs" (Proc. 1st. Int. Symp., Milano 1966), Garattini, S. and Dukes, M. N. G., Eds., Excerpta Medica Foundation, Amsterdam, p. 44.

Gyermek, L. and Possemato, C., (1960) Med. Exper. 3, 225.

Hanson, H. M., (1961) Fed. Proc. Fed. Amer. Soc. Exper. Biol. 20, 396.

Hartigan, G. P., (1963) Brit. J. Psychiat. 109, 810.

Haydu, G. G., Dhrymiotis, A., and Quinn, G. P., (1962) Amer. J. Psychiat. 119, 574.

Herlofsen, H. B., (1965) Norvegian Psychiatric Society Meeting, Oslo, September 1965.

Herrmann, B. and Pulver, R., (1960) Arch. Int. Pharmacodyn. Thér. 126, 454.

Hess, S., Weissbach, H., Redfield, B. G., and Udenfriend, S., (1958) J. Pharmacol. Exper. Ther. 124, 189.

Himwich, H. E., (1965) in "The Scientific Basis of Drug Therapy in Psychiatry," Marks, J. and Pare, C. M. B., Eds., Pergamon Press, Oxford.

Himwich, W. A., and Petersen, J. C., (1961) Fed. Proc. Fed. Amer. Soc. Exper. Biol. 20, 394.

Ho, A. K. S., Loh, H. H., Craves, F., Hitzemann, R. J., and Gershon, S., (1970) Europ. J. Pharmacol. 10, 72.

Hoenig, J. and Visram, S., (1964) Brit. J. Psychiat. 110, 840.

Hollister, L. E., Overall, J. E., Johnson, M., Pennington, V., Katz, G., and Shelton, J., (1964) J. Nerv. Ment. Dis. 139, 370.

Hordern, A., (1965) New England J. Med. 272, 1159.

Hordern, A., Burj, C. G., Gordon, W. F., and Holt, N. F., (1964) Brit. J. Psychiat. 110, 641.

Horovitz, Z. P., (1965) Psychosomatics 6, 281.

Horovitz, Z. P., (1967) in "Antidepressant Drugs" (Proc. 1st. Int. Symp., Milano 1966), Garattini, S. and Dukes, M. N. G., Eds., Excerpta Medica Foundation, Amsterdam, p. 121.

Horowitz, D. and Sjoerdsma, A., (1963) Ann. N. Y. Acad. Sci. 107, 1033.

Itoh, H. and Takaori, S., (1968) Jap. J. Pharmacol. 18, 344.

Jacobson, J. E., (1965) Amer. J. Psychiat. 122, 295.

Jarvik, M. E., (1965) in "The Pharmacological Basis of Therapeutics," Goodman, L. S. and Gilman, A., Eds., McMillan, New York.

Johnson, H. E. and Goldberg, M. E., (1965) J. Pharm. Pharmacol. 17, 54.

Jori, A., (1972) in "Aspetti Attuali di Farmacologia e Farmacoterapia," Bertelli, A., Ed., Tamburini Editore, Milano, p. 560.

Jori, A. and Garattini, S., (1965) J. Pharm. Pharmacol. 17, 480.

Jouvet, M., (1967) Res. Publs. Assoc. Res. Nerv. Ment. Dis. 45, 86.

Jouvet, M., Vimont, P., and Delorme, F., (1965) C. R. Soc. Biol. 159, 1595.

Katz, R. I., Chase, T. N., and Kopin, I. J., (1968) Science 162, 466.

Kiloh, L. G. and Garside, R. F., (1963) Brit. J. Psychiat. 109, 451.

Kivalo, E., Rinne, U. K., and Karinkanta, H., (1961) J. Neurochem. 8, 105.

Klerman, G. L. and Cole, J. O., (1965) Pharmacol. Rev. 17, 101.
Kline, N. S., Loomer, H. P., and Saunders, J. C., (1957) in "Psychochemotherapy," Remmen, E., Ed., Western Medical Publ., Los Angeles.
Kline, N. S. and Stanley, A. M., (1959) in "Neuropsychopharmacology, "Bradley, P. B., Deniker, P., and Radouco-Thomas, C., Eds., Elsevier Publ. Amsterdam, p. 612.
Koechlin, B. and Iliev, V., (1959) Ann. N. Y. Acad. Sci. 80, 864.
Kopin, I. J., (1966) Pharmacol. Rev. 18, 513.
Kornetsky, C., (1963) Pharmacologist 5, 239.
Kuehn, A. and Schallek, W., (1965) Fed. Proc. Fed. Amer. Soc. Exper. Biol. 24, 516.
Kuhn, R., (1957) Schweiz. Med. Wochenschr. 87, 1135.
Kuhn, R., (1958) Amer. J. Psychiat. 115, 459.
Kumadaki, N., Hitomi, M., and Kumada, S., (1967) Jap. J. Pharmacol. 17, 659.
Kuriyama, K. and Speken, R., (1970) Life Sci. (part 1) 9, 1213.
Lange, C., (1897) Hospitalstidende 5, 1.
Lapin, I. P., Osipova, S. V., Uskosa, N. V., and Stabrovski, E. M., (1968) Arch. Int. Pharmacodyn. Thér. 174, 37.
Le Gassicke, J., Boyd, W. D., and McPherson, F. M., (1964) Brit. J. Psychiat. 110, 267.
Lehmann, H. E., (1966a) in "Pharmacotherapy of Depression," Cole, J. O. and Wittenborn, J. R., Eds., C. C. Thomas Publ., Springfield, Ill., p. 3.
Lehmann, H. E., (1966b) in "Antidepressant Drugs of Non-MAO Inhibitor Type," Efron, D. H. and Kety, S. S., Eds., U. S. Dept. of Health, Education and Welfare, Bethesda, Md., p. 122.
Lehmann, H. E., Cahn, C. H., and De Verteuil, R., (1958) Can. Psychiat. Assoc. J. 3, 155.
Lewis, A. J., (1934) J. Ment. Sci. 80, 277.
Lewis, J. J. and Van Petten, G. R., (1963) Brit. J. Pharmacol. 20, 462.
Leyberg, J. T. and Denmark, J. C., (1959) J. Ment. Sci. 105, 1123.
Maggs, R., (1963) Brit. J. Psychiat. 109, 56.
Maxwell, D. R. and Palmer, H. T., (1961) Nature, London 191, 84.
Meek, J., Fuxe, K., and Andén, N. E., (1970) Europ. J. Pharmacol. 9, 325.
Modell, W., (1962) Clin. Pharmacol. Ther. 3, 97.
Morpurgo, C. and Theobald, W., (1965) Med. Pharmacol. Exper. 12, 226.
Nair, V., (1959) Biochem. Pharmacol. 3, 78.
Neff, N. H. and Costa, E., (1967) in "Antidepressant Drugs" (Proc. 1st. Int. Symp., Milano, 1966), Garattini, S. and Dukes, M. N. G., Eds., Excerpta Medica Foundation, Amsterdam, p. 28.
Oltman, J. E. and Friedman, S., (1961) Clin. Notes 1, 355.
Opitz, K. and Borchert, U., (1968) Arzneim.-Forsch. 18, 316.
Ostow, M., (1962) "Drugs in Psychoanalysis and Psychotherapy," Basic Books, New York.
Oswald, I., (1968) Pharmacol. Rev. 20, 273.
Platman, S. R. and Fieve, R. R., (1969) Arch. Gen. Psychiat. 20, 285.
Pletscher, A., (1963) in "The Clinical Chemistry of Monoamines," Varley, H. and Gowenlock, A. H., Eds., Elsevier Publ., Amsterdam, p. 191.
Pletscher, A., (1965) in "Psychopharmacology," Kline, N. S. and Lehmann, H. E., Eds., Little & Brown Publ., Boston.
Pletscher, A. and Gey, K. F., (1959) Helv. Physiol. Pharmacol. Acta 17, 35.
Prockop, D. J., Shore, P. A., and Brodie, B. B., (1959) Ann. N. Y. Acad. Sci. 80, 643.
Pscheidt, G. R., (1962) Biochem. Pharmacol. 11, 501.
Rathbun, R. C. and Slater, I. H., (1963) Psychopharmacologia (Berlin) 4, 114.
Robitzek, E. H., Selikoff, I. J., and Ornstein, G. G., (1952) Quart. Bull. Sea View Hosp. 13, 27.

Rose, J. T. and Westhead, T. T., (1964) Amer. J. Psychiat. 121, 496.

Ross, S. B. and Renyi, L., (1967) Europ. J. Pharmacol. 2, 181.

Sabelli, H. C. and Sinay, I., (1960) Arzneim.-Forsch. 10, 935.

Santi, R. and Fassina, G., (1965) J. Pharm. Pharmacol. 17, 596.

Sargant, W. and Slater, E., (1963) "An Introduction to Physical Methods of Treatment in Psychiatry," Livingstone Publ., Edinburgh.

Schaeppi, U., (1960) Helv. Physiol. Pharmacol. Acta 18, 545.

Schallek, W. and Kuehn, A., (1963) Proc. Soc. Exper. Biol. Med. 112, 813.

Schanberg, S. M., Schildkraut, J. J., and Kopin, I. J., (1967) Biochem. Pharmacol. 16, 393.

Scheckel, C. L. and Boff, E., (1964) Psychopharmacologia (Berlin) 5, 198.

Schiele, B. C., Vestre, N. M., and MacNaughton, D. V., (1963) Compr. Psychiat. 4, 66.

Schildkraut, J. J., (1965) Amer. J. Psychiat. 122, 509.

Schildkraut, J. J., Klerman, G. L., Hammond, R., and Friend, D. G., (1964) J. Psychiat. Res. 2, 257.

Schildkraut, J. J., Logue, M. A., and Dodge, G. A. (1969) Psychopharmacologia (Berlin) 14, 135.

Schildkraut, J. J., Schanberg, S. M., and Kopin, I. J., (1966) Life Sci. 5, 1479.

Schindler, W. and Häfliger, F., (1954) Helv. Chim. Acta 37, 472.

Schmitt, H., (1967) in "Antidepressant Drugs," (Proc. 1st. Int. Symp., Milano 1966), Garattini, S. and Dukes, M. N. G., Eds., Excerpta Medica Foundation, Amsterdam, p. 104.

Schou, M., (1956) Nord. Med. 55, 790.

Schou, M., (1958a) Acta Pharmacol. Toxol. 15, 85.

Schou, M., (1958b) Acta Pharmacol. Toxol. 15, 115.

Schou, M., (1959) Psychopharmacologia (Berlin) 1, 65.

Schou, M., (1963) Brit. J. Psychiat. 109, 803.

Schou, M., (1967) in "Antidepressant Drugs" (Proc. 1st. Int. Symp., Milano 1966), Garattini, S. and Dukes, M. N. G., Eds., Excerpta Medica Foundation, Amsterdam, p. 80.

Schou, M., Juel-Nielsen, N., Stromgren, E., and Voldby, H., (1954) J. Neurol. Neurosurg. Psychiat. 17, 250.

Selikoff, I. J., Robitzek, E. H., and Ornstein, G. G., (1952) J. Amer. Med. Assoc. 150, 973.

Shepherd, M., Lader, M., and Rodnight, T. R., (1968) "Clinical Psychopharmacology," The English Universities Press Ltd., London.

Shore, P. A., and Brodie, B. B., (1957) Proc. Soc. Exper. Biol. Med. 94, 433.

Sigg, E. B., (1959) Can. Psychiat. Assoc. J. (Suppl.) 4, 75.

Skou, Y. C., (1964) Progr. Biophys. Mol. Biol. 14, 133.

Snow, L. H. and Rickels, K., (1964) Psychopharmacologia (Berlin) 5, 409.

Sourkes, T. L., (1962) "Biochemistry of Mental Disease," Harper and Row, New York.

Stacey, R. S., (1961) Brit. J. Pharmacol. 16, 284.

Steffen, J., Adam, W., Knapowski, J., and Arasimowicz, C., (1962) Acta Med. Pol. 3, 121.

Stein, L., (1967) in "Antidepressant Drugs" (Proc. 1st. Int. Symp., Milano 1966), Garattini, S. and Dukes, M. N. G., Eds., Excerpta Medica Foundation, Amsterdam, p. 130.

Stein, L. and Seifter, J., (1961) Fed. Proc. Fed. Amer. Soc. Exper. Biol. 20, 395.

Stern, D. N., Fieve, R. R., Neff, N. H., and Costa, E., (1969) Psychopharmacologia (Berlin) 14, 315.

Stolt, G., (1965) Läkartidningen 62, 3018.

Strömgren, E. and Schou, M., (1964) Postgrad. Med. **35**, 83.

Sulser, F. and Dingell, J. V., (1966) in "Antidepressant Drugs of Non-MAO Inhibitor Type," Efron, D. H. and Kety, S. S., Eds., U. S. Dept. of Health, Education and Welfare, Bethesda, Md., p. 1.

Tedeschi, D. H., Tedeschi, R. E., and Fellows, E. J., (1959) J. Pharmacol. Exper. Ther. **126**, 223.

Theobald, W., Büch, O., Kunz, H. A., Morpurgo, C., Stenger, E. G., and Wilhelmi, G., (1964) Arch. Int. Pharmacodyn. Thér. **148**, 560.

Thiele, J. and Holzinger, O., (1899) Ann. Chim. **305**, 96.

Toyoda, J., (1964) Folia Psychiat. Neurol. Jap. **18**, 198.

Valzelli, L., (1967) in "Advances in Pharmacology," vol. 5, Garattini, S. and Shore, P. A., Eds., Academic Press, New York, p. 79.

Valzelli, L., (1969) Psychopharmacologia (Berlin) **15**, 232.

Valzelli, L., (1971) Actual. Pharmacol. **24**, 133.

Valzelli, L., and Bernasconi, S., (1971) Psychopharmacologia (Berlin) **20**, 91.

Valzelli, L., Giacalone, E., and Garattini, S., (1967) Europ. J. Pharmacol. **2**, 144.

Vernier, V. G., (1961) Dis. Nerv. Syst. **22**, 7.

Vernier, V. G., Alleva, F. R., Hanson, H. M., and Stone, C. A., (1962) Fed. Proc. Fed. Amer. Soc. Exper. Biol. **21**, 419.

Von Korff, R. W., (1953) J. Biol. Chem. **203**, 265.

Warnes, H., Lehmann, H. E., and Ban, T. A., (1967) Can. Med. Assoc. J. **96**, 1430.

Weissman, A., (1961) Pharmacologist **3**, 60.

West, E. D. and Dally, P. J., (1959) Brit. Med. J. **2**, 433.

Whittam, R. and Ager, M. E., (1964) Biochem. J. **93**, 337.

Wilson, S. P. and Tislow, R., (1962) Proc. Soc. Exper. Biol. Med. **109**, 847.

Wilson, I. C., Vernon, J. T., Guin, T., and Sandifer, M. G., Jr., (1963) J. Neuropsychiat. **4**, 331.

Wittenborn, J. R., (1962) J. Nerv. Ment. Dis. **134**, 117.

Wittenborn, J. R., (1967) ECDEU Meeting, Montreal.

Zeller, E. A., Barsky, J., Fouts, J. R., Kirchheimer, W. F., and Van Orden, L. S., (1952) Experientia **8**, 349.

Zetler, G., (1968) Int. J. Neuropharmacol **7**, 325.

Chapter XI

THE PSYCHOSTIMULANTS

The term psychostimulant refers to those drugs capable of inducing excitatory effects upon several higher brain structures and several complex cerebral functions. In this way such compounds exert their behavioral effects, which are generally manifested as an elevation of mood. This effect, however, is only part of a larger complex of potential changes, since many compounds within this category also act upon several subcortical areas and nuclei, as well as upon lower nervous structures and peripheral functions; such effects are specifically dose dependent.

Psychostimulants, generally, and particularly those which share properties with the psychodysleptics (also referred to as psychotomimetics, psychedelics, or mysticomimetics) may be considered as having limited utility in their therapeutic applicability; this is due both to the profound thought distortion processes that these drugs induce and to the possible onset of psychological dependency which may develop into a sustained and continuous self-administration of increasing dosages.

This latter problem has become particularly distressing over the last few years, due to the continuously increasing rate of abuse of many psychostimulant and psychodysleptic drugs among young people of varied nationalities and social stratus. An analysis of such a phenomenon, which seems to be rapidly becoming a new life style, should sufficiently enlarge the picture to include the entire processes of brain functional evolution, at the core of which lies the serious threat of an involuntary disintegration. This effect would appear dependent upon the release from those constraints of a social environment by the individual, such that he becomes increasingly more removed and depersonalized from reality. The continuous and prolonged stress associated with attempts to emerge from the context of a social group as an individual is uniformly great; the reduction of more traditional moral values, the anxious and somewhat compulsive denial of behavioral limitations and of family or group "taboos," without the concrete availability of any valid substitute, are only several of the manifold bases for the induction of strong feelings of frustration and inadequacy which can degenerate into a denial of reality, and a flight into the psychedelic experience in an attempt to search for the self.

From this background several premises have been evolved which, in spite of some questionable philosophical and literary referents, still support the operation of several active and prosporous commercial enterprises which have found an incredibly fertile ground in an ever increasing number of practitioners of the manifold psychedelic philosophies; the aim of this is, paradoxically, the demolition of the so-called consumer society. The jacket of a record collection issued some years ago, entitled "The Psychedelic Sounds of the 13th Floor Elevators," seems to be appropriately representative of such a commercially philosophical tendency, which is expressed in the following pretentious statement: "Recently, it has become possible for man to chemically alter his mental state and thus alter his point of view (i.e., his own basic relation with the outside world which determines how he stores his information). He then can restructure his thinking and change his language so that his thoughts bear more relation to his life and his problems, and therefore approach them more sanely. It is this quest for a pure sanity that forms the basis of the songs on this album" (CURRY, 1968).

However, apart from some obvious contradictions (how can it be possible to reach "a pure sanity" through a "chemical alteration" of the mental state?), the expressed concepts reflect a form of stating the problems of the individual, the resolution of which depends upon the use of certain drugs claimed to provide for the revelation of concealed intellectual capacities or capable of enhancing the faculties of "human mind." In this context, drugs are thought to be "divine helpers" to achieve new "mind dimensions." This is, fundamentally, the misunderstanding which serves to drive thousands of young people into the traps of drug abuse and servitude to various psychoanaleptic or psychodysleptic compounds, with the same irrational determination that may be observed in the periodic suicidal migrations of some rodents.

It then seems of considerable importance to emphasize, in accord with KOESTLER (1967), that it is fundamentally erroneous, to believe that drugs can gratuitously enrich the human mind, providing it with something which was not previously existent, so that neither mystical visions nor philosophical wisdom can be supplied by a pill or by an injection. In fact, the psychopharmacologist can add nothing to brain abilities but he may, in the best of the cases, be able to eliminate those obstacles and blocks that impair its more proper use. Consistent with KOESTLER's advice, the psychopharmacologist cannot improve us but he may, within limits, provide us with some normality; he cannot insert more circuits into our brain, but he can, once more within limits, ameliorate the coordination among existing ones, attenuate conflicts, prevent potential short circuits, and assure a constant energy supply.

These are the major and probably the most difficult goals of psychopharmacology.

A) PSYCHOANALEPTICS

The term psychoanaleptic includes all of those compounds incapable of elevating mood without compromising human performance capacity, altering reality, or modifying the accuracy of responses to environmental stimulation. These drugs, then, in contrast to the sedatives, reduce wakefulness, augment attention and concentration (ESPLIN and ZABLOCKA, 1965).

Other central stimulant drugs, such as *picrotoxin, strychnine, niketamide,* and *pentamethylenetetrazole* may be more properly considered as convulsants, as classically described in standard textbooks of pharmacology (GOODMAN and GILMAN, 1970; AIAZZI-MANCINI and DONATELLI, 1957; CROSSLAND, 1970), and have been accorded a minor importance in a formal psychopharmacological context. However, some recent data concerning such molecules may be found in an excellent review by ESSMAN (1971) in which their possible effect upon learning and memory processes has been considered.

The category of psychoanaleptics refers to the chemical family of xanthines of which trimethylxanthine or *caffeine* is the most active derivative; other xanthines, such as *theobromine* and *theophylline*, are in fact, qualitatively similar to caffeine but have quantitatively less stimulant properties. Psychomotor activation is more evident for caffeine, the action of which extends from the cerebral cortex to the spinal cord (Fig. 51), encompassing a series of effects, the intensity of which is extremely variable from one individual to another (GOLDSTEIN et al., 1965a); this applies to wakefulness, psychomotor coordination, and mood (GOLDSTEIN et al., 1965b).

Similar individual differences have also been described in laboratory animals wherein the effects of caffeine are influenced by age and sex (PETERS and BOYD, 1967a), a reduction of food intake (PETERS, 1966), the type of diet (PETERS and BOYD, 1967b), and by several other factors.

Recently it was shown that xanthine toxicity is increased by monoamine oxidase inhibitors (BERKOWITZ et al., 1971), suggesting the hypothesis that xanthines can interfere with neurochemical mediator metabolism; in fact, caffeine and theophylline increase the concentration of both 5-HT and 5-HIAA in the brain (BERKOWITZ and SPECTOR, 1971), decrease the turnover of this amine in the brain (CORRODI et al., 1972; VALZELLI, 1973), and release NE (BERKOWITZ et al., 1970). Brain NE and DA turnover are, respectively, increased and decreased by caffeine (CORRODI et al., 1972). Moreover, caffeine has been described as an inducer of microsomal enzyme system activity (MITOMA et al., 1968).

From the behavioral point of view, psychotic-like reactions in caffeine-

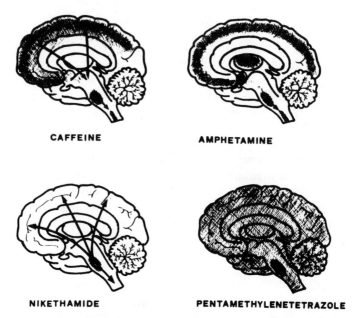

CAFFEINE   AMPHETAMINE

NIKETHAMIDE   PENTAMETHYLENETETRAZOLE

Fig. 51. Brain areas effected by some psychoanaleptic drugs.

intoxicated rats were reported by several investigators (Mc MANAMY and SCHUBE, 1936; PFEIFFER and GASS, 1962; BOYD et al., 1965; PETERS, 1967) who noticed self-mutilation of the feet or tail; in contrast, caffeine, in low doses, was able to counteract the aggressiveness induced in mice by isolation (VALZELLI, 1973). Moreover, caffeine exerts a time-dependent facilitative effect upon memory fixation of a discriminative avoidance response (ESSMAN, 1971). However, it should be pointed out that high doses of xanthines in man are capable of inducing insomnia, restlessness, and hyperexcitation eventuating in delirium and convulsions.

The major representative of the psychostimulants consist of *amphetamine* (Fig. 52) and a series of chemically related compounds, which even with certain distinct structural differences, exert similar functional effects; as a consequence, the latter have also been identified by the general term "amphetamines".

In the historical evolution of psychostimulants, a most important step is represented by the synthesis of epinephrine, the vasomotor principle of the

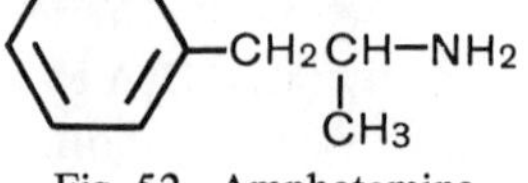

$$\text{—CH}_2\text{CH—NH}_2$$
$$\text{CH}_3$$

Fig. 52. Amphetamine.

suprarenal medulla, that was independently accomplished by STOLZ (1904) and by DAKIN (1905). Epinephrine, in turn, provided a basis for a series of other syntheses resulting in several aminate derivatives which were studied pharmacologically by BARGER and DALE (1910). However, seventeen years elapsed before ALLES (1927) described the typical stimulant effect of amphetamine upon the central nervous sytem. Other derivatives, such as *methylamphetamine* and *benzylamphetamine* were later utilized, so that this group of compounds became actively utilized (LEAKE, 1958), mainly for their euphoriant properties which, though transitory and poorly effective from a psychiatric point of view, had some therapeutic relevance for nonspecific elevation of mood and counteracting feelings of fatigue (SHEPHERD et al., 1968).

1) General Aspects

The *absorption* of psychostimulants and of amphetamines is generally very rapid so that the effects become evident by half an hour after oral administration and by about five minutes following parenteral administration (BAN, 1969); in constrast with other similar molecules that are more polar, such as the catecholamines, amphetamine crosses the blood-brain barrier very easily and rapidly reaches several brain structures (AXELROD, 1959).

Amphetamine *metabolism* is quite variable, depending upon the animal species. In fact, amphetamine can be inactivated by demethylation, deamination, or para-hydroxylation followed by conjugation with glucuronic acid (AXELROD, 1959) but, in the rat and, to a lesser extent, in the dog, the major metabolic pathway is prepresented by p-hydroxylation (AXELROD, 1954; ELLISON et al., 1966); in other animal species, such as the monkey and man, an oxidative deamination takes place (ELLISON et al., 1966; AXELROD, 1970). However, to a minor extent as compared with the rat, amphetamine is also p-hydroxylated in the cat (THOENEN et al., 1966) and in man (DRING et al., 1966), although in the latter case, a portion of the compound, when administered by the oral route, is eliminated in unaltered form (CARTONI and DE STEFANO, 1963) and as a N-demethylated product (UTENA et al., 1955; BECKETT and ROWLAND, 1965). All of these metabolic reactions are performed by liver microsomal enzymes. Recently, however, it was reported that in cat, rat, and man amphetamine can be hydroxylated in the β position by dopamine β-hydroxylase, which is present in the granules which store the catecholamines in the sympathetic nervous terminals (SJOERDSMA and VON STUDNITZ, 1963; KOPIN et al., 1965; MUSACCHIO et al., 1965; FISCHER et al., 1965; GUNNE and GALLAND, 1967); this metabolic transformation can be of relevance to those cerebral interactions between neuronal catecholamines and amphetamine.

The *excretion* of amphetamine and its metabolite from the body is essentially accomplished by urinary excretion; the intensity and rate of clearance are maximally dependent upon urinary pH, which acts positively in the acidic range and negatively at basic levels (BECKETT et al., 1965; ASATOOR et al., 1965).

Amphetamine *pharmacology* may be characterized as an intense stimulation of brain structures and functions resulting in excitation, hyperactivity, euphoria, insomnia, piloerection, and hyperthermia; at larger doses, tremors, motor and psychomotor incoordination, stereotypes, convulsions, and death may occur. This general picture basically represents a common paradigm for the activities of psychoanaleptics. Moreover, it should be emphasized that this class of compounds, and amphetamine in particular, are occasionally potentiated or inhibited by several factors partially related to environmental factors and partially to the species of animal utilized in the experiments. In fact, it is known that increased environmental temperature (HOHN and LASAGNA, 1960; ASKEW, 1961; FINK and LARSON, 1962), as well as auditory (CHANCE, 1946, 1947; COHEN and LAL, 1964), visual, and nociceptive stimulation (WEISS et al., 1961), and the number of animals present in the cage (CHANCE, 1946; BURN and HOBBS, 1957) can potentiate the toxicity of amphetamine; other variations, both in lethality and of the the effects induced by this substance depend upon age (CHERNOV et al., 1966; SOFIA, 1969), hormonal factors (CHANCE, 1947; FINK and LARSON, 1962), strain (WEAVER and KERLEY, 1962; DOLFINI and KOBAYASHI, 1967; DOLFINI et al., 1969), sex (GUPTA and HOLLAND, 1969), emotional level (CONSOLO et al., 1965a, c; GUPTA and HOLLAND, 1969; VALZELLI, 1969), and upon the previous experience of the animal employed (PORSOLT et al., 1970). Such situations are of particular relevance as they can experimentally reflect the role of so-called nonspecific factors and of possible personality-related variables in man as possible determinants of the behavioral response to amphetamine and to drugs in general (FORREST et al., 1967; FISHER, 1970).

The *neuropharmacology* of the amphetamines is characterized by several central effects including a decrease in the threshold to and an increase in the intensity of the alerting reaction in a manner similar to that experimentally induced by the direct stimulation of the afferent collateral fibers of the medulla or of the reticular formation (BRADLEY and KEY, 1958). In fact, amphetamine stimulates this activating system without exerting any direct effect upon the cerebral cortex (KILLAM, 1962).

Other neuropharmacological effects of amphetamine include those exerted on the hypothalamic nuclei, where this molecule stimulates the medial structures which are related to the inhibition of food intake (BROBECK et al., 1956) exerting an obvious anorectic effect common to many other amphetamine derivatives.

Moreover, amphetamines, to different and varying degrees, induce a series of sympathomimetic effects such as mydriasis, vasoconstriction, tachycardia, bronchodilatation, increased muscle tonus hyperglycemia, and, finally, a blocking of the autonomic ganglia (BAN, 1969).

The interactive effects of amphetamine on brain *neurochemical mediators* are also of relevance. In fact, the effect of amphetamine on brain serotonin content appears to be equivocal, having been described as both increasing (SMITH, 1963) and decreasing (LAVERTY and SHARMAN, 1965; LAL and CHESSIK, 1964), or even without any effect (PLETSCHER et al., 1964; BEAUVALLET et al., 1967b; DUHAULT and VERDA-VAINNE, 1967) upon the concentration of this biogenic amine. Many experimental observations have also sought to explain the activity of this drug in terms of brain catecholamine interaction (HALPERN et al., 1962; WEISSMAN et al., 1966; HANSON, 1967; LITTLETON, 1967; RANDRUP and MUNKVAD, 1966a; GLOWINSKY and AXELROD, 1965; SULSER et al., 1968).

Recently it was shown that the stereotaxic destruction of the brain serotoninergic system in rats did not affect the action of amphetamine in blocking food intake (SAMANIN et al., 1972), while a block of catecholamine synthesis by administration of alpha-methyl-p-tyrosine induced the disappearance of amphetamine activities (WEISSMAN et al., 1966; DINGELL et al., 1967; LITTLETON, 1967; MENNEAR and RUDZIK, 1968); some experimental observations have led to the conclusion that hyperthermia induced by amphetamine depends upon brain norepinephrine changes.

Amphetamine-dopamine interactions are more likely responsible for the motor activiation initiated by this psychostimulant drug (BEAUVALLET et al., 1967a) and also for the stereotyped behaviors that occur following the administration of amphetamine as well as of other psychostimulant drugs (RANDRUP and MUNKVAD, 1966b, 1967, 1968). Amphetamine acts on neuronal mechanisms in several ways: (1) directly stimulating catecholaminergic receptors (LITTLETON, 1967; SAMANIN et al., 1972); (2) releasing catecholamines from synaptic vesicles (CARLSSON et al., 1965, 1966; EVETTS et al., 1970); (3) impairing the catecholamine reuptake mechanism (GLOWINSKY and AXELROD, 1965); and (4) partially inhibiting monoamine oxidase activity (GLOWINSKY et al., 1966).

All of these effects (Fig. 53) result in a very pronounced stimulation of the catecholaminergic areas of the brain.

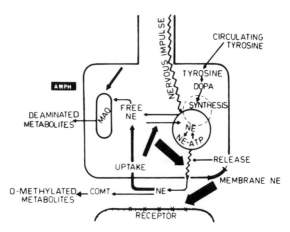

Fig. 53. Amphetamine activity upon synaptic mechanism.

The effects of amphetamine are largely dependent upon a previous level of neuronal activation or, upon the general activity level of the central nervous system (LITTLETON, 1967; WELCH and WELCH, 1967); this partially explains how an increase in environmental stimulation as well as increased emotional tension can potentiate psychoanaleptic drug activity and toxicity as previously reported.

2) Behavioral Effects

One of the most typical effects of amphetamine, and of psychoaneleptics in general, is an obvious increase in spontaneous *motor activity* (FROMMEL et al., 1960; VERNIER et al., 1962; HALLIWELL et al., 1964; LEWANDER, 1968; MANTEGAZZA et al., 1968). This effect is easily measurable and, to some extent, directly proportional to the dose administered (MANTEGAZZA et al., 1968); it is accompanied by hyperthermia (MORPURGO and THEOBALD, 1965; JORI and GARATTINI, 1965, VALZELLI et al., 1967a; MANTEGAZZA et al., 1968), as well as by stereotyped movements (RANDRUP et al., 1963), and eventuates, at higher doses, in motor incoordination, tremors and convulsions.

The toxicity of amphetamines, and other psychostimulant drugs such as *fencanfamine* (BRITTAIN et al., 1964), is more pronounced in aggressive mice than in normal animals (CONSOLO et al., 1965b, c). The difference in toxicity is not dependent upon differences in amphetamine concentration in the brain tissue of the two types of animals (CONSOLO et al., 1965a), but seems to depend upon both differences in emotionality between animals and on differences in microsomal enzyme activity induced in mice as a consequence of differential housing (ESSMAN et al., 1972).

Amphetamine seems to act paradoxically on *aggressiveness* induced *by isolation*; in one respect it acts as an antiaggressive drug, similar to other central stimulants that induce hyperexcitation capable of causing incoordination and reduced orienting and fighting behavior (VALZELLI et al., 1967b; VALZELLI, 1967; VALZELLI and BERNASCONI, 1971).

The *exploratory behavior* of normal mice is, to some extent, inhibited by amphetamine (BOISSIER et al., 1964; VALZELLI, 1969), probably as a function of the anxiogenic activity exerted by this compound (BRADY, 1956), whereas the exploratory activity of aggressive mice is improved (VALZELLI, 1969). This dual effect once more indicates the importance of emotional status for the determination of behavioral changes following the administration of central stimulant drugs.

The effects of amphetamine on *learning* processes are still unclear and controversial, mainly because the drug exerts hypothalamic effects, particularly in areas mediating hunger and/or thirst, so that the assessment of any behavior maintained under either motivational state creates a difficult methodological problem (ESSMAN, 1971). The distinction between psychomotor excitation, elevated performance level, or reduced fatigue effects appears to constitute the major interpretative considerations that apply to amphetamine-induced changes in learning and memory. Experimental evidence in man indicates that amphetamine decreases reaction time (BATTIG, 1963; TONINI et al., 1963) and that this effect is much more evident as the individual is affected by fatigue or decreased arousal (HAUTY and PAYNE, 1958; PAYNE et al., 1957). Similar results, in general defined as "antifatigue" effects, can be observed in animals previously submitted to conditioning techniques and then exhausted by numerous experimental sessions (BOVET and AMORICO, 1963; OLIVERIO, 1967; BOVET and OLIVERIO, 1967).

The results of experiments in which amphetamine was administered to rats with poor acquisition ability for a conditioned avoidance response are more consistent; in this situation, an improved rate of acquisition was shown (RECH, 1966). However, it appears, from a series of experiments, that if psychoanaleptic drugs can improve the learning process under some particular conditions, this occurs only with a low dosage limit, beyond which the effect may become negative depending upon prevailing hyperexcitatory effects producing psychomotor incoordination. This general picture can also be applied to man where there are still less clearly uniform relationships among the manifold psychological and characterological variables which may be intermittently activated and modulated by the stimulatory effects of these compounds. From the psychodynamic point of view, amphetamines are classified as "Egotonic" because their basal activity is believed to strengthen the ego functions (OSTOW, 1962).

The *pharmacological interactions* which take place among amphetamines and other drugs are quite numerous. Barbiturate and reserpine antagonism (BURTON et al., 1957) are well known; these are also present in man (GELDER and VANE, 1962), and the potentiation of antidepressant drugs, both of monoamine oxidase inhibitor and of tricyclic types, has also been documented.

3) Clinical Effects

Recently (COSTA and GARATTINI, 1970) it was concluded that amphetamine was void of any useful activity in the management of psychiatric illnesses. In fact, earlier claims for amphetamine and its congeners as effective antidepressant drugs (MYERSON, 1936; PEOPLES and GUTT-MANN, 1936; RUDOLF, 1949) were largely modified later with the conclusion that those results obtained in moderately and severely depressed patients were, at least, disappointing (KINROSS-WRIGHT, 1959; SHEP-HERD et al., 1968) and certainly irrelevant when compared with those induced by the tricyclic antidepressants.

Sometimes amphetamines exert a favorable sedative effect on adult men or children with a psychopathological personality characterized by recurrent aggressive outbursts, immaturity, hyperactivity, nosiy behavior, and electro-encephalographic abnormalities (HILL, 1947; BAN, 1969); this therapeutic and, to some extent, paradoxical activity, is generally accompanied by a peculiar resistance to amphetamines, which, however, exert their most intense clinical activity in those patients where the syndrome is sustained by an organic brain damage (LASAGNA and EPSTEIN, 1970).

Narcolepsy (PRINZMETAL and BLOOMBERG, 1935), *postencephalitic Parkinsonism,* and some enuretic syndromes (GWYNNE-JONES, 1960) represent other indications for amphetamine treatment which has also been employed in combination with psychotherapeutic approaches (SARGANT and SLATER, 1963).

Regardless of their very limited psychiatric indications, amphetamines have been and to some extent are still prescribed in many countries, with an excessive confidence shown by the general practitioner in these agents as general antifatigue compounds and as anorexiants in the course of weight control therapy (SEATON and DUNCAN, 1965; PATEL et al., 1963). These two areas, however, represent bases from which an uncontrolled source of psychostimulant drug use and abuse has derived with the appearance of several, sometimes severe, psychotic syndromes (KNOLL, 1970; ELLINWOOD, 1967; BREAMISH and KILOH, 1960; HAMPTON, 1961;

CONNELL, 1958). Moreover, every physician must be aware of the possible onset of both toxic consequences and of drug dependence (CONNELL, 1966; KILOH and BRANDON, 1962), as well as of the possibility of enhancing overt psychoses, depending upon an amphetamine-induced decompensation of functional behavior (ELLINWOOD, 1967). However, where diet control therapies are concerned, it is important to remember that there are other compounds currently available, such as chlorfentermine and fenfluramine, which provide a potent anorexic effect and corresponding weight loss without displaying any central stimulating activity (STRONG and LAWSON, 1970; PAWAN, 1970; WOODWARD, 1970; SOULAIRAC and SOULAIRAC, 1970; COSTA and GARATTINI, 1970).

4) Undesirable Effects

The least desirable effects brought about by the amphetamines are the possible onset of addiction and the emergence of psychotic syndromes (KNOLL, 1970). More commonly, however, anxious states, hyperirritability, tremors, tachycardia, hypertensive spikes, dryness of the mouth, anorexia, impotence, and insomnia have been observed (SHEPHERD et al., 1968). In this latter context, amphetamines delay the onset of sleep (KORNETSKY et al., 1959) and induce an obvious reduction in REM sleep cycles as well as providing for increased body movements during sleep (RECHTSCHAFFEN and MARON, 1964). Withdrawal of these compounds is followed by a clear rebound effect with a long-lasting increase of REM sleep cycles (OSWALD, 1968, 1970).

Finally, concerning the use of amphetamines in sporting events, aside from any ethical consideration, it is important to emphasize that emotional tension and muscular strain are both conditions which can seriously augment the negative effects of these compounds.

5) Other Psychoanaleptics

More recently, other derivatives, chemically unrelated to amphetamine but essentially amphetamine-like in their activity, have been synthesized; these include the piperidyl derivatives which have fewer unwanted side effects, especially upon the cardiovascular system. They also provide less frequently for addictive or dependence syndromes.

One of the most important derivatives of this class, *methylphenidate,* acts substantially as amphetamine; however, providing for more gradual onset and dissipation of effect (MEIER et al., 1954). Some investigators have demonstrated a facilitative effect of methylphenidate upon both memory retrieval and discriminative processes as well as an increased vigilance produced even during the course of prolonged therapy with anxiolytic or tranquilizing drugs (AYD, 1957; FERGUSON, 1956; GRUBER et al., 1956; PLUMMER and EARL, 1957; TICKTIN et al., 1958); its therapeutic effect in chronically anergic psychiatric patients is quite minimal (BHASKA-RAN and NAND, 1959; LEHMANN and BAN, 1964). Its effect upon neurotic depressions is also questionable (ROBIN and WISEBERG, 1958). Methylphenidate was reported to induce anhedonia and paranoid outbursts in psychotic, depressed subjects (BOJANOVSKY and CHLOUPKOVA, 1965) and to produce markedly hostile behavior when administered intravenously (FREED, 1958; HARTERT and BROWNE-MAYERS, 1958).

Similar to amphetamine, methylphenidate can be usefully employed to control hyperactive behavior in children (LYTTON and KNOBEL, 1959).

Another piperidyl derivative is *pipradol* which, like methylphenidate, acts through the stimulation of some hypothalamic structures and the brain stem reticular formation (COLE and GLEES, 1956; JOUVET and COUR-JON, 1959) to induce increased psychomotor activity and heightened reactivity to environmental stimuli (BROWN and WERNER, 1954; FABING, 1955).

The therapeutic activity of pipradol in the treatment of different depressive syndromes is somewhat questionable (FABING et al., 1955; FEDOTOV, 1958; HOUSTON, 1956), although it shows a good activity in attenuating the torpor and somnolence resulting from prolonged tranquilizer treatment (ANTOS, 1955; BUTTON, 1956; KISTNER and DUNCAN, 1956; KLINGMAN, 1962). However, BEGG and REID (1956) reported the appearance of some psychotic episodes during the treatment with low doses of pipradol.

Other compounds such as *deanol, centrophenoxine,* and *mephexamide* are not very different in their activity spectrum from those compounds considered.

Another psychostimulant, considered to be quite mild in its action, is *magnesium pemoline* (SCHMIDT, 1956); the activity of this compound has been reported to exert little or no sympathomimetic effect and to be of prolonged duration (PLOTNIKOFF et al., 1969). This substance has been mainly utilized in studies concerned with learning and memory processes (PLOTNIKOFF, 1966a, b; YUWILER et al., 1968; BIANCHI and MARAZZI-UBERTI, 1969; ESSMAN, 1971) and has been reported to be effective in facilitating learning and in antagonizing the retrograde amnesic effect of electroconvulsive shock both in animals (PLOTNIKOFF, 1966a, b, 1969) and in man (SMALL et al., 1968). These effects have been the subject of some controversy (SMITH, 1967; BURNS, et al., 1967), chiefly concerning a purported effect upon brain RNA metabolism (GLASKY and SIMON,

1966; PUIG-MUSET et al., 1967) and the metabolic events regulating RNA synthesis.

All these data still remain under critical discussion, primarily concerned with specificity of an effect of magnesium pemoline on memory; these have been recently reviewed (ESSMAN, 1971).

B) PSYCHODYSLEPTICS

The psychodysleptic drugs are quite numerous and may be classified within several chemical categories; they induce an intense variation of affective behavior, mood, thought processes, and perception at doses low enough not to induce obvious peripheral effects. In other words, such compounds show a peculiar selectivity of action on the central nervous system, mainly upon higher functions concerned with the modulation of personality variables.

From time to time, in accord with different scientific, philosophical, or literary treatments, the psychodysleptic compounds have been designated as hallucinogenics, psycholytics, psychotomimetics, phantastica, mysticomimetics, and by other varied descriptive terminology indicative of the convergence of varied interests in this area. Beyond the gradual evolution of man's scientific knowledge, there has been and still is a deep drive to potentiate his own intellectual abilities such as to exceed the limits of present knowledge and to expand his mind beyond the frontiers of reality. The roots of this feeling have suffused the entire evolution of mankind in its historical, philosophical and religious development; the methods utilized to achieve this goal have been notably different, but largely derive from the use of potions or preparations for magical rites or religious ceremonies.

From such mystical and superstitious tradition the belief was perpetuated that the use of particular drugs could extensively enhance the abilities of the mind to such an extent as to provide deep insight into the essence of life and to solve all the problems of existence. Such belief could be considered both as ingenuous and dangerous depending upon the type, manner, and frequency with which varied mixtures, potions, and drugs are used and abused.

Most of the psychodysleptic compounds can be divided into four main categories represented by (a) indole, (b) phenylethylamine, (c) piperidine, and (d) tetrahydrocannabinol derivatives; however, many other compounds of several different origins, capable of inducing psychodysleptic symptomatology, may also be added. The major portion of the active principle related to the classification derives mainly from several plants or vegetables traditionally employed by primitive peoples during their mystical ceremonies

(SCHULTES, 1969; FARNSWORTH, 1968). For instance, *mescaline,* for which DIXON (1898) first described the effects in man, is present in peytol (Lophophora Williamsii), a cactus employed by Aztec Indians in their religious ceremonies; *psilocybin,* chemically identified by HOFMANN et al., in 1958, is the active principle of some hallucinogenic mushrooms such as Psilocybe Mexicana and Stropharia Cubensis; *lysergic acid diethylamide* or LSD-25, which is the emblem of the psychedelic philosophy, is found in rye-ergot (Claviceps Purpurea) and it was initially synthesized and studied for its effect in man by STOLL (1947) and by STOLL and HOFMANN (1943) (Fig. 54).

As previously mentioned, the sources of psychodysleptic principles are manifold and continuously increasing so that an organic classification of the subject becomes virtually impossible. However, the symptoms induced by psychodysleptic compounds, even though they differ in intensity, duration, and deliriant effects, are sufficiently similar to allow for the formulation of a general framework within which activity reference-points for the action of these agents may be constructed.

1) General Aspects

Lysergic acid diethylamide (LSD) and some tryptamine derivatives such as *dimethyl-tryptamine* (SZARA, 1961), dimethyl-serotonin or *bufotenine*

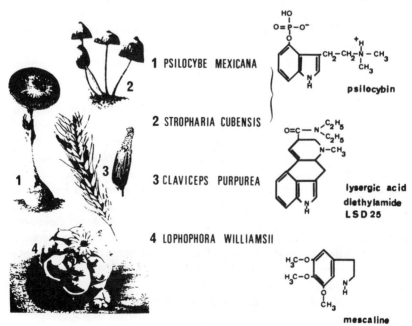

Fig. 54. Some sources of psychotomimetic drugs.

(AXELROD, 1961; FABING and HAWKINS, 1956), psilocybin, harmine derivatives (DOWNING, 1964), and adrenochromes (HOFFER et al., 1954) may all be classified as indole derivatives; mescaline, amphetamine and amphetamine-like drugs, some recent amphetamine derivatives such as 2,5-dimethoxy-4-methylamphetamine (STP or DOM) (SNYDER et al., 1967), and 2,5-dimethoxy-4-ethylamphetamine (DOET) (SNYDER et al., 1968), are the major representatives of the phenylethylamine class; *ditran, phencyclidine,* and *benactyzine* are central anticholinergic compounds with psychodysleptic activity (LUBY et al., 1959; COHEN, 1967); finally, Δ^1-tetrahydrocannabinol (GAONI and MECHOULAM, 1964; MECHOULAM and GAONI, 1965) and some of its isomers (WASKOW et al., 1970) were recently isolated and chemically synthesized, and represent the active principles of hashish and marijuana (SCARLATO and BONARETTI, 1959), obtained from the leaves of Cannabis Indica.

The *absorption* of psychodysleptic agents is, in general, quite rapid and they easily pass from the bloodstream to the different organs of the body, brain included. Lysergic acid diethylamide concentrates in a decreasing order, in bile, plasma, lungs, liver, kidneys, brain, intestine and easily and rapidly crosses the blood-brain barrier (AXELROD et al., 1957); in the brain, this drug is accumulated mainly in the hypothalamus, visual and auditory mesencephalic structures (corpora guadrigemina), limbic system and cerebral cortex, and in surprisingly large quantities, in the optic chiasma, hypophysis and pineal (SNYDER and REIVICH, 1966). Such a regional distribution of this drug provides sufficient bases for its psychodysleptic effects and for the "mystical visions and revelations" induced by this agent.

The *metabolism* of LSD by liver microsomes results in: (1) 2-oxy-LSD, which does not exert LSD-like effects, either in animals or in man (AXELROD et al., 1957); and (2) to β-glucuronides of hydroxy-LSD and hydroxy-iso-LSD (SLAYTOR and WRIGHT, 1962). Psilocybin is transformed into the O-phosphorylated ester of psilocin, which is rapidly hydrolized to *psilocin*; this has psychodysleptic activity closely resembling that of psilocybin (CERLETTI, 1959; WEIDMANN and CERLETTI, 1960). Mescaline, at least in the brain, is transformed directly to an inactive product, trimethoxyphenylacetic acid (NEFF et al., 1964). The *excretion* of many psychodysleptic derivatives occurs mainly as unchanged compounds (CHARALAMPOUS et al., 1966; BOYD, 1959; GIARMAN and FREEDMAN, 1965; HO et al., 1971).

The general *pharmacology* of hallucinogenic substances is characterized by a series of peripheral effects ranging from the stimulation of several smooth-muscle preparations, such as the isolated uterus, to the vasoconstrictor activity exerted on perfused dog hind-limb preparation by phencyclidine. Moreover, intense sympathomimetic effects provide for tachycardia, increased blood pressure, hyperglycemia, and exophthalmus. LSD, like amphetamine, exerts an anorexigenic activity (SHEPHERD et al., 1968), mydriasis, the evaluation of which has been proposed as a measure of the intensity of LSD effects (RINKEL et al., 1955), and an obvious analgesic effect of long duration (KAST and COLLINS, 1964).

The effects of hallucinogenic drugs upon the electrical activity of the brain has been less easily generalizable; LSD, similar to amphetamine, induces desynchronization of the electrocorticographic record but one major difference is that the arousal effect of LSD is abolished in the "cerveau isolé" preparation (BRADLEY and ELKES, 1953). This difference has been explained on the basis that amphetamine directly stimulates the reticular formation while LSD stimulates the afferent collateral fibers reaching the same structure (BRADLEY and KEY, 1958). Some experimental evidence indicates that psilocybin brings about an arousal reaction which may depend upon depressed electrical activity of the amygdala more than on a direct stimulation of the reticular formation (ADEY et al., 1962). Mescaline also induces desynchronization (TAKEO and HIMWICH, 1965; WIKLER, 1954) presumably by acting upon the mesodiencephalic activating system (HIMWICH et al., 1959).

High doses of some psychodysleptic agents have been reported to induce only minor variations in the concentration of putative *neurochemical mediators*. More precisely, LSD leads to slight increases in brain serotonin level and decreases in norepinephrine concentration similar to the effects of psilocybin treatment, while mescaline does not alter brain norepinephrine levels (FREEDMAN, 1963). A well-documented antagonism, initially observed by GADDUM (1953), has been noted between LSD and 5-HT in peripheral structures; this led to the hypothesis that such an interaction could occur in the brain, possibly explaining the autonomic and behavioral effects of LSD as well as some of the psychotomimetic features induced by this compound (BRODIE and COSTA, 1962; MIURA et al., 1957; WOOLLEY, 1958a, b; WOOLLEY and SHAW, 1957); however, COSTA (1960) stated that the psychotomimetic effects of LSD could not be strictly correlated with such an anti-5-HT activity. More recently it was reported that LSD increases 5-HT concentration both in nerve-ending particles and in microsomal fractions (ROSECRANS et al., 1967), decreases the brain 5-HT turnover (ROSECRANS et al., 1967; ANDÉN et al., 1968), increases brain norepinephrine but not dopamine turnover, and directly stimulates central 5-HT receptors (ANDÉN et al., 1968) and neurons (AGHAJANIAN, 1970), without excluding, at least in part, catecholamine mediation of its effects (DIXON, 1968). Moreover, LSD was reported to impair the rhythmic pulsatory movements of oligodendroglia, usually enhanced by 5-HT, and to induce a cell-vacualization and a chromatolysis of neuronal NISSL's substance (GEIGER, 1957, 1960).

Other psychodysleptics of the tryptamine class, such as N,N-diethyltryptamine, lead to transitory increases in hypothalamic 5-HT (SZARA, 1964). Mescaline, which has been shown to concentrate at the synapse (DENBER and TELLER, 1970), as well as another very potent psycho-tomimetic compound, *3,4-dimethoxyphenyl-ethylamine* (DMPEA), have been reported to consistently impair cerebral synaptic transmission in the cat (VACCA et al., 1968).

With respect to *brain biochemistry*, LSD exerts some effects on (1) phos-phate metabolism, (2) oxidative phosphorylation of brain mitochon-dria, (3) glucose transport, (4) protein turnover (GIARMAN and FREED-MAN, 1965), and (5) blocks brain cholinesterase activity (TONINI, 1955; FRIED and ANTOPOL, 1956, 1957; ZSIGMOND et al., 1960, 1961) to almost the same extent as eserine (GOLDENBERG and GOLDENBERG, 1956); mescaline (1) inhibits oxidative processes (QUASTEL and WHEAT-LEY, 1933) and, (2) at high dosages, increases brain alanine levels (DE ROPP and SNEDEKER, 1961).

2) Behavioral Effects

In laboratory animals psychodysleptics induce a dose-dependent reduc-tion in spontaneous *motor activity* (DELAY, 1953) along with an obvious hyperreactivity to environmental stimuli (LAGUTINA et al., 1964), mainly auditory (SPECK, 1957), and produce a bizarre behavior characterized by a backward gait and violent and repetitive head-shaking (WOOLLEY, 1955; KELLER and UMBREIT, 1956). Many of such compounds also induce a pseudotaming effect due both to a diminution of the sensitivity to painful stimuli (EVARTS, 1956) and to a stupor-like activity (FULLER, 1962; BARUK et al., 1962; WINTER and FLATAKER, 1957). An accurate evaluation of different behavioral activities indicates that both LSD and mescaline increase either offensive and defensive aggressiveness (NORTON, 1957; NORTON and TAMBURRO, 1958; ELDER and DILLE, 1962); cannabis extracts as well as marijuana, chronically administered to starved normal rats, induce strongly agressive behavior (CARLINI and KRAMER, 1965; CARLINI and MASUR, 1969; PALERMO-NETO and CARLINI, 1972) while such extracts have been reported to reduce the aggressiveness of isolated mice (SANTOS et al., 1966; SALUSTIANO et al., 1966); low doses of LSD are, however, ineffective in modifying the *aggressiveness* induced *by isolation* both in mice and rats (VALZELLI and BERNASCONI, 1971).

In the etiology of the symptomatology induced by psychotomimetics, a very important role is played by the limbic system and temporal lobes; for example, a bilateral temporal lobectomy in chimpanzees completely abolishes the behaviorally disruptive effects of LSD (BALDWIN et al., 1959).

Psychotomimetic drugs produce considerable increases in the emotional reactivity of animals (BRIMBLECOMBE, 1963), but clearly reduce the *exploratory behavior* of both normal and aggressive mice; the performance of such aggressive mice which characteristically show blocked exploration (blocked aggressive mice–VALZELLI, 1971) is, however, enhanced by psychotomimetic agents.

Numerous experiments have shown that *learning* ability appears to be consistently impaired with LSD, mescaline, and other psychodysleptic agents (LIBERSON et al., 1961, 1962; MARAZZI, 1962; RAY and MARAZZI, 1961, 1962; GROF et al., 1963; CHOROVER, 1961; WADA, 1962); this has been attributed to a drug-related limitation upon the discriminative skill of the animals (FURSTER, 1957; ANSFIELD and JOHNSON, 1961; KEY, 1961a, b). Such reports appear consistent with others in which hallucinogens disrupt temporal discrimination (MELGES et al., 1970a, b) and impair memory, as has, for example, been reported in man with marijuana (ABEL, 1970; TINKLENBERG et al., 1970).

Psychodysleptic agents also interfere with the specialized behavior of insects, so that LSD, adrenochrome, mescaline, and psilocybin can induce obvious asymmetries in spider web construction (WITT, 1951, 1952, 1956; CHRISTIANSEN et al., 1962), and can inhibit the normal motor activity of gastropods (ABRAMSON and JARVIK, 1955; JARVIK, 1957; SALANKI and KOSCHTOJANTZ, 1962).

With respect to pharmacological *interactions,* chlorpromazine can antagonize both the behavioral effects (JACOBSEN, 1963; DHAWAN, 1959) and the electroencephalographic changes (BRADLEY and HANCE, 1957) induced by LSD, whereas this latter compound does not act on the effects of the former (BRADELY and HANCE, 1957. Reserpine inhibits only the peripheral sympathomimetic effects of LSD, but only when it is administered two to four hours before LSD; in this way the amine depletion in the brain is practically complete, leading to impaired transmission of the effect of the central stimulation induced by LSD to the periphery. The simultaneous administration of the two substances, however, enhances sympathomimetic effects due to the stimulating effect of LSD and to the massive efflux of catecholamines on the receptors induced by reserpine (ELDER and SHELLENBERGER, 1962).

3) The Psychotomimetic Syndrome

Psychodysleptic activity in man varies depending on (1) dosage, (2) route of administration, and (3) individual sensitivity, while the psychological effects depend upon (1) real or apparent mental integrity of the subject, (2) intelligence, (3) cultural influences, (4) perspicacity, (5) descriptive skill and expectation, and, despite the emphasis placed upon the apparent capacity of such substances to promote the induction of pure states of contemplation (HUXLEY, 1960) or to induce an unlimited expansion of thought experiences and of self (MORTIMER, 1963), these phenomena, illusive enough in their essence, do not consistently occur.

From a general point of view, however, apart from the described sources of variation, the effects of LSD, mescaline, and psilocybin are quite similar (HOLLISTER and SJOBERG, 1964).

The onset of the *somatic effects* of psychodysleptics usually occur within half an hour after drug administration and most frequently consist of nausea, vomiting, severe stomach cramps, headache, dizziness, tremor of the extremities, hyperreflexia, incoordination, ataxia, chills and shivering. Blurring of vision, palpitations, increased blood pressure, pupillary dilatation, and hyperglycemia can also occur (SHEPHERD et al., 1968).

Such a symptomatologic pattern may be present to varying degrees during the action of the psychodysleptics, while nausea and ataxia generally subside with the onset of the perceptual effects.

Following the somatic effects of psychodysleptics, the *affective effects* occur; among these, the most common is anxiety which may reach such intensity that the entire drug experience is pervaded by a continuous feeling of dread. However, in other instances, the anxiety dissipates and may be followed by euphoria which can reach hypomanic exaltation and loss of contact with environmental characteristics and response to stimulation; suspicion and paranoid ideas may occur in other subjects giving rise to fear and flight reactions or clear aggressive outburst. All these different attitudes and reactions are largely dependent upon personality characteristics of the individual (SHEPHERD et al., 1968; HOFFER and OSMOND, 1967).

The alterations in *thought processes* brought about by psychodysleptics generally deteriorates further into indecision, distractability, difficulty in concentration, and slowness and poverty of thought content; these become less logical and discriminative and increase in frequency to the point where a continuous flow of ideative association intrudes upon reasoning (Mc KELLAR, 1963). The introspective tendencies increase to such a great extent that the ability of the subject to communicate his experiences is severely impaired, while a feeling develops that something of a mystical or metaphysical character, usually dependent upon the subject's previous experiences, is about to be revealed.

The *perceptual phenomena* generally complete the psychodysleptic syndrome, they may occasionally be absent (SHEPHERD et al., 1968). Auditory, gustatory, and olfactory hallucinations can all be present, but the most striking are the visual experiences (DENBER, 1958; MAYER-GROSS, 1959; FISCHER et al., 1969; HILL and FISCHER, 1970; HOFFER and

OSMOND, 1967); in this latter respect, figure-ground discrimination is severely distorted and may appear as continuously moving and rotating, shapes can appear as expanding or contracting, while colors become more vivid, continuously changing into one another while sometimes only a single color can dominate and monopolize visual experience and may be supported by sounds, which may appear distant or to be highly amplified in intensity. Distortion of body image has been commonly reported, such that the body may appear like that of a giant or, conversely, extremely tiny, while often the limbs appear as if in motion and detached from the body or transformed into paws and hooves; erotic sensations are less common. The disruption of the sense of time (MELGES et al., 1970a, b) with a feeling of timelessness is frequently experienced.

At average doses of psychodysleptic drugs the subject generally remains aware of the anomalies of his experience so that he may describe himself as divided into two entities; it is just such a dissociative reaction that sometimes is extremely accentuated, and leads from the psychotomimetic syndrome to a psychiatric state of depersonalization (OSMOND, 1957).

Piperidylbenzilate derivatives, such as ditran, induce a psychodysleptic syndrome that differs from the previous description in that it provides for an extremely marked distortion of space and time, which induces a severe disruption of thought processes to the point of incoherence and hallucinations with a complete loss of contact with the environment (ABOOD and BIEL, 1962); this picture, as a whole, resembles that of delirium tremens (HOLLISTER et al., 1960) with mydriasis, tachycardia, hypertension, restlessness, ataxia, rigidity, and tremors (OSTFELD et al., 1958).

The most characteristic symptoms induced by phencyclidine are dizziness, diminution of pain sensation, severe impairment of sensory discrimination, euphoria, difficulties in thinking and concentration, feelings of unreality, and distortion of the body image and of the sense of time (DOMINO, 1964).

Other psychodysleptic agents may provide for some differences from the symptoms reported above; a good account of such differences can be found in the volume "The Hallucinogens" by HOFFER and OSMOND (1967).

4) Clinical Effects

The earliest indications of a possible therapeutic use of psychodysleptic agents concerned peyotl extracts (LANDRY, 1889; PRENTISS and MORGAN, 1896). Presently, LSD is perhaps the unique compound that has sometimes been employed in the treatment of behavior disorders, mainly as a consequence of the work of BUSCH and JOHNSON (1950). More recently, SHAGASS and BITTLE (1967) suggested that LSD can be usefully employed in patients with specific disorders, such as chronic alcoholics (CHWELOS et al., 1959) and sexual deviates (BALL and ARMSTRONG, 1961), while ALNAES (1964) has stressed the importance of the psychedelic experience induced by LSD and psilocybin in the treatment of neurosis; moreover, the use of LSD and ditran was suggested in the management of the therapy-resistant schizophrenics (ITIL et al., 1969).

A use of LSD has been made in the treatment of alcoholism. In a study in which LSD was compared with dextroamphetamine in the treatment of alcoholism, slightly better early results were obtained with the former, but after six months, the two treatment groups did not differ (HOLLISTER et al., 1969). Other studies (LUDWIG et al., 1969) failed to confirm any advantage for LSD treatment over no therapy or millieu therapy in the treatment of alcoholism. An indication of short-term initial benefit from LSD therapy in the treatment of chronic alcoholism (KURLAND et al., 1971) was obtained when LSD was employed as an adjunct to psychotherapy and patients were followed for from six to eighteen months; those given a 450 μg dose showed a significant improvement over those given 50 μg—both in drinking behavior as well as in general adjustment. No significant differences in these measures, however, were apparent between groups after twelve to eighteen months following treatment. There is some indication that means for sustaining initial LSD-induced therapeutic gains in the treatment of alcoholism should be sought.

According to SHEPHERD et al., (1968) a lysergic acid treatment may be indicated in four overlapping categories: (a) for abreactive procedures, in which, however, it seems to be of no particular advantage when compared with amobarbital sodium and metamphetamine (ROBINSON et al., 1963); (b) for facilitating psychoanalytic sessions, particularly in "blocked" patients (SANDISON, 1963); (c) for use in individual or group psychotherapy; and (d) for inducing a single overwhelming psychedelic experience (RICKELS, 1962).

The potential therapeutic use of psychotomimetics remains rather strictly specialized and limited, particularly when it is considered that many doubts still remain concerning a true therapeutic efficacy of such derivatives for the treatment of mental illnesses (HOLLISTER, 1964).

5) Undesirable Effects

After a hasty review of the activity of psychodysleptic agents, it might appear somewhat pleonastic to consider the undesirable effects of these substances; however, it seems important to underline some issues that render the use and the abuse of the psychodysleptics extremely hazardous. In fact, during the phase of acute intoxication the subject may be of danger to himself or to others (ELKES et al., 1955), while psychotic reactions can be triggered off by LSD (COHEN, 1960; COHEN and DITMAN, 1963), by cannabis abuse and by STP (KEUP, 1970), and it has been clearly shown that idiosyncratic reactions can take place, so that in occasional individuals such psychotic episodes may occur at quite low dosages (ISBELL et al., 1967). Moreover, even prolonged adverse reactions (COHEN and DITMAN, 1963; KLEBER, 1967), persistent hallucinosis (ROSENTHAL, 1964), schizophrenic-like syndromes (LANGS and BARR, 1968), and stable chronic psychoses have been associated with long-term psychotomimetic drug abuse (GLASS and BOWERS, 1970). Occasionally prolonged states of severe depression and anxiety (STEVENSON and RICHARDS, 1959; BOER and SIPPRELLE, 1969), confusion, perceptual changes, and loss of the drives to self-affirmation (UNGERLIEDER et al., 1966) have occurred; some cases of homicide associated with the use of LSD have also been described (BARTER and REITE, 1969).

Moreover, COHEN et al. (1967) have reported chromosomal damages in human leucocytes induced by LSD, although subsequently WARKANY and TAKACS (1968) and ROUX et al. (1970) claimed that this substance lacks any teratogenic action in rats, mice and hamsters; still, many other studies have shown a teratogenic action of LSD on mice and monkeys (EGOZCUE and IRWIN, 1969) as well as in man (KATO and JARVIK, 1969; IRWIN and EGOZCUE, 1967; ABBO et al., 1968; EGOZCUE and FOWLIS, 1969; EGOZCUE et al., 1968; NIELSEN et al., 1968; JARVIK et al., 1968). In a double-blind, controlled study in 32 patients, lymphocyte chromosomes were studied in 72-hour cultures (TIJO et al., 1969). No definitive evidence for a pure LSD-induced chromosomal damage could be evolved from the data. Even marijuana extracts have been shown to induce malformations of brain, spinal cord, foreleg, and liver, as well as to produce edema of the head and spinal region, of fetal hamsters and rabbits from mothers injected subcutaneously with multiple doses (GEBER and SCHRAMM, 1969a, b).

As a final point, several dangers evolving from pharmacological toxicity can characterize many of the most recent psychodysleptic agents.

REFERENCES

Abbo, G., Norris, A., and Zellweger, H., (1968) Humangenetik 6, 253.
Abel, E. L., (1970) Nature, London 227, 1151.
Abood, L. G. and Biel, J. H., (1962) Int. Rev. Neurobiol. 4, 217.
Abramson, H. A. and Jarvik, M. E., (1955) J. Psychol. 40, 337.
Adey, W. R., Bell, F. R., and Dennis, B. J., (1962) Neurology 12, 591.
Aghajanian, G. K., (1970) Neurosci. Res. Program Bull. 8, 40.
Aiazzi-Mancini, M. and Donatelli, L., (1957) "Trattato di farmacologia," F. Vallardi Publ., Milan.

THE PSYCHOSTIMULANTS   231

Alles, G. A., (1927) J. Pharmacol. Exper. Ther. 32, 121.
Alnaes, R., (1964) Acta Psychiat. Scand. (suppl. 180) 40, 397.
Andén, N. E., Corrodi, H., Fuxe, K., and Hökfelt, T., (1968) Brit. J. Pharmacol. 34, 1.
Ansfield, P. J. and Johnson, J. I., Jr., (1961) Amer. Psychologist 16, 452.
Antos, R. J., (1955) Southwest. Med. 36, 166.
Asatoor, A. M., Galman, B. R., Johnson, J. R., and Milne, M. D., (1965) Brit. J. Pharmacol. 24, 293.
Askew, B. M., (1961) J. Pharm. Pharmacol. 13, 701.
Axelrod, J., (1954) J. Pharmacol. Exper. Ther. 110, 315.
Axelrod, J., (1959) Physiol. Rev. 39, 751.
Axelrod, J., (1961) Science 134, 343.
Axelrod, J., (1970) in "International Symposium on Amphetamines and Related Compounds" (Proc. Symp. Milan, 1969), Costa, E. and Garattini, S., Eds., Raven Press, New York, p. 207.
Axelrod J., Brady, R. O., Witkop, B., and Evarts, E., (1957) Ann. N. Y. Acad. Sci. 66, 435.
Ayd, F. J., (1957) Dis. Nerv. Syst. 18, 394.
Baldwin, M., Lewis, S. A., and Bach, S. A., (1959) Neurology 9, 469.
Ball, J. R. and Armstrong, J. J., (1961) Can. Psychiat. Assoc. J. 6, 231.
Ban, T. A., (1969) "Psychopharmacology," Williams and Wilkins, Baltimore.
Barger, G. and Dale, H. H., (1910) J. Physiol.. London 41, 19.
Barter, J. T. and Reite, M., (1969) Amer. J. Psychiat. 126, 113.
Baruk, H., Launay, J., Berges, J., and Perles, R., (1962) in "Annales Moreau de Tours," Baruk H. and Launay, J., Eds., Université de France, Paris, p. 275.
Battig, K., (1963) in "Psychopharmacological Methods," Votava, Z., Horvath, M., and Vinar, O. Eds., Pergamon Press, Oxford, p. 151.
Beauvallet, M., Fugazza, J., and Legrand, M., (1967a) C. R. Soc. Biol. 161, 2161.
Beauvallet, M., Legrand, M., and Fugazza, J., (1967b) C. R. Soc. Biol. 161, 1291.
Beckett, A. H. and Rowland, M., (1965) J. Pharm. Pharmacol. (suppl.) 17, 109s.
Beckett, A. H., Rowland, M., and Turner, P., (1965) Lancet 1, 303.
Begg, W. G. A. and Reid, A. A., (1956) Brit. Med. J. 1, 946.
Berkowitz, B. A. and Spector, S., (1971) Europ. J. Pharmacol. 16, 322.
Berkowitz, B. A., Spector, S., and Pool, W., (1971) Europ. J. Pharmacol. 16, 315.
Berkowitz, B. A., Tarver, J. H., and Spector, S., (1970) Europ. J. Pharmacol. 10, 64.
Bhaskaran, K. and Nand, D. S., (1959) Indian J. Med. Sci. 13, 117.
Bianchi, C. and Marazzi-Uberti, E., (1969) Psychopharmacologia (Berlin) 15, 9.
Boer, A. P. and Sipprelle, C. N., (1969) Psychother. Psychosom. 17, 108.
Boissier, J. R., Simon, P., and Lwoff, J. M., (1964) Thérapie 19, 571.
Bojanovsky, J. and Chloupkova, K., (1965) Activ. Nerv. Super. 7, 56
Bovet, D. and Amorico, L., (1963) C. R.- Séances Acad. Sci. 256, 3901.
Bovet, D. and Oliverio, A., (1967) J. Psychol. 65, 45.
Boyd, E. M., Dolman, M., Knight, L. M., and Sheppard, E. P., (1965) Can. J. Physiol. Pharmacol. 43, 995.
Boyd, E. S., (1959) Arch. Int. Pharmacodyn. Thér. 120, 292.
Bradley, P. B. and Elkes, J., (1953) J. Physiol., London 120, 13P.
Bradley, P. B. and Hance, A. J., (1957) Electroenceph. Clin. Neurophysiol. 9, 191.
Bradley, P. B. and Key, B. J., (1958) Electroenceph. Clin. Neurophysiol. 10, 97.
Brady, J. V., (1956) Science 123, 1033.
Breamish, P. and Kiloh, L., (1960) J. Ment. Sci. 106, 337.
Brimblecombe, R. W., (1963) Psychopharmacologia (Berlin) 4, 139.
Brittain, R. T., Jack, D., and Spencer, P. S. J., (1964) J. Pharm. Pharmacol. 16, 565.
Brobeck, B. Y. R., Larsson, S., and Reyes, E., (1956) J. Physiol., London 132, 358.

Brodie, B. B. and Costa, E., (1962) in "Monoamines et Système Nerveux Central" (Symp. Bel-Air, Genève), De Ajuriaguerra, J., Ed., Georg et Cie. S. A., Genève, p. 13.
Brown, B. B. and Werner, H. W., (1954) J. Pharmacol. Exper. Ther. 110; 180.
Burn, J. H. and Hobbs, R., (1957) Arch. Int. Pharmacodyn. Thér. 113, 290.
Burns, J. T., House, R. F., Fensch, F. C., and Miller, J. C., (1967) Science 155, 849.
Burton, R. M., Sodd, M. A., and Goldin, A., (1957) Arch. Int. Pharmacodyn. Thér. 112, 188.
Busch, A. K. and Johson, W. C., (1950) Dis. Nerv. Syst. 11, 241.
Button, J. C., (1956) J. Amer. Osteopath. Assoc. 55, 501.
Carlini, E. A. and Kramer, C., (1965) Psychopharmacologia (Berlin) 7, 175.
Carlini, E. A. and Masur, J., (1969) Life Sci. (Pt. 1) 8, 607.
Carlsson, A., Lindqvist, M., Dahlström, A., Fuxe, K., and Masuoka, D., (1965) J. Pharm. Pharmacol. 17, 521.
Carlsson, A., Lindqvist, M., Fuxe, A., and Hamberger, B., (1966) J. Pharm. Pharmacol. 18, 128.
Cartoni, G. P. and De Stefano, F., (1963) Ital. J. Biochem. 12, 296.
Cerletti, A., (1959) Deut. Med. Wochenschr. 84, 2317.
Chance, M. R. A., (1946) J. Pharmacol. Exper. Ther. 87, 214.
Chance, M. R. A., (1947) J. Pharmacol. Exper. Ther. 89, 289.
Charalampous, K. D., Walker, K. E., and Kinross-Wright, J., (1966) Psychopharmacologia (Berlin) 9, 48.
Chernov, H. J., Furness, P., Partyka, D., and Plummer, A. J., (1966) J. Pharmacol. Exper. Ther. 154, 346.
Chorover, S. L., (1961) J. Comp. Physiol. Psychol. 54, 649.
Christiansen, A., Baum, R., and Witt, P. N., (1962) J. Pharmacol. Exper. Ther. 136, 31.
Chwelos, N., Blewett, D. B., Smith, C. M., and Hoffer, A., (1959) Quart. J. Stud. Alc. 20, 577.
Cohen, M., (1967) Arch. Int. Pharmacodyn. Thér. 169, 412.
Cohen, M. and Lal, H., (1964) Nature, London 201, 1037.
Cohen, M. M., Marinello, M. J., and Back, N., (1967) Science 155, 1417.
Cohen, S., (1960) J. Nerv. Ment. Dis. 130, 30.
Cohen, S. and Ditman, K. S., (1963) Arch. Gen. Psychiat. 8, 475.
Cole, J. and Glees, P., (1956) Lancet 1, 338.
Connell, P. H., (1958) "Amphetamine Psychosis," Chapman & Hall Publ., London.
Connell, P. H., (1966) J. Amer. Med. Assoc. 196, 718.
Consolo, S., Garattini, S., Ghielmetti, R., and Valzelli, L., (1965a) J. Pharm. Pharmacol. 17, 666.
Consolo, S., Garattini, S., and Valzelli, L., (1965b) J. Pharm. Pharmacol. 17, 53.
Consolo, S., Garattini, S., and Valzelli, L., (1965c) J. Pharm. Pharmacol. 17, 594.
Corrodi, H., Fuxe, K., and Jonsson, G., (1972) J. Pharm. Pharmacol. 24, 155.
Costa, E., (1960) Int. Rev. Neurobiol. 2, 175.
Costa, E. and Garattini, S., Eds. (1970) "International Symposium on Amphetamines and Related Compounds" (Proc. Symp. Milan, 1969), Raven Press, New York.
Crossland, J., (1970) "Lewis's Pharmacology," 4th ed., Williams and Wilkins, Baltimore.
Curry, A. E., (1968) Clin. Toxicol. 1, 235.
Dakin, H. D., (1905) Proc. Roy. Soc. 76, 491.
Delay, J., (1953) Electroenceph. Clin. Neurophysiol. 5, 130.
Denber, H. C. B., (1958) in "Chemical Concepts of Psychosis," Rinkel, M. and Denber, H. C. B., Eds., McDowell Publ. New York, p. 120.

Denber, H. C. B. and Teller, D. N., (1970) Arzneim.-Forsch. 20, 903.
De Ropp, R. S. and Snedeker, E. H., (1961) Proc. Soc. Exper. Biol. Med. 106, 696.
Dhawan, B. N., (1959) Arch. Int. Pharmacodyn. Thér. 123, 186.
Dingell, J. V., Owens, M. L., Norwich, M. R., and Sulser, F., (1967) Life Sci. 6, 1155.
Dixon, A. K., (1968) Experientia 24, 744.
Dixon, W. E., (1898) Brit. Med. J. 2, 1060.
Dolfini, E., Garattini, S., and Valzelli, L., (1969) J. Pharm. Pharmacol. 21, 871.
Dolfini, E. and Kobayashi, M., (1967) Europ. J. Pharmacol. 2, 65.
Domino, E. F., (1964) Int. Rev. Neurobiol. 6, 303.
Downing, D. F., (1964) in "Psychopharmacological Agents," vol. 1, Gordon, M., Ed.,
    Academic Press, New York, p. 555.
Dring, L. G., Smith, R. L., and Williams, R. T., (1966) J. Pharm. Pharmacol. 18, 402.
Duhault, J. and Verdavainne, C., (1967) Arch. Int. Pharmacodyn. Thér. 170, 276.
Egozcue, J. and Fowlis, M. J., (1969) Acta Obstet. Gynecol. Hisp. Lus. 2, 135.
Egozcue, J. and Irwin, S., (1969) Humangenetik 8, 86.
Egozcue, J., Irwin, S., and Maruffo, C. A., (1968) J. Amer. Med. Assoc. 204, 214.
Elder, J. T. and Dille, J. M., (1962) J. Pharmacol. Exper. Ther. 136, 162.
Elder, J. T. and Shellenberger, M. K., (1962) J. Pharmcol. Exper. Ther. 136, 293.
Elkes, C., Elkes, J., and Mayer-Gross, W., (1955) Lancet 1, 719.
Ellinwood, E. H., (1967) J. Nerv. Ment. Dis. 144, 273.
Ellison, T., Gutzeit, L., and Van Loon, E. J., (1966) J. Pharmacol. Exper. Ther. 152,
    383.
Esplin, D. W. and Zablocka, B., (1965) in "The Pharmacological Basis of Therapeu-
    tics," 3rd ed., Goodman, L. S. and Gilman, A., Eds., MacMillan Publ., New York,
    p. 345.
Essman, W. B., (1971) Advan. Pharmacol. Chemother. 9, 241.
Essman, W. B., Heldman, E., Barker, L. A., and Valzelli, L., (1972) Fed. Proc. Fed.
    Amer. Soc. Exper. Biol. 31, 121.
Evarts, E. V., (1956) Arch. Neurol. Psychiat. 75, 49.
Evetts, K. D., Uretsky, N. S., Iversen, L. L., and Iversen, S. D., (1970) Nature, London
    225, 961.
Fabing, H. D., (1955) Dis. Nerv. Syst. 16, 10.
Fabing, H. D. and Hawkins, J. R., (1956) Science 123, 886.
Fabing, H. D., Hawkins, J., and Moulton, J., (1955) Amer. J. Psychiat. 111, 832.
Farnsworth, N. R., (1968) Science 162, 1086.
Fedotov, D. D., (1958) Zh. Nevropatol. Psikhiatim. S. S. Korsakov 58, 592.
Ferguson, R. S., (1956) J. Ment. Sci. 102, 30.
Fink, G. B. and Larson, R. E., (1962) J. Pharmacol. Exper. Ther. 137, 361.
Fischer, J. E., Horst, W. D., and Kopin, I. J., (1965) Brit. J. Pharmacol. 24, 477.
Fischer, R., Hill, R. M., and Warshay, D., (1969) Experientia 25, 166.
Fisher, S., (1970) in "Clinical Handbook of Psychopharmacology," Di Mascio, A. and
    Shader, R. J., Eds., Science House Publ., New York, p. 17.
Forrest, G. L., Bortner, T. W., and Bakker, C. B., (1967) J. Psychiat. Res. 5, 281.
Freed, H. (1958) Amer. J. Psychiat. 114, 944.
Freedman, D. X., (1963) Amer. J. Psychiat. 119, 843.
Fried, G. H. and Antopol, W., (1956) Anat. Rec. 125, 610.
Fried, G. H. and Antopol, W., (1957) J. Appl. Physiol. 11, 25.
Frommel, E., Fleury, C., and Schmidt-Ginzkey, J., (1960) Schweiz. Med. Wochenschr.
    90, 830.
Fuller, J. L., (1962) Ann. N. Y. Acad. Sci. 96, 199.
Furster, J. M., (1957) Fed. Proc. Fed. Amer. Soc. Exper. Biol. 16, 43.

Gaddum, J. H., (1953) J. Physiol., London 121, 15P.

Gaoni, Y. and Mechoulam, R., (1964) J. Amer. Chem. Soc. 86, 1646.

Geber, W. F. and Schramm, L. C., (1969a) Arch. Int. Pharmacodyn. Thér. 177, 224.

Geber, W. F. and Schramm, L. C., (1969b) Toxicol. Appl. Pharmacol. 14, 276.

Geiger, R. S., (1957) Fed. Proc. Fed. Amer. Soc. Exper. Biol. 16, 44.

Geiger, R. S., (1960) J. Neuropsychiat. 1, 185.

Gelder, M. G. and Vane, J. R., (1962) Psychopharmacologia (Berlin) 3, 231.

Giarman, N. J. and Freedman, D. X., (1965) Pharmacol. Rev. 17, 1.

Glasky, A. J. and Simon, J. N., (1966) Science 151, 702.

Glass, G. S. and Bowers, M. B., (1970) Arch. Gen. Psychiat. 23, 97.

Glowinski, J. and Axelrod, J., (1965) J. Pharmacol. Exper. Ther. 149, 43.

Glowinski, J., Axelrod, J., and Iversen, L. L., (1966) J. Pharmacol. Exper. Ther. 153, 30.

Goldenberg, H. and Goldenberg, V., (1956) J. Hillside Hosp. 5, 246.

Goldstein, A., Warren, R., and Kaizer, S., (1965a) J. Pharmacol. Exper. Ther. 149, 165.

Goldstein, A., Kaizer, S., and Warren, R., (1965b) J. Pharmacol. Exper. Ther. 150, 146.

Goodman, L. S. and Gilman, A., (1970) "The Pharmacological Basis of Therapeutics," 4th ed., MacMillan Publ., New York.

Grof, S., Vojtechovsky, M., Vitek, V., and Prankova, S., (1963) J. Neuropsychiat. 5, 33.

Gruber, K., Illig, H. H., and Pflanz, M., (1956) Deut. Med. Wochenschr. 81, 1130.

Gunne, L. M. and Galland, L., (1967) Biochem. Pharmacol. 16, 1374.

Gupta, B. D. and Holland, H. C., (1969) Psychopharmacologia (Berlin) 14, 95.

Gwynne-Jones, H., (1960) in "Behavior Therapy and the Neuroses," Eysenck, H. J., Ed., Pergamon Press, Oxford.

Halliwell, G., Quinton, R. M., and Williams, F. E., (1964) Brit. J. Pharmacol. 23, 330.

Halpern, B. N., Drudi-Baracco, C., and Bessirard, D., (1962) C. R. Soc. Biol. 156, 769.

Hampton, W. H., (1961) Bull. N. Y. Acad. Med. 37, 167.

Hanson, L. C. F., (1967) Psychopharmacologia (Berlin) 10, 289.

Hartert, D. and Browne-Mayers, A. N., (1958) J. Amer. Med. Assoc. 166, 1982.

Hauty, G. T. and Payne, R. B., (1958) in "Vistas in Austronautics," vol. 1, Alpernin, M. and Stern, J., Eds., Pergamon Press, Oxford, p. 304.

Hill, D., (1947) Brit. J. Addict. Alc. 44, 50.

Hill, R. M. and Fischer, R., (1970) Pharmacopsychiat. Neuropsychopharmacol. 3, 256.

Himwich, H. E., Van Meter, W. G., and Owens, H. (1959) in "Biological Psychiatry," Masserman, J. H., Ed., Grune and Stratton Publ., New York, p. 27.

Ho, B. T., Estevez, V., and Fritchie, G. E., (1971) Brain Res. 29, 166.

Hoffer, A. and Osmond, H., (1967) "The Hallucinogens," Academic Press, New York.

Hoffer, A., Osmond, H., and Smythies, J., (1954) J. Ment. Sci. 100, 29.

Hofmann, A., Heim, R., Brack, A., and Kobel, H., (1958) Experientia 14, 107.

Hohn, R. and Lasagna, L., (1960) Psychopharmacologia (Berlin) 1, 210.

Hollister, L. E., (1964) Ann. Rev. Med. 15, 203.

Hollister, L. E., Shelton, J., and Krieger, G. A., (1969) Amer. J. Psychiat. 125, 1352.

Hollister, L. E., Prusmack, J. J., Paulsen, A., and Rosenquist, N., (1960) J. Nerv. Ment. Dis. 131, 428.

Hollister, L. E. and Sjoberg, B. M., (1964) Compr. Psychiat. 5, 170.

Houston, F., (1956) Brit. Med. J. 1, 949.

Huxley, A., (1960) "The Doors of Perception," Chatto & Windus Publ., London.

Irwin, S. and Egozcue, J., (1967) Science 157, 313.
Isbell, H., Gorodetzsky, C. W., Jasinski, D., Claussen, U., u. Spulak, F., and Korte, F., (1967) Psychopharmacologia (Berlin) 11, 184.
Itil, T. M., Keskiner, A., and Holden, J. M. C., (1969) Dis. Nerv. Syst. (GWAN Suppl.) 30, 93.
Jacobsen, E., (1963) Clin. Pharmacol. Ther. 4, 480.
Jarvik, M. E., (1957) "Transaction 3rd. Conference Neuropharmacology," Josiah Macy, Jr. Foundation, New York.
Jarvik, L. F., Kato, T., Saunders, B., and Moralishvili, E., (1968) in "Psychopharmacology, A Review of Progress 1957-1967," Efron, D. H., Ed., Public Health Service Publ. no. 1836, Washington, D. C., p. 1247.
Jori, A. and Garattini, S., (1965) J. Pharm. Pharmacol. 18, 481.
Jouvet, M. and Courjon, J., (1959) Arch. Int. Pharmacodyn. Thér. 119, 189.
Kast, E. C. and Collins, V. J., (1964) Anesth. Analg., Cleveland 43, 285.
Kato, T. and Jarvik, L. M., (1969) Dis. Nerv. Syst. 30, 42.
Keller, D. L. and Umbreit, W. W., (1956) Science 124, 723.
Keup, W., (1970) Dis. Nerv. Syst. 31, 119.
Key, B. J., (1961a) Psychopharmacologia (Berlin) 2, 352.
Key, B. J., (1971b) in "Neuropsychopharmacology" (Proc. 2nd CINP Congress, Basle 1960), vol. 2, Rothlin, E., Ed., Elsevier Publ., Amsterdam, p. 158.
Killam, E. K., (1962) Pharmacol. Rev. 14, 175.
Kiloh, L. G. and Brandon, S., (1962) Brit. Med. J. 2, 40.
Kinross-Wright, J., (1959) J. Amer. Med. Assoc. 170, 1283.
Kistner, R. W. and Duncan, C. J., (1956) New England J. Med. 254, 507.
Kleber, H. D., (1967) J. Nerv. Ment. Dis. 144, 308.
Klingman, W. O., (1962) in "Psychosomatic Medicine," Nodine, J. H. and Moyer, J. H., Eds., Lea & Febiger Publ., Philadelphia.
Knoll, J., (1970) in "International Symposium on Amphetamines and Related Compounds" (Proc. Symp. Milan, 1969), Costa, E. and Garattini, S., Eds., Raven Press, New York, p. 761.
Koestler, A., (1967) "The Ghost in the Machine," Hutchinson Publ., London.
Kopin, I. J., Fischer, J. E., Musacchio, J. M., Horst, W. D., and Wiese, V. K., (1965) J. Pharmacol. Exper. Ther. 147, 186.
Kornetsky, C., Mirsky, A. I., Kessler, E. K., and Dorff, J. E., (1959) J. Pharmacol. Exper. Ther. 127, 46.
Kurland, A., Savage, C., Pahnke, W. N., Grof, S., and Olsson, J. E., (1971) Pharmakopsychiat. 4, 83.
Lagutina, N. I., Laricheva, K. A., Milshtein, G. I., and Norkina, L. N., (1964) Fed. Proc. Fed. Amer. Soc. Exper. Biol. 23, T737.
Lal, H. and Chessik, R. D., (1964) Life Sci. 3, 381.
Landry, S. F., (1889) Ther. Gaz. 13, 16.
Langs, R. J. and Barr, H. L., (1968) J. Nerv. Ment. Dis. 147, 163.
Lasagna, L. and Epstein, L. C., (1970) in "International Symposium on Amphetamines and Related Compounds" (Proc. Symp. Milan, 1969), Costa, E. and Garattini, S., Eds., Raven Press, New York, p. 849.
Laverty, R. and Sharman, D. F., (1965) Brit. J. Pharmacol. 24, 758.
Leake, C. D., (1958) "The Amphetamines; Their Actions and Uses," C. C. Thomas Publ., Springfield, Ill.
Lehmann, H. E. and Ban, T. A., (1964) Can. Psychiat. Assoc. J. 9, 28.
Lewander, T. (1968) Europ. J. Pharmacol. 5, 1.

Liberson, W. T., Ellen, P., Schwartz, E., Wilson, A., and Gagnon, V.P., (1962) J. Neuropsychiat. 3, 298.
Liberson, W. T., Kafka, A., and Schwartz, E., (1961) Biochem. Pharmacol. 8, 15.
Littleton, J. M., (1967) J. Pharm. Pharmacol. 19, 415.
Luby, E. D., Cohen, B., and Rosenbaum, G., (1959) Arch. Neurol. Psychiat., Chicago 81, 363.
Ludwig, A., Levine, J., Stark, L., and Lazar, R., (1969) Amer. J. Psychiat. 126, 59.
Lytton, G. J. and Knobel, M., (1959) Dis. Nerv. Syst. 20, 334.
Mantegazza, P., Naimzada, K. M., and Riva, M., (1968) Europ. J. Pharmacol. 5, 10.
Marazzi, A. S., (1962) Ann. N. Y. Acad. Sci. 96, 211.
Mayer-Gross, W., (1959) Amer. J. Psychiat. 115, 673.
McKellar, P., (1963) in "Hallucinogenic Drugs and Their Psychotherapeutic Use," Crocket, R., Sandison, R. A., and Walk A., Eds., Lewis Publ., London.
McManamy, M. C. and Schube, P. G., (1936) New England J. Med. 215, 616.
Mechoulam, R. and Gaoni, Y., (1965) J. Amer. Chem. Soc. 87, 3273.
Meier, R., Gross, F., and Tripod, J., (1954) Klin. Wochenschr. 32, 445.
Melges, F. T., Tinklenberg, J. R., Hollister, L. E., and Gillespie, H. K., (1970a) Arch. Gen. Psychiat. 23, 204.
Melges, F. T., Tinklenberg, J. R., Hollister, L. E., and Gillespie, H. K., (1970b) Science 168, 1118.
Mennear, J. H., and Rudzik, A. D., (1968) Life Sci. 7, 213.
Mitoma, C., Sorich, T. J. II., and Neubauer, S. E., (1968) Life Sci. 7, 145.
Miura, T., Tsujiyama, Y., Makita, K., Nakazawa, T., Sato, K., and Nakahara, M., (1957) in "Psychotropic Drugs," Garattini, S. and Ghetti, V., Eds., Elsevier Publ., Amsterdam, p. 478.
Morpurgo, C. and Theobald, W., (1965) Med. Pharmacol. Exper. 12, 226.
Mortimer, R., (1963) in "Hallucinogenic Drugs and Their Psychotherapeutic Use," Crocket, R., Sandison, R. A., and Walk, A., Eds., Lewis Publ., London.
Musacchio, J. M., Kopin, I. J., and Wiese, V. K., (1965) J. Pharmacol. Exper. Ther. 148, 22.
Myerson, A., (1936) Arch. Neurol. Psychiat. Chicago 36, 816.
Neff, N., Rossi, G. V., Chase, G. D., and Robinowitz, J., (1964) J. Pharmacol. Exper. Ther. 144, 1.
Nielsen, J., Friedrich, U., Jacobsen, E., and Tsuboi, T., (1968) Brit. Med. J. 2, 801.
Norton, S., (1957) in "Psychotropic Drugs," Garattini, S. and Ghetti, V., Eds., Elsevier Publ., Amsterdam, p. 73.
Norton, S. and Tamburro, J., (1958) J. Pharmacol. Exper. Ther. 122, 57A.
Oliverio, A., (1967) Farmaco, Ed. Sci. 22, 159.
Osmond, H., (1957) Ann. N. Y. Acad. Sci. 66, 418.
Ostfeld, A. M., Abood, L. G., and Marcus, D. A., (1958) Arch. Neurol. Psychiat., Chicago 79, 317.
Ostow, M., (1962) "Drugs in Psychoanalysis and Psycotheraphy," Basic Books Inc., New York.
Oswald, I., (1968) Pharmacol. Rev. 20, 273.
Oswald, I., (1970) in "International Symposium on Amphetamines and Related Compounds" (Proc. Symp. Milan, 1969), Costa, E. and Garattini, S., Eds., Raven Press, New York, p. 865.
Palermo-Neto, J. and Carlini, E. A., (1972) Europ. J. Pharmacol. 17, 215.
Patel, N., Mock, D. C., and Hagans, J. A., (1963) Clin. Pharmacol. Ther. 4, 330.
Pawan, G. L. S., (1970) in "International Symposium on Amphetamines and Related Compounds" (Proc. Symp. Milan, 1969), Costa, E. and Garattini, S., Eds., Raven Press, New York, p. 641.

Payne, R. B., Hauty, G. T., and Moore, E. W., (1957) J. Comp. Physiol. Psychol. 146, 50.

Peoples, S. A. and Guttmann, E., (1936) Lancet 1, 1107.

Peters, J. M., (1966) Toxicol. Appl. Pharmacol. 9, 390.

Peters, J. M., (1967) Arch. Int. Pharmacodyn. Thér. 169, 139.

Peters, J. M. and Boyd, E. M., (1967a) Can. J. Physiol. Pharmacol. 45, 305.

Peters, J. M. and Boyd, E. M., (1967b) Toxicol. Appl. Pharmacol. 11, 121.

Pfeiffer, C. J. and Gass, G. H., (1962) Can. J. Biochem. Physiol. 40, 1473.

Pletscher, A., Bartholini, G., Bruderer, H., Burkard, W. P., and Gey, K. F., (1964) J. Pharmacol. Ther. 145, 344.

Plotnikoff, N., (1966a) Science 151, 703.

Plotnikoff, N., (1966b) Life Sci. 5, 1495.

Plotnikoff, N., (1969) Psychonom. Sci. 17, 180.

Plotnikoff, N., Will, F., and Ditzler, W., (1969) Arch. Int. Pharmacodyn. Thér. 181, 441.

Plummer, A. M. and Earl, A. E., (1957) Amer. J. Med. Sci. 233, 719.

Porsolt, R. D., Joyce, D., and Summerfield, A., (1970) Nature, London 227, 286.

Prentiss, D. W. and Morgan, F. P., (1896) Ther. Gaz. 20, 4.

Prinzmetal, M. and Bloomberg, W., (1935) J. Amer. Med. Assoc. 105, 2051.

Puig-Muset, P., Ramia, J., and Martin-Esteve, J., (1967) Nature, London 215, 522.

Quastel, J. H. and Wheatley, A. H. M., (1933) Biochem. J. 27, 1609.

Randrup, A. and Munkvad, I., (1966a) Nature, London 211, 540.

Randrup, A. and Munkvad, I., (1966b) Acta Psychiat. Scand. (suppl. 191) 42, 193.

Randrup, A. and Munkvad, I., (1967) Psychopharmacologia (Berlin) 11, 300.

Randrup, A. and Munkvad, I., (1968) Pharmakopsychiat. Neuropharmacol. 1, 18.

Randrup, A., Munkvad, I., and Udsen, P., (1963) Acta Pharmacol. Toxicol. 20, 145.

Ray, O. S. and Marazzi, A. S., (1961) Amer. Psychologist 16, 453.

Ray, O. S. and Marazzi, A. S., (1962) Fed. Proc. Fed. Amer. Soc. Exper. Biol. 21, 415.

Rech, R. H., (1966) Psychopharmacologia (Berlin) 9, 110.

Rechtschaffen, A. and Maron, L., (1964) Electroenceph. Clin. Neurophysiol. 16, 438.

Rickels, K., (1962) in "Psychosomatic Medicine," Nodine, J. H. and Moyer, J. H., Eds., Lea & Febiger Publ., Philadelphia.

Rinkel, M., Hyde, R., and Solomon, H. C., (1955) Dis. Nerv. Syst. 16, 229.

Robin, A. and Wiseberg, S., (1958) J. Neurol. Neurosurg. Psychiat. 21, 55.

Robinson, J. T., Davies, L. S., Sack, E. L., and Morrissey, J. D., (1963) Brit. J. Psychiat. 109, 46.

Rosecrans, J. A., Lovell, R. A., and Freedman, D. X., (1967) Biochem. Pharmacol. 16, 2011.

Rosenthal, S. H., (1964) Amer. J. Psychiat. 121, 238.

Roux, C., Dupuis, R., and Aubry, M., (1970) Science 169, 588.

Rudolf, G. M., (1949) J. Ment. Sci. 95, 920.

Salanki, J. and Koschtojantz, C. S., (1962) Acta Physiol. Hung. 20, 45.

Salustiano, J., Hoshino, K., and Carlini, E. A., (1966) Med. Pharmacol. Exper. 15, 153.

Samanin, R., Ghezzi, D., Valzelli, L. and Garattini, S., (1972) Europ. J. Pharmacol. 13, 318.

Sandison, R. A., (1963) in "Hallucinogenic Drugs and Their Psychotherapeutic Use," Crocket, R., Sandison, R. A., and Walk, A., Eds., Lewis Publ., London.

Santos, M., Sampaio, M. R. P., Fernandes, N. S., and Carlini, E. A., (1966) Psychopharmacologia (Berlin) 8, 437.

Sargant, W. and Slater, E., (1963) "An Introduction to Physical Methods of Treatment in Psychiatry," Livingston Publ., Edinburgh.

Scarlato, G. and Bonaretti, T., (1959) Minerva Med. 50, 3458.

Schmidt, L., (1956) Arzneim.-Forsch. 6, 423.

Schultes, R. E., (1969) Science 163, 254.

Seaton, D. A. and Duncan, L. J., (1965) Brit. J. Clin. Pract. 19, 89.

Shagass, C. and Bittle, R. M., (1967) J. Nerv. Ment. Dis. 144, 471.

Shepherd, M., Lader, M., and Rodnight, R., (1968) "Clinical Psychopharmacology," The English Universities Press Ltd., London.

Sjoerdsma, A. and Von Studnitz, W., (1963) Brit. J. Pharmacol. 20, 278.

Slaytor, M. B. and Wright, S. E., (1962) J. Med. Pharm. Chem. 5, 483.

Small, I. F., Sharpley, P., and Small, J. G., (1968) Amer. J. Psychiat. 125, 149.

Smith, C. B., (1963) J. Pharmacol. Exper. Ther. 142, 343.

Smith, R. G., (1967) Science 155, 603.

Snyder, S. H., Faillace, L., and Hollister, L., (1967) Science 158, 669.

Snyder, S. H., Faillance, L. A., and Weingartner, H., (1968) Amer. J. Psychiat. 125, 357.

Snyder, S. H. and Reivich, M., (1966) Nature, London 209, 1093.

Sofia, R. D., (1969) Arch. Int. Pharmacodyn. Thér. 182, 139.

Soulairac, A. and Soulairac, M. L., (1970) in "International Symposium on Amphetamines and Related Compounds" (Proc. Symp. Milan, 1969), Costa, E. and Garattini, S., Eds., Raven Press, New York, p. 819.

Speck, L. B., (1957) J. Pharmacol. Exper. Ther. 119, 78.

Stevenson, I. and Richards, T. W., (1959) Psychopharmacologia (Berlin) 1, 214.

Stoll, W. A., (1947) Schweizer. Arch. Neurol. Psychiat. 60, 279.

Stoll, W. A. and Hofmann, A., (1943) Helv. Chim. Acta 26, 944.

Stolz, F., (1904) Ber. Deut. Chem. Ges. 37, 4149.

Strong, J. A. and Lawson, A. A. H., (1970) in "International Symposium on Amphetamines and Related Compounds" (Proc. Symp. Milan, 1969), Costa, E. and Garattini, S., Eds., Raven Press, New York, p. 673.

Sulser, F., Owens, M. L., Norvich, M. R., and Dingell, J. V., (1968) Psychopharmacologia (Berlin) 12, 322.

Szara, S., (1961) Fed. Proc. Fed. Amer. Soc. Exper. Biol. 20, 885.

Szara, S., (1964) in "Neuropsychopharmacology" (Proc. 3rd. CINP Congress, Munich 1962), vol. 3, Bradley P. B., Flügel, F., and Hoch, P. H., Eds., Elsevier Publ. Amsterdam, p. 412.

Takeo, Y. and Himwich, H. E., (1965) Science 150, 1309.

Thoenen, H., Hürlimann, A., Gey, K. F., and Haefely, W., (1966) Life Sci. 5, 1715.

Ticktin, H., Epstein, J., Shea, J., and Fazekas, J., (1958) Neurology 8, 267.

Tinklenberg, J. R., Melges, F. T., Hollister, L. E., and Gillespie, H. K., (1970) Nature, London 226, 1171.

Tjio, J-H., Pahnke, W. N., and Kurland, A. A., (1969) J. Amer. Med. Assoc. 210, 849.

Tonini, G., (1955) Boll. Soc. Ital. Biol. Sper. 31, 768.

Tonini, G., Riccioni, M. L., Babbini, M., and Missere, G., (1963) in "Psychopharmacological Methods," Votava, Z., Horvath, M., and Vinar, O., Eds., Pergamon Press, Oxford, p. 106.

Ungerlieder, J. T., Fisher, D. D., and Fuller, M., (1966) J. Amer. Med. Assoc. 197, 389.

Utena, H., Ezoe, T., and Kato, N., (1955) Psych. Neurol. Jap. 57, 124.

Vacca, L., Fujimori, M., Davis, S. H., and Marrazzi, A. S., (1968) Science 160, 95.

Valzelli, L., (1967) in "Advances in Pharmacology," vol. 5, Garattini, S. and Shore, P. A., Eds., Academic Press, New York, p. 79.

Valzelli, L., (1969) Psychopharmacologia (Berlin) 15, 232.

Valzelli, L., (1971) Psychopharmacologia (Berlin) 19, 91.

Valzelli, L., (1973) Pharm., Biochem. Behav., in press.

Valzelli, L. and Bernasconi, S., (1971) Psychopharmacologia (Berlin) 20, 91.

Valzelli, L., Consolo, S., and Morpurgo, C., (1967a) in "Antidepressant drugs" (Proc. 1st. Int. Symp. Milan 1966), Garattini, S. and Dukes, M. N. G., Eds., Excerpta Medica Foundation, Amsterdam, p. 61.

Valzelli, L., Giacalone, E., and Garattini, S., (1967b) Europ. J. Pharmacol. 2, 144.

Vernier, V. G., Alleva, F. R., Hanson, H. M., and Stone, C. A., (1962) Fed. Proc. Fed. Amer. Soc. Exper. Biol. 21, 419.

Wada, J. A., (1962) Ann. N. Y. Acad. Sci. 96, 227.

Warkany, J. and Takacs, E., (1968) Science 159, 731.

Waskow, I. E., Olsson, J. E., Salzman, C., and Katz, M. M., (1970) Arch. Gen. Psychiat. 22, 97.

Weaver, L. C. and Kerley, T. L., (1962) J. Pharmacol. Exper. Ther. 135, 240.

Weidmann, H. and Cerletti, A., (1960) Helv. Physiol. Pharmacol. Acta 18, 174.

Weiss, S., Laties, V. G., and Blanton, F. L., (1961) J. Pharmacol. Exper. Ther. 132, 366.

Weissman, A., Koe, B. K., and Tenen, S. S., (1966) J. Pharmacol. Exper. Ther. 151, 339.

Welch, B. L. and Welch, A. S., (1967) J. Pharm. Pharmacol. 19, 841.

Wikler, A., (1954) J. Nerv. Ment. Dis. 120, 157.

Winter, C. A. and Flataker, L., (1957) J. Pharmacol. Exper. Ther. 119, 194.

Witt, P. N., (1951) Experientia 7, 310.

Witt, P. N., (1952) Behavior 4, 172.

Witt, P. N., (1956) "Die Wirkung von Substanzen auf den Netsban der Spinne als biologischer Test," Springer Verlag, Berlin.

Woodward, E., Jr., (1970) in "International Symposium on Amphetamines and Related Compounds" (Proc. Symp. Milan, 1969), Costa, E. and Garattini, S., Eds., Raven Press, New York, p. 685.

Woolley, D. W., (1955) Proc. Nat. Acad. Sci. 41, 338.

Woolley, D. W., (1958a) Res. Publ. Assoc. Res. Nerv. Ment. Dis. 33, 381.

Woolley, D. W., (1958b) in "Chemical Concepts of Psychosis," Rinkel, M. and Denber, H. C. B., Eds., McDowell, Obolensky Publ., New York, p. 176.

Woolley, D. W. and Shaw, E. N., (1957) Ann. N. Y. Acad. Sci. 66, 649.

Yuwiler, A., Greenough, W., and Geller, E., (1968) Psychopharmacologia (Berlin) 13, 174.

Zsigmond, E. K., Foldes, F. F., and Foldes, V., (1960) Fed. Proc. Fed. Amer. Soc. Exper. Biol. 19, 266.

Zsigmond, E. K., Foldes, F. F., and Foldes, V. M., (1961) J. Neurochem. 8, 72.

AUTHOR INDEX

241

SUBJECT INDEX

Syndrome, 226
Undesirable effects, 229, 230
 chromosomal damage, 230
 homicide, 230
 persistent hallucinosis, 230
 psychotic reactions, 230
 schizophrenic-like syndromes, 230
 severe depression, 230
Psycholytics, 221
Psychoneuroses, 139, 165, 171, 174,
 189, 198
 Anxious, 165, 171, 174
Psychopathological personality, 218
Psychopharmacology, 59
 Clinical, 59
 Experimental, 59
 Goals, 210
 Methods, 59
Psychoses, 107, 139
 Affective, 138, 183, 194, 200
 Brain amines, 107
 Cyclophrenic, 197
 Depressive, 145, 189
 Involutional, 145, 189
 Posttraumatic, 139
 Toxic, 139, 173, 190, 198, 211, 212,
 219
Psychosomatic syndromes, 165, 171, 174
Psychostimulants, 116, 117, 209
Psychotic reactions, 230
 Syndromes, 230
Psychotomimetic syndrome, 226
 Affective effects, 227
 Components, 226
 Perceptual phenomena, 227
 Somatic effects, 227
 Thought processes, 227
Psychotomimetics, 209, 221
Psychotropic drugs, 113
 Abuse, 113
 Activity spectrum, 117
 Antipsychotic effect and hypnogenic
  activity, 118, 119
 Anxiolytics, 119
 Classification, 114
  antidepressants, 116
  neuroleptics, 116, 131
  psychostimulants, 116, 117
  sedatives, 115, 116
  tranquilizers, 116, 131
 Clinical application, 118, 119, 120

Definition, 113
Dependence, 113, 114, 117, 161
Differential activity, 71
Problems, 113, 114
Thymeretics, 119
Thymoleptics, 119
Punishment, 74
Pyramidal pathways, 5
Rage and noradrenaline, 105
Rauwolfia Serpentina, 132
REM, 18
Reserpic acid, 141
Reserpine, 132, 141
 Behavioral effects, 144
  aggressiveness by isolation, 144
  anticonvulsant effect, 144
  conditioned avoidance responses,
   144
  electroencephalogram, 144
  endocrine effects, 144
  exploratory behavior, 144
  hyperemotional rats, 144
  interactions, 145
   monoamine oxidase inhibitors,
    145
   potentiation of barbiturate,
    145
   tricyclic antidepressants, 145
  learning, 144
  proconvulsant effect, 144
  REM phases, 145
  spontaneous motor activity, 144
  taming effect, 144
 Clinical effects, 145
  depressive disorders, 145
  epilepsy, 145
  hypertension, 146
  involutional psychoses, 145
  neuroses, 145
  schizophrenia, 145, 146
 General aspect, 141
  absorption, 141
  brain biochemistry, 141-144
   adenosinetriphosphate-
    adenosinediphosphate
    ratio, 144
   glycolysis, 144
   phosphocreatine, 144
  excretion, 142
  metabolism, 141
  neurochemical mediators, 143